# BI■MECHANICAL
## SYSTEMS TECHN■L■GY

GENERAL ANATOMY

**BIOMECHANICAL SYSTEMS TECHNOLOGY**
**A 4-Volume Set**
**Editor:** Cornelius T Leondes *(University of California, Los Angeles, USA)*

Computational Methods
ISBN-13 978-981-270-981-3
ISBN-10 981-270-981-9

Cardiovascular Systems
ISBN-13 978-981-270-982-0
ISBN-10 981-270-982-7

Muscular Skeletal Systems
ISBN-13 978-981-270-983-7
ISBN-10 981-270-983-5

General Anatomy
ISBN-13 978-981-270-984-4
ISBN-10 981-270-984-3

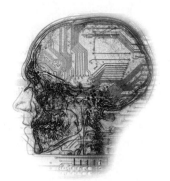

A 4-VOLUME SET

# BI■MECHANICAL
# SYSTEMS TECHN■L■GY

## GENERAL ANATOMY

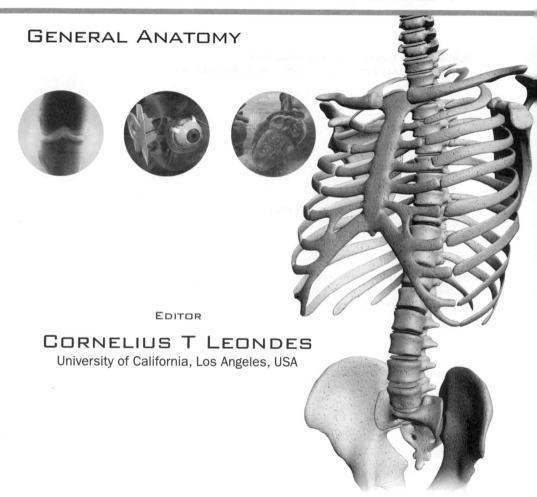

EDITOR

# CORNELIUS T LEONDES
University of California, Los Angeles, USA

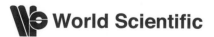 **World Scientific**

NEW JERSEY · LONDON · SINGAPORE · BEIJING · SHANGHAI · HONG KONG · TAIPEI · CHENNAI

*Published by*

World Scientific Publishing Co. Pte. Ltd.

5 Toh Tuck Link, Singapore 596224

*USA office:* 27 Warren Street, Suite 401-402, Hackensack, NJ 07601

*UK office:* 57 Shelton Street, Covent Garden, London WC2H 9HE

**British Library Cataloguing-in-Publication Data**
A catalogue record for this book is available from the British Library.

**BIOMECHANICAL SYSTEMS TECHNOLOGY**
**A 4-Volume Set**
**General Anatomy**

ISBN-13 978-981-270-798-7   (Set)
ISBN-10 981-270-798-0        (Set)

ISBN-13 978-981-270-984-4
ISBN-10 981-270-984-3

Typeset by Stallion Press
Email: enquiries@stallionpress.com

Printed in Singapore by World Scientific Printers (S) Pte Ltd

# PREFACE

Because of rapid developments in computer technology and computational techniques, advances in a wide spectrum of technologies, and other advances coupled with cross-disciplinary pursuits between technology and its applications to human body processes, the field of biomechanics continues to evolve. Many areas of significant progress can be noted. These include dynamics of musculosketal systems, mechanics of hard and soft tissues, mechanics of bone remodeling, mechanics of implant-tissue interfaces, cardiovascular and respiratory biomechanics, mechanics of blood and air flow, flow-prosthesis interfaces, mechanics of impact, dynamics of man-machine interaction, and many more. This is the fourth of a set of four volumes and it treats the area of General Anatomy in biomechanics.

The four volumes constitute an integrated set. The titles for each of the volumes are:

- Biomechanical Systems Technology: Computational Methods
- Biomechanical Systems Technology: Cardiovascular Systems
- Biomechanical Systems Technology: Muscular Skeletal Systems
- Biomechanical Systems Technology: General Anatomy

Collectively they constitute an MRW (Major Reference Work). An MRW is a comprehensive treatment of a subject area requiring multiple authors and a number of distinctly titled and well integrated volumes. Each volume treats a specific but broad subject area of fundamental importance to biomechanical systems technology.

Each volume is self-contained and stands alone for those interested in a specific volume. However, collectively, this 4-volume set evidently constitutes the first comprehensive major reference work dedicated to the multi-discipline area of biomechanical systems technology.

There are over 120 coauthors from 18 countries of this notable MRW. The chapters are clearly written, self contained, readable and comprehensive with helpful guides including introduction, summary, extensive figures and examples with comprehensive reference lists. Perhaps the most valuable feature of this work is the breadth and depth of the topics covered by leading contributors on the international scene.

The contributors of this volume clearly reveal the effectiveness of the techniques available and the essential role that they will play in the future. I hope that practitioners, research workers, computer scientists, and students will find this set of volumes to be a unique and significant reference source for years to come.

# CONTENTS

# CHAPTER 1

# ACOUSTICAL SIGNALS OF BIOMECHANICAL SYSTEMS

EUGENIJUS KANIUSAS

*Institute of Fundamentals and Theory of Electrical Engineering,*
*Bioelectricity & Magnetism Lab, Vienna University of Technology,*
*Gusshausstrasse 27-29/E351, A-1040 Vienna, Austria*
*kaniusas@tuwien.ac.at*

Traditionally, acoustical signals of biomechanical systems show a high clinical relevance when auscultated on the body skin. The heart and lung sounds are applied to the diagnosis of cardiac and respiratory disturbances, respectively, whereas the snoring sounds have been recently acknowledged as important symptoms of the airway obstruction. This chapter aims at the simultaneous consideration of all three types of body sounds from a biomechanical point of view. That is, the respective generation mechanisms are outlined, showing that the vibrations of different tissue structures and air turbulences manifest as regionally concentrated or distributed sound sources. The resulting acoustical properties and mutual interrelations of the body sounds are commented. The investigation of the sound propagation demonstrates an inhomogeneous and frequency-dependant attenuation of sounds within the body, yielding a specific spatial and regional distribution of the sound intensity inside the body and on the body skin (as the auscultation region), respectively. The presented issues pertaining to the biomechanical generation and transmission of the body sounds not only reveal clinically relevant correlations between the physiological phenomena under investigation and the registered biosignals, but also offer a solid basis for both proper understanding of the biosignal relevance and optimization of the recording techniques.

## 1. Introduction

In many ways, the body sounds of human biomechanical systems have remained timeless since Laennec, inventor of the stethoscope,[a] improved the audibility of

---

[a]The stethoscope (greek *stetos* chest and *skopein* explore) is a basic and widely established medical instrument, viewed by many as the very symbol of medicine, for conduction of the sounds generated inside the body between the body surface and the ears. The auscultation of the body sounds was employed more than 20 centuries ago, as suggested in Hippocrates work "de Morbis": "If you listen by applying the ear to the chest...".[1] The inventor of the original stethoscope, R. T. H. Laennec, made in 1816 an epoch making observation with a wooden cylinder which was primarily sought to avoid embarrassment. "I was consulted," says Laennec, "by a young woman who presented some general symptoms of disease of heart... On account of the age and sex of the patient, the common modes of exploration (immediate application of the ear) being inapplicable, I was led to recollect a well known acoustic phenomenon...." Later, in 1894, A. Bianchi introduced a rigid diaphragm over the part of the cylinder that was applied to the chest. Today, the modern stethoscope consists of a bell-type chestpiece for sound amplification, a rubber tube for sound transmission, and earpieces for conducting the sound into ears.[2,3]

heart and lung sounds with the stethoscope. These sounds have conveyed meaningful signals to the examiner looking for cardiorespiratory disturbances. Recently, medical interest has also been focused on snoring sounds, the relevance of which has been acknowledged, for instance, as a warning sign that normal breathing is not taking place during sleep or even as the first sign of the sleep apnea syndrome.[b]

Obviously the stethoscope has continued to be the most relevant instrument for the auscultation (latin *auscultare* the act of listening) of the body sounds since its invention nearly two centuries ago. A modern version of the stethoscope is shown in Fig. 1, which demonstrates a body sounds sensor, i.e. a chestpiece of the stethoscope combined with a microphone. The chestpiece diaphragm being in close contact with the skin vibrates with the skin which, in turn, follows the vibrations induced by the mechanical forces of the body sounds. The vibrations of the diaphragm create acoustic pressure waves traveling into the bell and further to the microphone. The latter acts as an electro-acoustic converter to establish a body sounds signal $s$ for the signal processing.

The physical properties of the arising acoustic transmission path within the body sounds sensor have strong implications on the transmission characteristics of the body sounds. In particular, the resonant characteristics of the chestpiece (= Helmholtz resonator[1,7]) play a significant role concerning the non-linear filtering and amplification characteristics of the body sounds sensor.[1-3,8-10]

## 2. Body Sounds — An Overview

A brief outline of the body sounds is given below, including their biomechanical generation mechanisms and acoustical properties. In particular, it will be shown that the vibrations of tissues, valves inside the heart, blood, walls of airways, and air turbulences manifest as the body sounds which are accessible through the auscultation on the skin (Fig. 1). From an acoustical point of view, the body sounds are normally impure tones or noises, and therefore are composed of a conglomeration of frequencies of multitudinous intensities. As already mentioned, the body sounds include (Fig. 1)

It is worth mentioning that the introduction of the stethoscope forced physicians to a cardinal reorientation, for the stethoscope had altered the physician's perception of acoustical body sounds and his relation to both disease and patient. Despite the clear superiority of the instrument in sound auscultation, it was accepted with some antagonism even by prominent chest physicians.[4] The amusing critics included "The stethoscope is largely a decorative instrument... Nevertheless, it occupies an important place in the art of medicine..." or even complaints of physicians that "they heard too much."

[b]The sleep apnea syndrome represents a complex medical problem characterized by a cessation of effective respiration during sleep. In particular, the so-called obstructive apneas are of great interest, which are characterized by an obstruction of the upper airways and obstructive snoring, i.e. intermittent, loud and irregular snoring. The minimum prevalence of the apneas is about 1%, the apneas causing a severe deterioration of quality of life, excessive daytime somnolence, decreased life expectancy, and negative effects on other family members.[5,6]

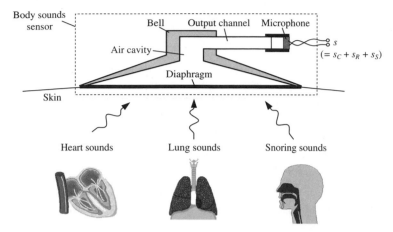

Fig. 1.   Recording of the heart, lung, and snoring sounds by means of the body sounds sensor — a microphone attached to a chestpiece (component of the stethoscope) by a plastic tube. The cross section of the chestpiece is shown, which depicts the diaphragm and the bell with its output channel.

- cardiac component $s_C$,
- respiratory component $s_R$, and
- snoring component $s_S$.

## 2.1. *Heart sounds*

The heart sounds are perhaps the most traditional sounds, as indicated by the fact that the stethoscope was primarily devoted to the auscultation of the heart sounds. These sounds are related to the contractile activity of the cardiohemic system[c] and particularly yield direct information on myocardial and valvular deterioration or on hemodynamic abnormalities.[11,12]

The normal and abnormal heart sounds are generated within the heart (Fig. 2) and may include the following sounds, [11,13–15] as schematically demonstrated in Fig. 3:

(i)    the first sound,
(ii)   the second sound,
(iii)  the third sound,
(iv)   the fourth sound,
(v)    ejection sounds,
(vi)   opening sounds, and
(vii)  murmurs.

---

[c]The cardiohemic system represents the heart and blood together and may be compared to a fluid-filled balloon, which, when stimulated at any location, vibrates as the whole and thus emits the heart sounds.[11]

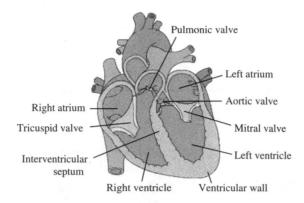

Fig. 2.   Heart anatomy relevant for the generation of the heart sounds.

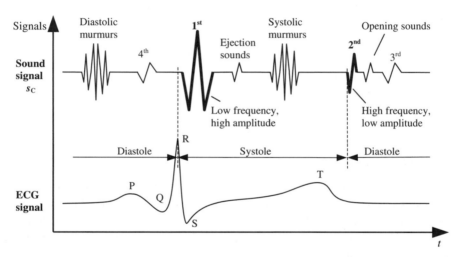

Fig. 3.   Schematic representation of the heart sounds in relation to electrocardiogram (ECG) signal with indicated positions of typical waves P, Q, R, S and T. The amplitude and frequency of the sounds are qualitatively indicated, and the normal sounds are drawn in bold.

**The first sound:** This sound is initiated at the onset of ventricular systole and is related to the close of the atrioventricular valves, i.e. the mitral and the tricuspid valve. Abrupt tension of the valves, deceleration of the blood, and jerky contraction of the ventricular muscles yield vibrations which manifest as the first heart sound. It is the loudest and the longest of all the heart sounds and consists of a series of vibrations of low frequencies. The sound duration is about 140 ms. The frequency spectra of the first heart sound has a peak about 30 Hz with a $-18$ dB/octave decrease in intensity, whereas the intensity decrease in the range $[10,100]$ Hz is about 40 dB.

**The second sound:** It is generated by the closure of the semilunar aortic and pulmonic valves when the interventricular pressure begins to fall. Analogous to the first heart sound, the vibrations occur in the arteries due to deceleration of blood; the ventricles and atria also vibrate due to transmission of vibrations through the blood and the valves. The sound is of shorter duration of about 110 ms ($<$ 140 ms) and lower intensity, and has a more snapping quality than the first heart sound, as will be demonstrated later. The reason for the shorter duration is that the semilunar valves are much tauter than the atrioventricular valves and thus tend to close much more rapidly. As a result of the short duration, the second sound is composed of high frequency vibrations. Contrary to the first heart sound, the second sound does not show any consistent spectral peak, but rolls off more gradually as a function of frequency with an intensity decrease of only 30 dB ($<$ 40 dB) over the range [10,100] Hz.

**The third sound:** It occurs in early diastole, just after the second heart sound, during the time of rapid ventricular filling when the ventricular wall twitches. The vibrations are of very low frequency because the walls are relaxed. The sound is abnormal if heard in individuals over the age of 40.

**The fourth sound:** This sound is an abnormal diastolic sound which occurs at the time when the atria contract during the late diastolic filling phase, displacing blood into the distended ventricles. The fourth heart sound is heard just before the first heart sound and is a low frequency sound.

**Ejection sounds:** They are produced by the opening of the semilunar aortic or pulmonic valves, in particular, when one of these valves is diseased. The sounds arise shortly after the first heart sound with the onset of ventricular ejection. The ejection sounds are high frequency clicky sounds.

**Opening sounds:** They are most frequently the result of a sudden pathological arrest of the opening of the mitral or tricuspid valve. The sounds occur after the second heart sound in early diastole and represent short high frequency sounds.

**Murmurs:** These sounds, by definition, are sustained noises that are audible during the time periods of systole (= systolic murmurs) and diastole (= diastolic murmurs). Basically, the murmurs are abnormal sounds and are produced by

(a)  backward regurgitation through a leaking valve,
(b)  forward flow through a narrowed or deformed valve,
(c)  high rate of blood flow (= turbulent flow) through a normal or abnormal valve, and
(d)  vibration of loose structures within the heart.

The systolic and diastolic murmurs consist principally of high frequency components in the range[d] [120,600] Hz, occasionally ascending to 1000 Hz.

---

[d]In particular, the systolic murmurs of aortic insufficiency and the mitral diastolic murmurs fall in the range [20,115] Hz.[1,2] The aortic diastolic murmurs and pericardial rubs occur at higher frequencies in the range [140,600] Hz. The presystolic murmurs lay, for the most part, in the range below 140 Hz, but may contain components up to 400 Hz.

In normal subjects, only the first and the second heart sound are audible (Fig. 3), as the other sounds are normally of very low intensity. Concerning the spectral region of both normal heart sounds, early studies[1] found that the energy components above 110 Hz are negligible. The main frequency components were found to fall in the approximate range [20,120] Hz.[2] However, the second heart sound includes more high frequency components than the first sound,[14] which complies with the respective origin of the sounds, as discussed above. Furthermore, the second heart sound is not confined to a narrow frequency bandwidth lacking in concentrated energy which is also contrary to the first heart sound.

Figure 4 demonstrates the normal cardiac sounds for a healthy subject during breath hold, as registered by the body sounds sensor (Fig. 1).[5] It consists of $s_C$, which shows cardiac rate $f_C$ close to 0.9 Hz. According to the spectrogram, the first and the second heart sound are mainly characterized by short-term frequency components of up to approximately 100 Hz, with weak harmonics of up to approximately 500 Hz. In the intermediate time intervals, the spectrum is restricted to about 50 Hz. It can be observed that the second heart sound shows slightly higher spectral amplitudes and is shorter in duration ($\Delta t_1 > \Delta t_2$, Fig. 4), which is in full agreement with the discussed behavior of the first and the second heart sound.

Obviously, the frequency components of the heart sounds overlap with those of the breath sounds (Sec. 2.2), especially with the low frequency components of the breath sounds spectrum.[15] The particular interference of the heart sounds in the breathing sounds recorded on the neck was investigated by Lessard and Jones.[14] The authors have shown that the contribution of the heart sounds cannot be neglected even at frequencies above 100 Hz. The first sound was shown to contribute to the acoustic power in the frequency band [75,125] Hz during expiration and to band [175,225] Hz during inspiration. The second heart sound appeared to contribute

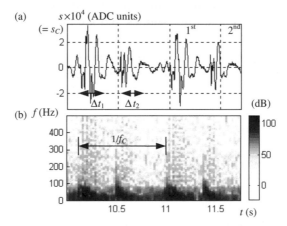

Fig. 4. Heart sounds during breath hold. (a) Sound signal $s$ in the time domain, restricted to the cardiac component $s_C$ including first and second heart sounds. (b) The spectrogram shows higher spectral amplitudes of the second heart sound ($\Delta t_1 > \Delta t_2$).

to the acoustic power in the more extended bands, namely [75,325] Hz during expiration and [75,425] Hz during inspiration. It should be noted that the latter observation is consistent with the aforementioned intensity decreases of the first and the second heart sound.

## 2.2. *Lung sounds*

Unlike the heart sounds, the situation with the respiratory induced lung sounds is considerably more complicated, though devaluated by some physicians 30 years ago as "the sound repertoire of a wet sponge such as the lung is limited."[16] Today, the most promising application areas of the lung sounds are in the upper airway diagnostics, e.g. monitoring of apneas,[b] in the lower airway diagnostics, e.g. registration of asthma, and in the registration of regional ventilation.

Generally, the lung sounds are caused by air vibrations within the lung and its airways that are transmitted through the lung tissue (= lung parenchyma) and thoracic wall[e] to the recording site.[4] The lung sounds depend upon several factors, such as airflow, inspiration and expiration phases, site of recording, and degree of voluntary control, and are spread over a wide frequency band,[17] as will be discussed in the following.

The status of the lung sounds nomenclature is best viewed in terms of a historical fact that Laennec, inventor of the stethoscope (refer to footnote a), noted that the lung sounds heard were easier to distinguish than to describe.[f] No doubt, high variability of the lung sounds yielded at that time and yields up to now difficulties in the reproducibility of observations. However, the lung sounds can be roughly categorized into

- normal sounds which are characteristic for healthy subjects and
- abnormal sounds heard in pathological cases only.

The most common classification of the normal lung sounds is based on their location, i.e. their auscultation region.[4,15–19] Three following types of the normal sounds can be distinguished:

(i)   tracheobronchial sounds,
(ii)  vesicular sounds, and
(iii) bronchovesicular sounds.

---

[e]The vibration amplitude may be less than $10\,\mu m$ depending on the method of recording. For instance, mechanical loading by a massive chestpiece (compare Fig. 1) would limit the amplitude of the skin surface motion, for the stress of the skin beneath the chestpiece is increased.
[f]To accommodate the difficulties in describing the lung sounds, familiar sounds (at that time) were chosen to clarify the distinguishing characteristics.[4] Descriptive and illustrative sounds were used as "crepitation of salts in a heated dish," "noise emitted by healthy lung when compressed in the hand," or even "cooing of wood pigeon."

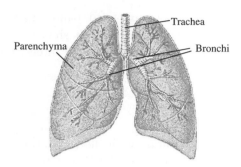

Fig. 5.   Lung and adjacent airways relevant for the generation of the lung sounds.

**Tracheobronchial sounds:** The bronchial and tracheal breath sounds are heard over the large airways (4 mm and larger), e.g. on the lateral neck. The generation region of these sounds is situated centrally and is primarily related to the turbulent airflow in the upper airways, i.e. the trachea and bronchi (Fig. 5). The high air velocity[g] and turbulent airflow induce vibrations in the airway gas and airway walls. The vibrations that reach the neck surface are then recorded as the tracheobronchial sounds. These sounds show hollow character, are loud, and contain frequency components up to about 1 kHz, the spectral response curve falling sharply to reach the base line levels in the range [1.2,1.8] kHz.[17] Furthermore, a typical characteristic of these sounds is a silent gap[h] between inspiration and expiration.

**Vesicular sounds:** These sounds are heard on the thorax in the peripheral lung fields through alveolar tissue. They mainly arise due to air movements into the small airways of the lung parenchyma (Fig. 5) during inspiration. The air branches into smaller and smaller airways as it moves to the alveoli, and turbulences are created as the air hits these branches of the airways. These turbulences are suspected of producing the vesicular sounds. Contrary to the inspiration, the air flows during the expiration from small airways to much larger less confining ones and does not contact the airway surfaces. Thus there is much less turbulence created during the expiration and therefore less sound. At the expiration also the tracheobronchial sounds (with their central source) significantly contribute to the relatively weak surface sounds on the thorax. As a result, the sounds during the inspiration are produced in the locally distributed sources in the periphery of the lung and show relatively high amplitudes and high frequency maxima; during the expiration the sounds originate more centrally and are relatively weak because of long transmission paths. The latter behavior is demonstrated in Fig. 6(a) showing that the vesicular sounds, as recorded by the body sounds sensor (Fig. 1), occur mainly during the inspiration. For instance, Fachinger[19] reports that the inspiratory sounds show

---

[g]The airflow of lower velocity is laminar in type and is therefore silent.
[h]The reason for this gap is that the tracheobronchial sounds come only from the largest airways, the trachea and bronchi, the sounds disappearing temporally at the end of inspiration because at this moment the flow of air passes through the peripheral part of the lung.[20]

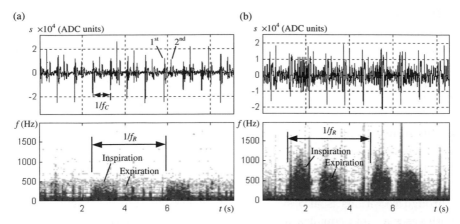

Fig. 6. Lung sounds during normal breathing. (a) Vesicular sounds in the time and spectral domain when recorded on the chest. (b) Tracheobronchial sounds recorded on the neck.

twice as large intensity on the anterior chest as that of the expiratory sounds. Generally, the vesicular sounds are clearly distinguishable at about 100 Hz but the amplitude fall-off to baseline values at about 1 kHz is much more rapid than for the tracheobronchial sounds,[17] as can also be observed in Fig. 6.

Thus, in comparison with the tracheobronchial sounds (Fig. 6(b)), the vesicular sounds (Fig. 6(a)) show lower intensity, smaller spectral range, and more rapid amplitude fall-off with increasing frequency. These differences can be mainly attributed to the fact that the vesicular sounds, when transmitted to the periphery, are filtered to a greater extent than the tracheobronchial sounds. The vesicular sounds have longer transmission paths with more inertial (= damping) components (Sec. 4). For instance,[4] the normal lung sounds with frequencies higher than 1 kHz were more clearly detected over the trachea than on the chest wall.

**Bronchovesicular sounds:** These are breath sounds intermediate in characteristics between the tracheobronchial and vesicular sounds.

The abnormal (or adventitious) sounds are heard in pathological cases only and can be classified[1,4,16,20–23] into

(i)   continuous sounds with a duration of more than 250 ms and
(ii)  discontinuous sounds arising for a time period of less than 20 ms.

**Continuous sounds:** These sounds show a musical character and exhibit a larger deviation from the Gaussian distribution than the discontinuous sounds. A further subdivision is commonly used:

(a) **Wheezes:** The generation mechanism appears to involve central and lower airways walls interacting with the gas moving through the airways. In particular, narrowing and constriction of the airways as well as narrowing to the point where opposite walls touch one another cause the wheezes. Wheezes are high frequency, musical noises.

(b) **Rhonchi:** These sounds are caused by large airways becoming narrowed or constricted, for instance, due to secretions that are moving through the large bronchioles and bronchi. The sounds are sonorous and are like rapidly damped sinusoids of low frequency.

(c) **Stridors:** These sounds are musical wheezes that suggest obstructed trachea or larynx.

**Discontinuous sounds:** This type of sounds arises due to explosive reopening of a succession of small airways or fluid-filled alveoli, previously held closed by surface forces during expiration. The abnormal closure is due to an increased lung stiffness or excessive fluid within the airways. On the other hand, bubbling of the air through secretions is also suspected of generating the discontinuous sounds. In both cases a rapid equalization of gas pressures and a release of tissue tensions occur, which cause a sequence of implosive noise-like sounds. A further subdivision is also used:

(a) **Coarse crackles:** These are low frequency sounds usually indicative of large fluid accumulation in the alveoli.

(b) **Fine crackles:** They show shorter duration than the coarse crackles and are high frequency sounds.

(c) **Squawks:** These explosive sounds represent a combination of the wheezes and crackles, which arise from an explosive opening and fluttering of the unstable airways.

Figure 7 shows vesicular sounds during normal breathing with respiratory rate $f_R$ close to 0.2 Hz, the sounds being recorded by the body sounds sensor (Fig. 1).[5] It can be seen that $s$ in this case (Fig. 7(a)) is similar to $s_C$ in the case of breath holding (Fig. 4(a)), as the signal level of $s_R$ is about 30 dB lower than that of $s_C$ (compare with Fig. 17 in Sec. 5), thus $s_R$ being completely overlaid by $s_C$. However, during inspiration we recognize that $s_R$ is slightly superimposed on $s_C$, as demonstrated in the left fragment of the sum signal $s$ (Fig. 7(a)), but not during expiration, as shown in the right fragment. This difference related to the phases of inspiration and expiration is in full agreement with the aforementioned generation mechanisms of the vesicular sounds.

A clear manifestation of the respiratory activity is restricted to the spectrogram, as one can observe in Fig. 7(b). Here, inspiration appears with a basic frequency $f_{R1}$ close to 250 Hz and a second harmonic at 500 Hz, the value of $f_{R1}$ varying between patients. The expiration is characterized by a noise-like spectrum of even lower intensity (about −15 dB) in the range up to about 500 Hz.

From a practical point of view, one of the most important characteristics of the normal lung sounds is that their intensity reflects the strength of the respiratory airflow $F$. That is, the amplitude and the frequency maxima of the normal lung sounds increase as $F$ rises, particularly during inspiration.[17]

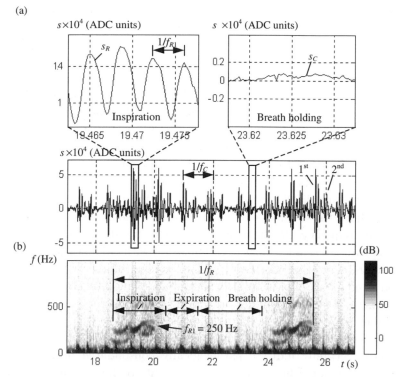

Fig. 7. Vesicular lung sounds during normal breathing. (a) Sensor signal $s$ dominated by $s_C$ (first and second heart sounds). Details are given for the instant of inspiration (left upper figure) and for the break between expiration and next inspiration (right upper figure). (b) The spectrogram with indicated basic oscillation frequency $f_{R1}$.

For instance, the regional intensity of the vesicular sounds varies with the regional distribution of ventilation;[4,24] thus the sound intensity is a potentially good measure of regional pulmonary ventilation. The amplitude of $s_R$ could be approximated by an exponential relationship, to give

$$s_R \propto F^n, \tag{1}$$

where $n$ is the power index. The reported values of $n$ were 1.75 and 2 according to Fachinger[19] and Pasterkamp *et al.*,[16] respectively.

Similar to the vesicular sounds, measurements of mean amplitudes and mean frequencies of the tracheobronchial sounds provide a linear measure for $F$ ($n = 1$ in Eq. (1)), in particular, when sounds at higher frequencies are analyzed, e.g. at frequencies above 1 kHz.[16,25] Dalmay *et al.*[17] confirm this linear relationship, however, for a different frequency range [100,800] Hz. In addition, the latter authors report that the maximum frequency values are shifted upwards as $F$ increases.

It should be noted that the intensity of the lung sounds, especially, of the vesicular sounds and the wheezes, shows a strong inverse relation to the severity of airflow obstruction.[16] In other words, reduced sound intensity indicates obstructive pulmonary disease while increased intensity is considered indicative of lung expansion.[24]

The aforementioned high variability of the lung sounds should be addressed in some depth. As shown in many studies,[16–18,24] sound amplitudes vary greatly from one subject to another, even from sitting to lying position, the variability being more significant during expiration than during inspiration. The variability is mainly due to the strong influence of individual airway anatomy[16] and lung–muscle–fat ratios.[18] An abolishment of this variability was shown to be unsuccessful for identical $F$ or even by an introduction of correction for physical characteristics of subjects, e.g. weight or age of subjects.[17] As a result of the high variability, flagrant disparities can be observed in published quantitative data on the lung sounds.

For instance, the infants exhibit increased vesicular sound intensity and higher median frequency, the differences being attributed, respectively, to acoustic transmission through smaller lungs in combination with thinner chest walls (Sec. 4) and to a different resonance behavior of the smaller thorax.[16,24] Contrary to the infants and adults, elderly patients show decreased sound intensity due to restricted lung volume, i.e. restricted ventilation. However, the decrease in sound intensity towards higher frequencies is similar at all ages.

The tracheobronchial sounds if heard instead of or in addition to the vesicular sounds almost certainly indicate pathologically consolidated lung.[4,17,26] This is because the consolidated lung acts like an efficient conducting medium that does not attenuate the transmission of the centrally produced tracheobronchial sounds, as does the inflated normal lung.

## 2.3. *Snoring sounds*

Unlike the heart and lung sounds, medical interest has only been recently focused on the snoring sounds. These arise mainly during the inspiration,[27] may constitute excessive noise exposure, and may even cause hearing problems.[28] Epidemiological studies[6] have shown that 36% of males and 19% of females were snorers, whereby the prevalence increases significantly after the age of 40, with 50% of elderly population being habitual snorers.[29]

Generally, the snoring is preceded by a temporal decrease in the diameter of the oropharynx which can be reduced even to a slit, the reduced diameter yielding an increase in the supraglottic resistance.[27,30] Further narrowing of the oropharynx may lead to not only louder snoring, but also labored breathing. Finally, yet further narrowing can cause complete occlusion of the airways, which manifests as the sleep apnea (refer to Footnote b).

The snoring sounds are mainly generated by high frequency oscillations (= vibrations) of the soft palate and pharyngeal walls, as shown in Fig. 8, as well as by the turbulence of air.[29,31] Usually the sounds energy is negligible above 2 kHz.[31]

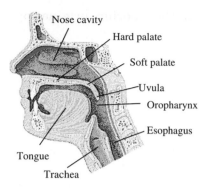

Fig. 8.   Pharyngeal airways and surrounding structures relevant for the generation of the snoring sounds.

The rate of appearance of repetitive sound structures during snoring coincides with the time course of airway wall motions and the collapsibility of the upper airways.[32] Generally, the characteristics of snoring are determined by the relationship between $F$ and pressure in the upper airways as well as by the airway collapsibility.

Mainly two complementing theories exist, which describe the sound generation mechanisms[31]:

- flutter theory and
- relaxation theory.

The so-called "flutter theory" is devoted to the explanation of the steady continuous forms of the snoring sounds in the time domain. According to this theory, the continuous sounds are produced by the oscillations of the airway walls when the airflow is forced through a collapsible airway and can interact with the elastic walls.

The "relaxation theory" is dedicated to the explosive snoring sounds which are produced by collapsible airways. That is, the low frequency oscillations of the airway walls yield complete or partial occlusion of the lumen with the point of maximum constriction moving upstream along the airway. The repetitive openings of the airway lumen with abrupt pressure equalization generate the explosive sounds.

Similar to the lung sounds (Sec. 2.2), the diversity and the variability of the snoring sounds are extremely large. The snoring sounds may change even from one breath to another. As a result, there is a large number of possibilities to classify the snoring sounds, each of them relying on different bases,

- snoring origination region,
- type of snoring generation, and
- snoring signal waveform.

Obviously, the above classification possibilities are non-exclusive, i.e. some types of the snoring sounds may be described by the use of two or more bases from the above.

**Classification based on the snoring origination region,**[27,31] i.e. snoring through

(i)   nose,
(ii)  mouth, or
(iii) nose and mouth.

**Nasal snoring:** In this case the soft palate remains in close contact with the back of the tongue, and only the uvula yields high frequency oscillations, the oscillation frequency being about 80 Hz.[27] In the frequency domain, the snoring has been demonstrated to show discrete sharp peaks at about 200 Hz, the peaks corresponding to the resonant peaks (= formants) of the resonating cavities of the airways and suggesting a single sound source.[31]

**Oral snoring:** This type of snoring is characterized by an ample oscillation of the whole soft palate. The oscillation frequency of about 30 Hz[27] is lower than that during the nasal snoring because the oscillating mass of the soft palate is larger than that of the uvula.

**Oronasal snoring:** These snoring sounds include both nasal and oral snoring. The corresponding spectrum shows a mixture of sharp peaks and broad-band white noise in the [400,1300] Hz range.[31] The large number of peaks may reflect two or more segments oscillating with different frequencies.

**Classification according to the type of generation,**[27,29,31,32] i.e.

(i)   normal snoring,
(ii)  obstructive snoring, and
(iii) simulated snoring.

**Normal snoring:** It is always preceded by the airflow limitation.[27,31,32] The narrowing of the pharyngeal diameter is thought to be produced by the negative oropharyngeal pressure generated during the inspiration or sleep-related fall[i] in the tone of upper airway muscles, which yields a passive collapse of the upper airways. Furthermore, the supraglottic pressure and $F$ show 180° out-of-phase oscillations[j] and a relatively small hysteresis.[27] The snoring sounds show a regular rattling character[31] with significant spectral components in the frequency range [100,600] Hz and minor components of up to 1000 Hz.[29] The normal snoring most likely pertains to the aforementioned "flutter theory."

**Obstructive snoring:** This pathological type of snoring is associated with high frequency oscillations of the soft palate. In particular, a strong narrowing of the

---

[i]The pharyngeal muscle tone can be reduced by not only sleep, but also alcohol, sedatives, or neurological disorders.[6]

[j]The 180° out-of-phase relationship between the supraglottic pressure (= pressure drop across the supralaryngeal airway) and $F$ could be explained by successive partial closings and openings of the pharynx by the soft palate, resulting in opposite changes in the supraglottic pressure and $F$.[27]

airways and even their temporal occlusion[27] occur due to high compliance of the airway walls.[31] The hysteresis between the supraglottic pressure and $F$ is much larger than that during the normal snoring. The obstructive snoring sounds are louder than the normal snoring sounds, exhibit fricative and high frequency sounds, and show intermittent and highly variable patterns. They show an irregular white noise with a broad spectral peak of about 450 Hz and another around 1000 Hz. Furthermore, the ratio of cumulative power above 800 Hz to power below 800 Hz is higher for the obstructive snoring when compared to the normal snoring. The obstructive snoring likely pertains to the already described "relaxation theory," in contrast to the normal snoring.

**Simulated snoring:** Contrary to the normal and obstructive snoring, the simulated snoring is not preceded by the air flow limitation.[27] The narrowing of the pharyngeal diameter could be produced by voluntary active contraction of the pharyngeal muscles. According to Beck *et al.*,[29] the simulated snoring could be characterized as complex waveform snoring (see below).

**Classification accounting for the distinct signal waveform patterns,**[29] i.e.

(i)   complex waveform snoring and
(ii)   simple waveform snoring.

**Complex waveform snoring:** In the time domain, these snores are characterized by repetitive, equally spaced train of structures which start with a large deflection and end up with a decaying amplitude. The sound structures arise with the frequencies in the [60,130] Hz range showing internal oscillations of up to 1000 Hz. In the frequency domain, a comb-line spectrum with multiple peaks can be observed. The complex waveform snoring may result from colliding of the airway walls with an intermittent closure of the lumen.

**Simple waveform snoring:** Contrary to the complex waveform snoring, the simple waveform snoring shows a nearly sinusoidal waveform of higher frequency with negligible secondary oscillations. Thus the frequency domain exhibits only 1 up to 3 peaks in the [180,300] Hz range, of which the first is the most prominent. This type of snoring results probably from the vibration of the airway walls around a neutral position without actual closure of the lumen.

Figure 9 shows typical experimental results for different types of snoring which were recorded by the body sounds sensor (Fig. 1).[5] The variability of snoring proved to be very high, with significant changes in the time and frequency domain being possible even from one breath to the next. Nevertheless, there is an evident difference between the normal and obstructive snoring.

As can be seen in Fig. 9(a), the normal snoring is characterized by distinct heart sound peaks, $s_S$ not appearing clearly in the time domain, which is similar to the appearance of the heart and lung sounds (Figs. 4 and 7). However, the snoring becomes evident in the spectrogram. The given case shows a basic harmonic line $f_{R1} \approx 140$ Hz which also clearly appears in the depicted time domain fragment

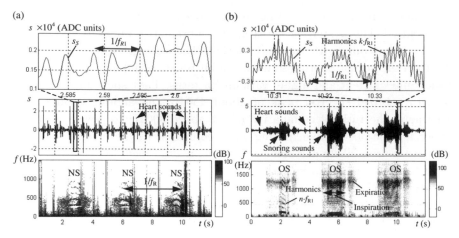

Fig. 9. Snoring sounds including a fragment (upper figure) and the corresponding spectrogram (lower figure). (a) Sensor signal $s$ during normal snoring (NS) from a non-apneic patient, dominated by the heart sounds. (b) Obstructive snoring (OS) dominated by the snoring events from a patient with obstructive sleep apnea.

(upper figure of Fig. 9(a)). Furthermore, we find a series of harmonics up to almost 1000 Hz. This means that compared to the lung sounds during normal breathing, the spectrum proves to be wider here and shows higher intensity, according to the stronger gray tones.

Figure 9(b) shows the obstructive snoring. Contrary to the normal snoring (Fig. 9(a)), the obstructive snoring is not characterized by heart sound peaks in the time domain. Component $s_S$ exhibits much higher amplitudes, the difference being up to approximately 20 dB. The snoring events are also predominant in the spectrogram. Inspiration shows the series of harmonics up to 1000 Hz. It is followed by a noise-like structure which may exceed 1500 Hz and which also appears with lower amplitude during expiration. It can be deduced from the above description that the observed normal snoring (Fig. 9(a)) shows properties of the oronasal and normal snoring, whereas the observed obstructive snoring (Fig. 9(b)) is intermediate in characteristics between oronasal, obstructive, and complex waveform snoring.

A few words should be dedicated to the intensity levels of the snoring sounds, in comparison with the normal lung sounds (Sec. 2.2). Generally, the background noise level in test rooms could reach 50 dB SPL,[k] and normal breathing levels could go up to 54 dB SPL.[32] The normal breathing levels are in the [40,45] dB SPL range (or [17,26] dBA[l]).[34,35]

---

[k] Abbreviation dB SPL stays for sound pressure measurements in decibels using the reference sound pressure level (SPL) of 20 $\mu$Pa and a flat response network in the frequency domain (compare Footnote 1). For instance, a normal conversation yields about 60 dB SPL, whereas a vacuum cleaner and a pneumatic drill exhibit in a distance of a few meters about 70 dB SPL and 100 dB SPL, respectively.[33]

The snoring sound level has spikes in intensity greater than 60 dB SPL[32,36] or even greater than 68 dB SPL[34] and may reach levels of more than 100 dB SPL (according to diverging reports) in a distance of less than 1 m from the head of the patient. According to Schäfer,[34] women show reduced snoring sound levels by about 10 dB SPL, whereas Wilson *et al.*[28] report about the men–women difference of only about 3 dBA, which translates into a substantially different sound intensity perception. Furthermore, the latter authors report average snoring sound intensities in the [50,70] dBA range of patients with the obstructive snoring, the levels being more than 5 dBA higher for apneic snoring than for non-apneic snoring. An overview[35] refers to snoring sound levels up to 80 and 94 dBA for non-apneic snoring and apneic snoring, respectively.

Analogous to the lung sounds (Sec. 2.2), there are reports about the relationship between the snoring sounds and $F$. As reported by Beck *et al.*,[29] the highest and sharpest amplitude deflections of the snoring sounds occur when the amplitude of $F$ is at its highest (compare Eq. (1)).

Similar to the lung sounds, the snoring sounds also show the aforementioned high variability.[37] In particular, the variability of the obstructive snoring is very high; the sound characteristics may strongly change even from one breath to the next.[29] As suggested by Perez-Padilla *et al.*,[31] the high variability may arise due to

(i)  changing characteristics of the resonant airway cavities, e.g. pharynx or mouth cavities,
(ii)  variations of the site of collapse of the airway, or
(iii)  varying upper airway resistance since the airways geometry varies from occluded to fully dilated.

It should be noted that the snoring, especially the obstructive snoring, may be related to increased morbidity, systemic hypertension, cerebrovascular diseases, stroke, severe sleep abnormalities, and even impaired cognitive functions.[6,28,32] As a physiologic example, the duration of the snoring seems to be positively correlated to the strength of oxygen desaturation in blood.[38]

As already mentioned, there is strong evidence that the obstructive snoring may also be an intermediate in the natural history of sleep apnea syndrome (refer to Footnote b) and thus may be applied for the detection of apneas.[m] As shown in Fig. 10, the pathologically narrowed airways can periodically interrupt the snoring by respiratory arrests, followed by sonorous breathing resumptions as apneic gasps

---

[l]Analogous to the definition of dB SPL (compare Footnote k), abbreviation dBA stays for the sound pressure measurements in decibels, however, employing the A-weighting network that yields the response of the human ear. This network attenuates disproportionately the very low frequencies, e.g. −30 dB SPL at 50 Hz and 0 dB SPL at 1 kHz.[33]
[m]An overview of the available literature discloses a number of possibilities for the detection of apneas by the use of the body sounds. In particular, the detection procedures can be roughly classified into three groups, i.e. detection by (i) trained physicians,[39] (ii) total sound intensity,[16,36,38,40–43] and (iii) partial sound intensity within restricted spectral region.[25,43–48]

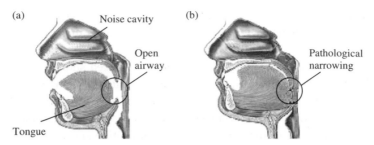

Fig. 10.   Pharyngeal airways and surrounding structures (compare Fig. 8) for (a) a non-apneic patient and (b) an apneic patient.

for air.[29] Indeed, the snoring is considered as a primary symptom for the sleep apnea[41]; however, the snoring is not specific for the apnea.[28]

Lastly, the physiologic and social factors which favor the snoring should be shortly discussed. Obviously, small pharyngeal area, as demonstrated in Fig. 10, and pharyngeal floppiness (= distensibility), i.e. strong changes in the pharyngeal area in response to externally applied positive pressure, favor the snoring.[6,41] In addition, cervical position, obesity (= high values of the obesity index, the so-called body mass index BMI[n]), large neck circumference, presence of space occupying masses impinging on the airway, e.g. soft palate (or uvula) hypertrophy or tumors, and pathological restriction of the nasal airway, e.g. rhinitis, assist the snoring in a disadvantageous way.[49,50] Among the social factors supporting the occurrence of the snoring, stress, tiredness and alcohol intake are worth to be mentioned. Finally, subjective factors as home environment or sleep lab influence the severity of the snoring, which tends to be higher in the sleep lab.[32]

## 3. Mutual Interrelations of Body Sounds

One can expect that the different body sounds, as described in Secs. 2.1–2.3, are not fully independent, and so the sound components $s_C$, $s_R$, and $s_S$ are interdependent. Thus the signal characteristics of the latter components show specific relationships, as schematically demonstrated in Fig. 11, which can be generally attributed to mechanical, neural and functional interrelations between the respective sound generation sources.

We start with the respiratory induced effects on $s_C$ (Sec. 2.1), i.e. with a dependence of $s_C$ on $s_R$ (Fig. 11). During inspiration, these effects can be summarized as follows:

[n]The BMI is an anthropometric measure defined as weight in kilograms divided by the square of height in meters. Usually BMI $> 30$ indicates obesity.

Heart sounds ($s_C$)

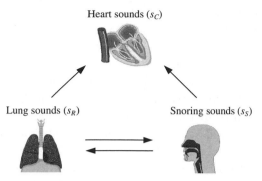

Lung sounds ($s_R$)          Snoring sounds ($s_S$)

Fig. 11. Mutual interrelations of the different body sounds with indicated direction of influence.

(i)   the second heart sound is split,
(ii)  the right-sided heart sounds are intensified while the left-sided heart sounds are slightly attenuated, and
(iii) the rate of the heart sounds ($= f_C$) is increased.

The first two effects arise because the heart is in the immediate anatomical vicinity of the lung, which suggests a rather strong mechanical interrelation between the sources of $s_C$ and $s_R$. Here the source of $s_R$, in particular, the changing volume of the lung, influences the pressure conditions within the heart and those close to the heart over the respiration cycle. During inspiration, the intrathoracic pressure is decreased, allowing air to enter the lungs, which yields an increase of the right ventricular stroke volume (of the venous blood)[o] and a simultaneous decrease of the left ventricular stroke volume (of the arterial blood).[p]

The reason for the split heart sound during inspiration (the first effect) can be especially attributed to the temporal increase of the right ventricular stroke volume, which causes the pulmonic valve (Fig. 2) to stay open longer during ventricular systole (Fig. 3). The delayed closure of the pulmonic valve gives rise to a delayed sound contribution to the second heart sound, whereas the preceding contribution

---

[o]In particular, the right ventricular stroke volume is increased during inspiration because of the respiratory pump mechanism.[51] That is, the intrathoracic pressure decreases, and the pressure gradient between the peripheral venous system and the intrathoracic veins increases.[52] This causes blood to be drawn from the peripheral veins into the intrathoracic vessels, which increases the right ventricular stroke volume.
[p]The decreased left ventricular stroke volume during inspiration can be mainly attributed to three effects[51-55]:

(i) the increased capacity in the pulmonary vessels (see Footnote o) reduces mechanically the left ventricular stroke volume due to leftward displacement of the interventricular septum (Fig. 2),

(ii) corresponding to the mechanism of the respiratory sinus arrhythmia (see Footnote q), an increase of $f_C$ during inspiration reduces the diastolic filling time of the heart and contributes to the decrease of the left ventricular stroke volume, and

(iii) the decreased intrathoracic ($=$ pleural) pressure during inspiration lowers the effective left ventricular ejection pressure and impedes the left ventricular stroke volume ($=$ reverse thoracic pump mechanism).

to this sound results from a slightly earlier closure of the aortic valve (Sec. 2.1). In analogy, the earlier closure can be attributed to the decreased left ventricular stroke volume. As a result, the second heart sound is split more strongly during inspiration than during expiration.

The dominance of the right-sided heart sounds during inspiration (the second effect) can be also explained by the increased right ventricular stroke volume. Since these sounds are generated by the closure of the right-sided tricuspid and pulmonic valve (Fig. 2), the increased volume of the decelerated right-sided blood tends to increase the intensity of the right-sided sounds. On the other hand, the amount of blood entering the left-sided chambers of the heart is decreased, which causes the left-sided heart sounds (generated by the closure of the left-sided mitral and aortic valve, Fig. 2) to generally decrease in intensity.

In contrast to the first two effects as discussed above, the third effect is not governed by the mechanical interrelations between the sources of $s_C$ and $s_R$, but by a neural interrelation in between. Corresponding to the mechanism of the respiratory sinus arrhythmia,[q] the value of $f_C$ increases temporally during inspiration, whereas the reverse is true for expiration. In addition, the degree of the variation of $f_C$ is also significantly controlled by impulses from the baroreceptors in the aorta and carotid arteries since the blood pressure also changes over the breathing cycle.[55]

Obviously, the mutual interrelation between $s_R$ and $s_S$ is very strong (Fig. 11), for the respective sources are governed by the same breathing activity. This intrinsic dependence yields identical respiratory and snoring rate (= $f_R$); nonetheless, the signal properties of $s_R$ and $s_S$ are very different (Secs. 2.2 and 2.3). In addition, one can also expect an indirect interrelation between $s_R$ and $s_S$. For instance, the obstructive snoring may intermittently occlude the upper airways, which could temporally alter the resonance characteristics of the upper airways and thus the spectral content of $s_R$.

At last, the dependence of $s_C$ on $s_S$ will be shortly addressed (Fig. 11). In healthy subjects, this dependence equals the discussed dependence between $s_C$ and $s_R$, for both $s_R$ and $s_S$ are of the respiratory origin. However, in pathological cases the obstructive snoring may strongly influence $s_C$ since the obstruction overloads the heart, favoring cardiovascular diseases (compare Sec. 2.3). In particular, the influence on $s_C$ gets stronger when the obstructive snoring occurs in combination with the intermittent closures of the airway lumen, i.e. with the intermittent apneas (see Footnote b).

Figure 12 exemplifies the discussed relationship between $s_C$ and $s_R$, the latter components assessed by the body sounds sensor (Fig. 1). The depicted envelope in Fig. 12(a) demonstrates the intensification of the heart sounds (= $s_C$) during

---

[q]The respiratory sinus arrhythmia occurs through the influence of breathing on the sympathetic and vagus impulses to the sinoatrial node which initiates the heart beats.[52,55] During inspiration, the vagus nerve activity is impeded, which increases the force of contraction and raises $f_C$, whereas during expiration this pattern is reversed.

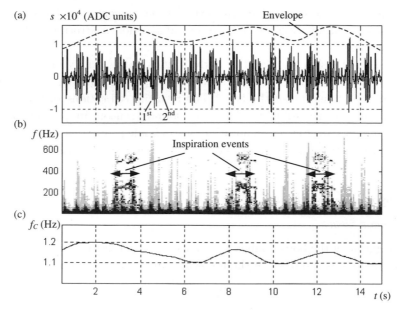

Fig. 12. Mutual dependence of the heart and lung sounds. (a) Sensor signal $s$ with prevailing $s_C$ (first and second heart sounds) and the respiratory induced envelope. (b) The corresponding spectrogram. (c) Variation of the heart rate $f_C$ over respiration cycles.

inspiration, the inspiratory events ($= s_R$) being recognizable in the spectral domain (Fig. 12(b)). Furthermore, Fig. 12(c) shows that the values of $f_C$ increase temporally during the phases of inspiration, which is in full agreement with the aforementioned effect of the respiratory sinus arrhythmia (see Footnote q) on $f_C$.

It can be deduced from the latter experimental observation that the amplification of the right-sided heart sounds during inspiration is stronger than the concurrent attenuation of the left-sided heart sounds, since the total intensity of the heart sounds raises. In addition, an identical tendency of the amplitude of $s_C$ to increase during inspiration can be observed in Fig. 7(a) which depicts a different experimental data set. However, the observed dominance of the amplification of the right-sided heart sounds versus the non-dominant attenuation of the left-sided heart sounds during inspiration may not be generally valid. This is because there are published data[56] that demonstrate the opposite behavior, namely the intensity of the heart sounds was observed to increase during expiration.

## 4. Transmission of Body Sounds

The total acoustical path of the body sounds begins with a vibrating structure which may be given by vibrating valves yielding the heart sounds or air turbulences in the upper airways accounting partially for the lung and snoring sounds (Secs. 2.1–2.3). These mechanically generated vibrations propagate within the body tissues along many paths toward the skin surface. However, a large percentage of the sound energy never reaches the surface because of spreading, absorption, scattering, reflection, and refraction losses.

Arrived to the skin surface, the body sounds cause skin vibrations of three different waveforms: transversal (or shear) waves, longitudinal (or compression) waves, and a combination of the two.[3] The resulting vibrations of the skin serve as a sound source accessible to the body sounds sensor, in particular, to the chestpiece diaphragm (Fig. 1). In addition, viscoelastic properties[r] of the skin make the interaction between the sounds and the skin even more complex.

## 4.1. *Propagation of sounds*

### 4.1.1. *General issues*

The propagation of the body sounds as well as any other acoustic waves in the time and space domain is a subject of the following simple relationship:

$$\lambda = \frac{v}{f}. \tag{2}$$

Here, symbol $\lambda$ is the sound wavelength, $v$ is the sound velocity, and $f$ is the sound frequency. In particular, the above equation describes the interrelation between the spatial sound characteristic $\lambda$ and the time-related characteristic $f$ by the use of the time-spatial characteristic $v$. The value of $v$ is determined through physical properties of the propagation medium, to give

$$v = \sqrt{\frac{\kappa}{\rho}} = \sqrt{\frac{1}{\rho \cdot D}}. \tag{3}$$

Here, $\kappa$ is the module of the volume elasticity, $\rho$ is the density of the propagating medium, and $D$ $(= 1/\kappa)$ is the compliance or adiabatic compressibility. In the case of gases, e.g. air, $\kappa$ is expressed as the product of adiabatic coefficient and gas pressure.

Obviously, Eqs. (2) and (3) account for the sound propagation in any type of homogeneous medium, including the biological tissue. Table 1 summarizes the values of $v$ and $\lambda$ for the most relevant types of biologic media involved in the transmission of the body sounds. One can observe that the lung parenchyma for which $\rho$ and $D$ are given by the mixture of the tissue and the air yields a relatively low $v$ in the order of only 50 m/s (23 m/s up to 60 m/s[18]), the value depending strongly on air content.[s] This value is much lower as compared with $v$ in the tissue ($\approx$ 1500 m/s) or

---

[r]The viscoelastic material demonstrates both viscous and elastic behavior under applied sound wave pressure which yields internal stress. That is, the material requires a finite time to reach the state of deformation appropriate to the stress and a similar time to regain its unstressed shape. In particular, the viscoelastic material exhibits hysteresis in the stress–strain curve, shows stress relaxation, i.e. step constant strain causes decreasing stress, and shows creeping, i.e. step constant stress causes increasing strain.[57,58]

Table 1. Approximate values of the sound velocity in air, water, muscle,[7] large airways, tissue,[18] tallow,[59] and lung.[18,26,60] Corresponding wavelengths are calculated according to Eq. (2). Approximate absorption coefficients are given according to the classical absorption theory.[59,61]

| | Sound velocity $v$ (m/s) | Wavelength at 1 kHz $\lambda$ (m) | Classical absorption coefficient at 1 kHz $\alpha_F + \alpha_T$ (1/m) |
|---|---|---|---|
| Air | 340 | 0.34 | $10^{-5}$ |
| Large airways (diameter $> 1\,$mm) | 270 | 0.27 | $10^{-5}$ |
| Water | 1400 | 1.4 | $10^{-8}$ |
| Tissue ($\approx$ water) | 1500 | 1.5 | $10^{-8}$ |
| Muscle ($\approx$ water) | 1560 | 1.56 | $10^{-8}$ |
| Tallow ($\approx$ fat) | 390 | 0.39 | $10^{-4}$ |
| Lung parenchyma | 50 | 0.05 | $> 10^{-5}$ |

in the large airways ($\approx 270\,$m/s) alone. As a result, the lung parenchyma accounts for the lowest values of $\lambda$ ($\approx 5\,$cm at 1 kHz) which certainly decrease even more with increasing $f$ (Eq. (2)).

It is worth to discuss shortly the influence of temperature $\vartheta$ and humidity on $v$ (and $\lambda$, Eq. (2)) from a physiological point of view. It is well known[7] that $v$ in air tends to increase with increasing $\vartheta$, the increase rate $\Delta v / \Delta \vartheta$ being of about 0.6 m/s per °C. Since inspiration brings cold air (usually room air) with $\vartheta < 37$°C into the airways and expiration delivers the warmed air with $\vartheta \approx 37$°C, the value of $v$ in the large airways decreases and increases, respectively. As a result, $v$ oscillates by a few percents over the breathing cycle. The respiratory induced humidity changes in the large airways can also be expected to influence the effective value of $v$; however, the influence is practically negligible. To give an example, a humidity change from 80% during inspiration to 100% during expiration yields an increase in $v$ of only about 0.2% (or 0.7 m/s) at $\vartheta = 37$°C.

---

[s]The value of $v$ in the lung parenchyma can be theoretically estimated by Eq. (3) considering air content. If we assume that the volumetric portion of the air is 75% and the rest is the tissue,[26] then $\rho_L$ and $D_L$ of the lung (= composite mixture) can be estimated as

$$\rho_L = 0.75 \cdot \rho_A + 0.25 \cdot \rho_T \approx 0.25 \cdot \rho_T$$

and

$$D_L = 0.75 \cdot D_A + 0.25 \cdot D_T \approx 0.75 \cdot D_A,$$

where $\rho_A$ (1.3 kg/m$^2$) and $\rho_T$ (1000 kg/m$^2$) are the densities of the air and tissue, respectively. Correspondingly, $D_A$ (7000 1/GPa) and $D_T$ (0.5 1/GPa) are the compliances of the air and tissue, respectively. Here, the value of $D_A$ was estimated by the use of Eq. (3) with $v$ of the air (Table 1) and $\rho_A$ as parameters. The values of $\rho_T$ and $D_T$ were approximated by the corresponding characteristics of the water, for the tissue consists mainly of water.

As a result, Eq. (3) yields $v$ 28 m/s for the lung parenchyma with $\rho_L$ and $D_L$ from the above, the calculated value fitting well the reported [23,60] m/s range.[18]

### 4.1.2. *Spreading of sounds*

If the calculated values of $\lambda$ in Table 1 are put into relation with distance $r$ from the body sound sources (e.g. heart valves or upper airways) to a possible auscultation site on the chest (Fig. 13), then it becomes obvious that primarily the near field condition ($r < 2 \cdot \lambda$) prevails on the auscultation site. That is, the relevant relation $r < 2 \cdot \lambda$ is supported by the scaled real cross-section of the thorax, as shown in Fig. 13(a). It demonstrates that the practically relevant values of $r$ are in the $[0.2,0.3]$ m range. On the other hand, the size of the body sound sources is in the order of $\lambda$, which also supports the assumption of the near field.

One would observe that $r$ is smaller or at least equal to $\lambda$ in all types of the propagating media but not in the lung parenchyma (Table 1). The high frequency body sounds traveling through the parenchyma ($\lambda \approx 2.5$ cm at $f = 2$ kHz) would not meet the near field condition from the above. However, as will be shown in Sec. 4.1.3, the high frequency body sounds tend to take the airway bound route within the airway-branching structure but not the way bound to the inner mediastinum and parenchyma.

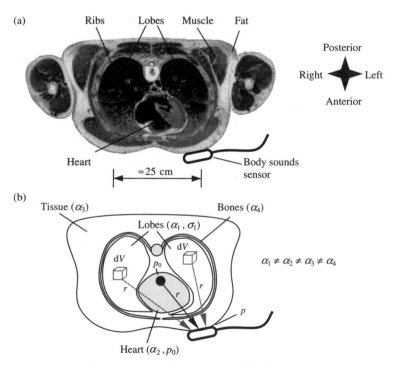

Fig. 13.   Propagation of the body sounds in the thorax. (a) Cross-section of the thorax[62] in the height of the heart showing highly heterogeneous propagation medium. (b) Contribution of the point source of sound (origin sound pressure $p_0$, Eq. (4)) and the distributed sources of sound (volume elements $dV$ with the respective volume density $\sigma$ of the distributed sound pressure, Eqs. (5) and (6)) to the acoustic pressure $p$ at the applied body sounds sensor as a function of the propagation distance $r$ and the attenuation coefficients $\alpha$.

In order to discuss the propagation phenomena of the body sounds and their absorption from a more theoretical point of view, two types of prevailing sound sources can be assumed:

(i) point source of sound, as approximately given in the case of the heart sounds (Sec. 2.1), tracheobronchial lung sounds (Sec. 2.2), and snoring sounds (Sec. 2.3); and

(ii) distributed sources of sound, as given for the vesicular lung sounds (Sec. 2.2).

In the case of the point source of sound, the sound intensity of the radially propagating sound waves will obey the inverse square law[t] under free-field conditions, i.e. without reflections or boundaries. This law yields that the sound intensity at $2 \cdot r$ has one-fourth of the original intensity at $r$, which can be considered as spreading losses. In addition to the latter intensity decrease, the propagation medium absorbs the sound intensity with increasing $r$ in terms of absorption losses (Sec. 4.2).

Given both phenomena from the above and assuming that the sound intensity is proportional to the square[u] of the sound wave pressure $p$, the amplitude of $p$ can be approximated as a function of $r$ according to

$$p(r) = k \cdot \frac{p_0}{r} \cdot e^{-\alpha(r) \cdot r}. \tag{4}$$

Here, $k$ is the constant, $p_0$ is the sound pressure amplitude of the point source at $r = 0$, and $\alpha(r)$ is the sound absorption coefficient (Sec. 4.2.1) as a function of $r$. Here, the geometrical damping factor[v] $1/r$ comes from the inverse square law and looses its weight with increasing $r$ while the original radial wave mutates into the plain wave.

Whereas Eq. (4) accounts for $p(r)$ from the point source of sound, the aforementioned distributed sources of sound can be considered by a modified version of Eq. (4), to give

$$p(r) = k \cdot \int_V \frac{\sigma(r)}{r} \cdot e^{-\alpha(r) \cdot r} \cdot dV \tag{5}$$

---

[t]The inverse square law comes from strict geometrical considerations. The sound intensity at any given radius $r$ is the source strength divided by the area of the sphere ($= 4 \cdot \pi \cdot r^2$) which increases proportional to $r^2$.[7]

[u]The assumption of the proportionality between the sound intensity ($= p^2/Z$ with $Z$ as the sound radiation impedance) and $p^2$ is strictly held only under far-field conditions ($r > 2 \cdot \lambda$).

[v]Generally, different assumptions regarding the geometrical damping factor can be found in literature. For instance, the damping factor $1/r$ in Eq. (4) was neglected completely by Wodicka et al.,[26] i.e. the authors assumed plain wave conditions for the propagation of the sound intensity ($\propto p^2$, compare Footnote u) in the lung parenchyma. On the other hand, the studies by Kompis et al.[18,63] assumed an even stronger geometrical damping factor of $1/r^2$ for the assessment of the spatial distribution of $p$ within the thorax region.

with

$$p_0 = \int_V \sigma(r) \cdot dV. \tag{6}$$

Here, $p_0$ from Eq. (4) is substituted by $\sigma(r)$ which represents the volume $V$ density of the distributed sound pressure (Eq. (6)).

Figure 13 demonstrates schematically the integration procedure for the highly heterogeneous thorax region (Fig. 13(a)), showing inhomogeneously distributed $\alpha(r)$ (Fig. 13(b)). The point source of sound with $p_0$ in the heart region and the distributed sources with local sound pressure $\sigma(r) \cdot dV$ in the lung parenchyma contribute to $p$ at the auscultation site, i.e. the application region of the body sounds sensor.

### 4.1.3. Frequency dependant propagation

The peculiarities of the propagation pathway of the body sounds should be shortly addressed. In particular, the propagation pathway of the lung sounds differs with varying frequency. At relatively low frequencies, i.e. below 300 Hz according to Pasterkamp et al.[16] or in the frequency range [100,600] Hz according to Wodicka et al.,[26] the transmission system of the lung sounds possesses primarily two features:

(i)    The large airway walls vibrate in response to intraluminal sound, allowing sound energy to be coupled directly into the surrounding parenchyma and inner mediastinum via wall motion.

(ii)   The entire air branching networks behave approximately as non-rigid tubes which tend to absorb sound energy and thus to impede the sound traveling further into the branching structure.

As a result of the transmission peculiarities from the above, the propagation pathway at the lower frequencies is primarily bound to the inner mediastinum, the sounds exiting the airways via wall motion. According to Rice,[60] the lung parenchyma acts nearly as an elastic continuum to audible sounds which travel predominantly through the bulk of the parenchyma but not along the airways.

Contrary to the case of lower frequencies, the airway walls become rigid at the higher frequencies because of their inherent mass, allowing more sound energy to remain within the airway lumen and travel potentially further into the branching structure. Thus, the sounds at the higher frequencies tend to take the airway bound route within the airway-branching structure.

Given the varying pathway of the sound propagation for different frequencies and the dependence of $v$ on the propagation medium (Table 1), it can be deduced that $v$ of the lung sounds at the lower frequencies is lower than $v$ at the higher frequencies. This is because the sounds of the lower frequencies are bound to the parenchymal tissue with $v \approx 50\,\text{m/s}$ and the sounds of the higher frequencies propagate primarily through the airways with $v \approx 270\,\text{m/s}$. Furthermore, the varying propagation pathway has strong implications on the asymmetry of the sound transmission, as will be discussed in Sec. 5.

Various experimental data confirm the changing transmission pathway and changing $v$ over the frequency of sounds. For instance, an overview[16] shows that the sound transmission from the trachea to the chest wall occurs with a phase delay of about 2.5 ms at 200 Hz (low frequencies), whereas at 800 Hz (higher frequencies) sound traverses a faster route with a phase delay of only 1.5 ms.[w]

Finally, it should be mentioned that an experimental estimation of the transmission characteristics of the sounds can lead even to diagnoses and categorization of diseases, for different diseases affect the transmission in a unique way. For instance, as shown by Iyer *et al.*,[23] this could be achieved in terms of the autoregressive modeling of the lung sounds with the aim to identify one or a combination of the hypothetical sound sources (e.g. random white noise sequence, periodic train of impulses, and impulsive bursts) and to characterize the prevailing sound transmission characteristics.

## 4.2. *Attenuation of sounds*

Besides attenuation of the body sounds due to the spreading losses (see geometrical damping factor $1/r$ in Eq. (4)), the ability of sounds to travel through matter depends upon the intrinsic attenuation within the propagation medium. Generally, the attenuation phenomena includes the following effects which will be discussed within the scope of the present chapter:

(i)   volume effects, e.g. absorption and scattering, and
(ii)  inhomogeneity effects, e.g. reflection and refraction.

### 4.2.1. *Volume effects*

Obviously, the most important volume effects are the absorption and scattering which account for the loss or transformation of sound energy while passing through a material. The absorption process is represented quantitatively by $\alpha$ in Eq. (4) (compare Fig. 13) and accounts for the influence of all three[26,59,61,64]:

(i)    inner friction,
(ii)   thermal conduction, and
(iii)  molecular relaxation.

---

[w]The hypothesis of the parenchymal propagation at the lower frequencies is also supported by the fact that the inhalation of a helium oxygen mixture only weakly affects (= reduces) the phase delay of the sound transmission from the trachea to the chest wall at the lower frequencies.[16] In contrast, the phase delays are significantly reduced at the higher frequencies by the helium oxygen mixture in comparison with the air; a reduction of about 0.7 ms can be observed at 800 Hz with practically no reduction at 200 Hz. Since the inhaled gas mixture shows higher value of $v$ than the air, the above observation proves a more airway bound sound route in the case of the higher frequencies.

*The inner friction* arises because of the differences in the local sound particle velocities. The friction strength is proportional to the ratio of the dynamic viscosity $\eta$ to $\rho$, which shows that the transmission pathways with inertial components yield larger damping. The corresponding friction-related component $\alpha_F$ of $\alpha$ can be calculated as

$$\alpha_F = \frac{8 \cdot \pi^2 \cdot \eta}{3 \cdot \rho \cdot v^3} \cdot f^2 . \tag{7}$$

The value of $\alpha_F$ in water is extremely low, e.g. $\alpha_F \approx 10^{-8}\,\mathrm{m}^{-1}$ at $1\,\mathrm{kHz}$. The latter value is also approximately applicable to the tissue which consists mainly of water (Table 1). To give an example, the value of $p$ decreases by about $1\,\mathrm{dB}$ after $10{,}000\,\mathrm{km}$ sound traveling at $1\,\mathrm{kHz}$ in water if only $\alpha_F$ is considered. In the air and large airways $\alpha_F$ increases by a factor of 1000 up to $10^{-5}\,\mathrm{m}^{-1}$, which yields a decrease of $p$ by about $1\,\mathrm{dB}$ after $5\,\mathrm{km}$ sound traveling in air.

*The thermal conduction* can be interpreted as diffusion of kinetic energy. Since the propagation of the sound wave is linked with the local variations of temperature, the local balancing of these variations by the thermal conduction withdraws the energy from the sound wave. Coefficient $\alpha_T$ accounting for the above energy losses can be calculated as

$$\alpha_T = \left(\frac{c_P}{c_V} - 1\right) \cdot \frac{2 \cdot \pi^2 \cdot v}{c_P \cdot \rho \cdot v^3} \cdot f^2, \tag{8}$$

where $c_P$ and $c_V$ are the specific heat capacities at constant pressure and volume, respectively, and $v$ is the heat conductivity. In water, the value of $\alpha_T$ is lower than $\alpha_F$ by a factor of 1000, whereas in air $\alpha_T$ is in some order as $\alpha_F$.

*The molecular relaxation* contributes also to the acoustic absorption in the tissue. This phenomenon is based on the fact that the rapidly submitted energy from the sound field is primarily stored as rotational energy of atoms of involved molecules and, on the other hand, as translational energy which is proportional to gas pressure. In contrast to the above energies, the vibrations of the molecules themselves start with some delay at the expense of rotational and translational energies. Thus a thermal equilibrium arises with a time constant $\tau$ (= relaxation time) between these three types of energies. However, the delayed setting of this equilibrium yields energy losses, accounted by the absorption coefficient $\alpha_M$,

$$\alpha_M = \left(1 - \frac{v_0^2}{v_\infty^2}\right) \cdot \frac{2 \cdot \pi^2 \cdot \tau}{v \cdot (1 + (f/f_M)^2)} \cdot f^2 . \tag{9}$$

Here, $f_M$ ($= 1/(2 \cdot \pi \cdot \tau)$) is the molecular relaxation frequency determined by the molecular properties, and $v_0$ and $v_\infty$ ($>\ v_0{}^\times$) are the sound velocities before

---

[×]The value of $v_0$ is lower than $v_\infty$ because the compressibility at lower frequencies before the relaxation ($f \ll f_M$) is higher than that at higher frequencies ($f \gg f_M$); compare the influence of $D$ on $v$ in Eq. (3).[61]

relaxation ($f \ll f_M$) and after relaxation ($f \gg f_M$), respectively. In particular, the energy losses show a maximum at $f = f_M$ concerning the product $\alpha_M \cdot \lambda$. In water, $f_M$ shows a very high value of about 100 GHz. This high value of $f_M$ ($\gg 2$ kHz) induces a very small $\alpha_M$ of about $10^{-8}$ m$^{-1}$ and a strong frequency dependence of $\alpha_M$ ($\propto f^2$) in the frequency range of the body sounds (Sec. 2). In water, the resulting value of $\alpha_M$ is in the range of $\alpha_F$. Contrary to the case of water, the value of $f_M$ in air is in the human acoustic range, the relaxation induced mainly by oxygen molecules ($f_M \approx 10$ Hz) and water molecules, the content of which is given by the air humidity. Thus $\alpha_M$ in air is relatively large and amounts to about $10^{-3}$ m$^{-1}$ at 1 kHz.

It is important to observe from Eqs. (7) and (8) that the sound absorption increases with increasing $f$, in particular, $\alpha_F$ and $\alpha_T$ are proportional to $f^2$. The total absorption $\alpha$, as used in Eq. (4), can be given as the sum of the discussed absorption coefficients, to give

$$\alpha = \alpha_F + \alpha_T + \alpha_M. \tag{10}$$

Table 1 compares $\alpha_F$ and $\alpha_T$ for the relevant types of biologic media involved in the sound transmission. It can be observed that the adipose tissue is the strongest absorber, followed by the air and airways, if only the inner friction and thermal conduction are considered. However, it should be stressed that $\alpha_F$ and $\alpha_T$ represent only the lowest threshold of the real absorption coefficient,[y] the component $\alpha_M$ in Eq. (10) being usually larger than the sum $\alpha_F + \alpha_T$ by a few orders of magnitude.

The scattering is the second volume effect being relevant for the attenuation of the propagating body sounds. Generally, the sound energy is scattered, i.e. redirected in random directions, when the sound wave encounters small particles.[z] If the size of particles is much smaller[aa] than $\lambda$, then the Rayleigh scattering occurs, whereas for larger particles the Mie scattering is the relevant phenomenon.[bb] Since the dimensions of the inner body structures, e.g. heart, lung lobes, and bones (Fig. 13(b)), are in the same order as $\lambda$ (Table 1), the scattering can be expected — from a qualitative point of view — to contribute significantly to the attenuation of the propagating body sounds. Furthermore, it is important to note that the scattering can be quantitatively assessed by a scattering coefficient which is defined in a similar way as $\alpha$ in Eq. (4).

---

[y] For instance, the absorption in gases is well accounted by the inner friction, thermal conduction, and molecular relaxation. That is, the observed absorption is only slightly higher than the predicted one. However, the real absorption in water is much higher than would be expected on these grounds. The excess absorption can be explained as due to a structural relaxation and a change in the molecular arrangement during the passage of the wave.[65]

[z] Generally, the scattering of acoustic waves in the tissue is due to the chaotic variation in the refractive index at macroscopic scale resulting in dispersion of the acoustic waves in all directions.

[aa] The scattering of sound waves around small obstacles (dimensions $\leq \lambda$) is also coined as wave diffraction.

[bb] The Rayleigh scattering presents isotropic scattering (scatters in all directions), while the Mie scattering is of anisotropic nature (forward directed within small angles of the beam axis).

If we consider the volume effects (absorption and scattering) from a more practical point of view, the following observations can be made. An early paper[1] suggests that if the effects of the inner friction ($\approx \eta$, Eq. (7)) are small, as in the case with water, air, and bone, the sound energy may be transmitted with remarkably little loss. In other media, such as fatty breast tissue, the sound waves are almost immediately suppressed (compare Table 1). The flesh of the chest acts also as a significant damping medium since the obesity might completely mask the low frequency heart sounds,[1] as will be demonstrated by own experimental data at the end of this chapter.

Regarding the mentioned theoretical frequency dependence of $\alpha (\propto f^2)$, it must be noted that experimental data for the biological tissue suggest a slightly different frequency dependence. That is, Erikson *et al.*[64] report that $\alpha$ is approximately proportional to $f$, whereas individual tissues may vary somewhat in between, e.g. hemoglobin has $\alpha$ proportional to $f^{1.3}$. In addition, there are publications[4,15] which report that the energy of the vesicular sounds (Sec. 2.2) declines exponentially with increasing $f$, which would imply the proportionality between $\alpha$ and $f$ either.

The obvious consequence of the frequency dependence of $\alpha$ is that the transmission efficiency of the lung parenchyma and the chest wall deteriorates with increasing $f$, i.e. the tissues act as a lowpass filter which transmit sounds mainly at low $f$.[26,66,67] For instance, a model-based estimation of the acoustic transmission has shown a sound attenuation in the $[0.5, 1]$ dB/cm range at 400 Hz,[18] the attenuation being negligible at 100 Hz and increasing to approximately 3 dB/cm at 600 Hz.[26] It can be derived from the preceding data that $\alpha$ is about $10 \, \mathrm{m}^{-1}$ according to Eq. (4). That is, the estimated $\alpha$ is higher than $\alpha_F + \alpha_T$ of the tissue according to Table 1 by orders of magnitude, which confirms that $\alpha_F$ and $\alpha_T$ represent only the lowest theoretical threshold of $\alpha$.

Because of the frequency dependence of $\alpha$ the higher frequency sounds do not spread as diffusely or retain as much amplitude across the chest wall as do lower frequencies. The high frequency sounds are thus more regionally restricted and play an important role in localizing, for instance, the breath sounds to underlying pathology.[cc]

The non-continuous porous structure[dd] of the lung parenchyma is of special importance regarding the frequency dependence of the sound absorption. As already

---

[cc]For instance, pathologically consolidated lung tissue yields a reduction of the attenuation of the high frequency components and thus a higher amount of high pitched sounds. This is because the intrinsic lowpass filtering characteristics of the lung are pathologically altered, which yields a decrease of the corresponding cut-off frequency. This behavior offers the ability to localize the regions of consolidated lung tissue, and it is the high frequencies of the lung sounds (Sec. 2.2) that facilitate this. To give another example of application, the non-linear spectral characteristics of the sound transmission help to localize also the cardiovascular sounds (Sec. 2.1) to their points of origin.

[dd]Homogenous materials tend to absorb the acoustic energy mainly because of the inner friction, i.e. due to inner local deformations of the material. Contrary to the homogenous materials, porous materials as the lung parenchyma tend to absorb the acoustic energy also in terms of outer friction, i.e. the friction between the oscillating air particles and porous elements of the material.[7]

mentioned in Sec. 4.1.1, the parenchyma is dominated by the components of tissue and air.[16,18] That is, the alveoli in the parenchyma act as elastic bubbles in water, whose dynamic deformation due to oscillating $p$ dissipates the sound energy.[61] As long as $\lambda$ (Table 1) is significantly greater than the alveolar size (diameter $< 1$ mm), the losses are relatively low. In this case, the losses due to the thermal conduction are considerably larger[ee] in magnitude than those associated with the inner friction and scattering effects.[26] If the value of $\lambda$ approaches the alveolar size, i.e. $f$ is increasing (Eq. (2)), the absorption exhibits very high losses.[16] However, it is important to note that the spectral range up to 2 kHz, i.e. the relevant spectral range of the body sounds (Sec. 2), yields values of $\lambda$ which are still significantly larger than the alveolar diameter. For instance, the alveolar size of $\lambda$ in the lung parenchyma is approached earliest at $f \approx 23$ kHz with $v = 23$ m/s from Sec. 4.1.1.

Indeed, own experimental data gained with the body sounds sensor (Fig. 1) support the findings from the above that the attenuation of the body sounds is significantly influenced by the volume effects. That is, the chest acts as a significant damping medium, and the obesity tends to attenuate significantly the investigated heart sounds (Sec. 2.1). Figure 14 shows a regression analysis for the heart sounds, i.e. the regression between the amplitude of $s_C$ and BMI (see Footnote n). Data of 20 patients were analyzed; in total nine patients had apnea (see Footnote b). It can be deduced from the regression that increasing BMI is linked to the decreasing amplitude of $s_C$, an increase from 24 to 38 kg/m$^2$ causing about 60% loss of the amplitude, the cross-correlation coefficient being about $-0.6$. This might indicate that the increasing thickness of tissue and increasing amount of adipose tissue (in patients with higher BMI) yield a strong damping of $s_C$.

Furthermore, the regression lines in Fig. 14 indicate that the amplitude of $s_C$ is slightly higher for the non-apnea patients in comparison with the apnea patients. This is in full agreement with the clinical signs of apnea, including the risk of apnea

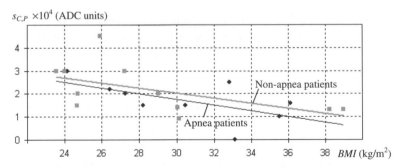

Fig. 14. Relationship between the peak amplitude $s_{C,P}$ of the cardiac component $s_C$ and the body mass index BMI for apnea patients (black) and non-apnea patients (gray), including corresponding linear regression lines.

---

[ee]This relation was shown by modeling the lung parenchyma as air bubbles in water, the bubbles being compressed and expanded by the acoustic wave.[26]

that is strongly interrelated with the increased values of BMI and thus the decreased values of $s_C$.

Finally, it should be noted that a significant variability of the amplitude of $s_C$ was observed among patients (Fig. 14) but not over the recording time of a single patient. A relatively small amplitude variation of up to 40% over the recording time was mainly caused by the respiratory dependence of the cardiac activity (compare Fig. 12(a)). Contrary to the variability of $s_C$, the amplitude variability of $s_R$ and $s_S$ (Secs. 2.2 and 2.3) was considerably high among patients as well as over the recording time. This is due to the fact that both $s_R$ and $s_S$ are directly influenced by highly varying strength and type of the respiration among patients as well as over the recording time.

### 4.2.2. Inhomogeneity effects

The inhomogeneity effects, namely the reflection and refraction, also play an important role within the scope of the body sound attenuation. The spatial heterogeneity of the thorax that reflects the underlying anatomy, as demonstrated in Fig. 13(a), indicates the relevance of the intrathoracic sonic reflections and refractions. In addition, the tubelike resonances[ff] of the respiratory tract influence the attenuation of the body sounds.[16]

The reflection phenomenon describes the relationship between the reflected and incident waves. If the reflection of the inner body sounds is considered on the skin (simplified tissue-air interface), as shown in Fig. 15, then the reflection law yields the following: the reflection angle to the normal matches the incident angle $\beta_T$ to the normal, and the reflection coefficient $R$, i.e. the ratio of the reflected and incident $p$ in the tissue, can be given as

$$R = \frac{Z_A - Z_T}{Z_A + Z_T}. \tag{11}$$

Here, $Z_A$ and $Z_T$ are the sound radiation impedances ($= \rho \cdot v$) of air and tissue, respectively. The calculation yields $Z_A \approx 340 \, \mathrm{kg \, m^{-2} \, s^{-1}}$ and $Z_T \approx 1.4 \times 10^6 \, \mathrm{kg \, m^{-2} \, s^{-1}}$, whereas the physical properties of the tissue were approximated by those of water. Given the values from the above, Eq. (11) yields $R \approx -0.998$. This very high value of $R$ indicates that more than 99% of the incident $p$ is reflected and less than 1% is transmitted through the skin if the simplified tissue–air interface is assumed.

---

[ff]The tubelike resonances can be attributed to the phenomenon of standing waves within the respiratory tract, which, in approximation, resembles a tube. For instance, the standing waves occur when the open tube length $l$ matches half-wavelength $\lambda/2$ of the acoustic wave passing through it, for the acoustic pressure nodes arise at both open ends of the tube. The resulting harmonic eigenfrequencies $f_n$

$$f_n = \frac{v}{\lambda} \cdot n = \frac{v}{2 \cdot l} \cdot n$$

with $n$ ($= 1,2,3,\ldots$) as the ordinal number of eigenoscillation provide frequencies at which the transmission efficiency reaches its maximum (compare Eq. (2)).

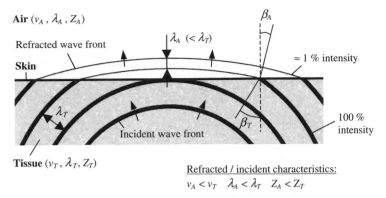

Fig. 15. Reflection losses and refraction of the body sounds when leaving the tissue. The decreasing thickness of the propagating wave front indicates the decreasing intensity due to the reflection losses.

A few restrictions should be mentioned regarding the above estimation of the reflection (and transmission). The first restriction is that the human skin is a true multilayer consisting approximately of three layers: the inmost subcutaneous fat tissue, followed by the dermis, and the outer epidermis. Actually, the transmission of the body sounds through this multilayer would tend to yield a higher transmission rate compared with the simplified tissue–air interface. It is because of the assumption that the respective two neighboring layers would show a less difference in their sound radiation impedances $Z_2$ and $Z_1$ than the difference between $Z_A$ and $Z_T$. As a result, term $|Z_2 - Z_1|$ from Eq. (11) would exhibit a lower value than term $|Z_A - Z_T|$, which would yield a lower $R$ for the respective neighboring layers and thus a higher total transmission rate.

The second restriction is that the reflection law holds only when $\lambda$ of the sound is small compared to the dimensions of the reflecting surface; otherwise the scattering laws (Sec. 4.2.1) govern the reflection phenomena. Indeed, in the case of the body sounds, the application of the reflection law is limited, since $\lambda$ (Table 1) and the dimensions of the reflecting surface (Fig. 13) are in the same order. In spite of the above restrictions, the estimated low transmission efficiency ($< 1\%$) underlines the importance of an optimal sound auscultation region, as will be discussed in Sec. 5.

The second inhomogeneity effect is the refraction which describes the bending of acoustic waves when they enter a medium where their $v$ is different. Given the aforementioned simplified tissue–air interface, as demonstrated in Fig. 15, the refracted angle $\beta_A$ to the normal and $\beta_T$ obey the Snell's refraction law

$$\frac{v_A}{v_T} = \frac{\sin(\beta_A)}{\sin(\beta_T)}, \tag{12}$$

where $v_A$ and $v_T$ are the sound velocities in air and tissue, respectively. Given the values from Table 1, it can be deduced that $\beta_A < \beta_T$. This means that the refracted wave front of the body sounds is bent toward the normal of the skin, which yields a more flat wave front in air than in the tissue (Fig. 15). From a practical point of view, the flattened wave front in air favors the sounds auscultation, for the wave front is bunched and redirected toward the body sounds sensor on the skin (Fig. 1). Lastly, it should be mentioned that the discussed restrictions pertaining to the reflection also apply to the refraction phenomenon.

### 4.3. *Coupling of sounds*

In addition to the discussed effects of the sound attenuation within the body (Sec. 4.2), the coupling of the body sounds by the body sounds sensor (Fig. 1) should be addressed, since it can be expected to affect the sound attenuation or the gain of $p$ at the microphone diaphragm. As demonstrated in Fig. 16(a), the coupling of the sounds through numerous interfaces within the body sounds sensor, namely from the skin into the chestpiece diaphragm, from the diaphragm into the air within the bell, and finally from the air into the microphone diaphragm, contributes to the sound attenuation.

From a technical point of view, the mechanical/acoustical impedance mismatch in the above interfaces of the sensor accounts for the sound attenuation, for matched impedances would not yield any sound attenuation due to coupling (compare Eq. (11) with $Z_A = Z_T$). The issue of the impedance mismatch can be qualitatively addressed by the use of the electromechanic analogy[gg] of the resulting skin–diaphragm–air–diaphragm interface, as shown in Fig. 16(b).

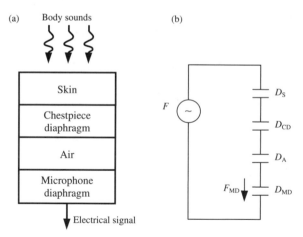

Fig. 16.   Coupling of the body sounds by the body sounds sensor (Fig. 1). (a) Sound coupling from the skin, through the chestpiece diaphragm, the air in the cavity of the bell into the microphone diaphragm. (b) Corresponding first electromechanic analogy.

[gg]Formally, the first electromechanic analogy is used here, which sets the mechanical force analogous to electrical voltage, the sound particle velocity to electrical current, the mechanical compliance to electrical capacity, the mass to electrical inductivity, and the frictional resistance to electrical resistance.[7] In addition, the first analogy yields electrical circuits which are reciprocally equivalent to mechanical circuits.

For the sake of simplicity, only compliances $D$ of the involved materials are considered here, not accounting for the mass and frictional resistance. It is important to note that the compliances (= feathers) are approximately connected in parallel in terms of mechanical connections because the feathers work against the same sensor housing which is not involved in the oscillations of $p$. Given the first electromechanic analogy implying a reciprocal electrical circuit, a series connection of the involved $D$ as capacitors results as a model for the sound coupling, as shown in Fig. 16(b). Here, index S of $D$ denotes the skin, index CD stays for the chestpiece diaphragm, index A for the air in the bell, and index MD for the microphone diaphragm.

The interesting quantity within this theoretical investigation is the resulting force $F_{MD}$ on the microphone diaphragm. It represents $p$ acting on the diaphragm and thus accounts for the output voltage of the microphone[hh] and the output signal $s$ of the body sounds sensor (Fig. 1). According to Fig. 16(b), the value of $F_{MD}$ (or in analogy, the voltage on the capacitor with value $D_{MD}$) can be then approximated as

$$F_{MD} = F \cdot \frac{D_S \| D_{CD} \| D_A}{D_S \| D_{CD} \| D_A + D_{MD}}. \tag{13}$$

Here, $F$ is the total force pertinent to the body sounds entering the skin, and operator $\|$ denotes the relevant calculation rule for the series connection of the capacitors. Expression $D_S \| D_{CD} \| D_A$ indicates the total capacity of the series connection of the capacitors with values $D_S$, $D_{CD}$, and $D_A$. In analogy with the mechanical circuit, term $D_S \| D_{CD} \| D_A$ represents the total compressibility of all three: the skin, the chestpiece diaphragm, and the air.

It is obvious that the material of both diaphragms is less compressible than the tissue of the skin, whereas the skin is less compressible than the air. As a rough estimation, the diaphragm material can be approximated by acrylic glass (= plexiglass) and the skin tissue by water. Then the following compliance values result: $D_{CD} = D_{MD} = 0.3 \ 1/\text{GPa}$, $D_S = 0.5 \ 1/\text{GPa}$, and $D_A = 7000 \ 1/\text{GPa}$ (see Footnote s). With the obvious relation $D_A \gg (D_{CD}, D_{MD}, D_S)$ and the above-mentioned values, the value of $F_{MD}$ can be estimated as

$$F_{MD} \approx F \cdot \frac{D_S \| D_{CD}}{D_S \| D_{CD} + D_{MD}} \approx F \cdot 0.4. \tag{14}$$

---

[hh]The used microphone within the body sounds sensor (Fig. 1) is an electroacoustic transducer (the Sell capacitor[7]) which converts the pressure $p$ variations at its diaphragm into an electrical sensor signal $s$. The microphone comprises a metallic diaphragm as a first electrode, spaced at a very short distance from a parallel fixed plate which acts as a second electrode. Both electrodes operate as a capacitor which is charged through the charging potential provoked by the permanent polarizing dielectric material in between the electrodes. The variations of $p$ at the microphone diaphragm yield its excursions, which change the capacity in between the electrodes and thus the voltage across the electrodes. As a result, a current through the capacitor is induced, which yields an output voltage (= $s$) on an external resistor.

The above equation shows that about 40% of the acoustical forces pertinent to the body sounds entering the skin are transmitted to the microphone diaphragm if only the coupling losses are roughly considered. However, this theoretical estimation yields a rather maximum value of the transmission efficiency since neither frictional resistance nor mass was considered.

In addition, the discussed electromechanic analogy allows an important insight into the phenomena of sound coupling. That is, the sound transmission from a medium of low compressibility, e.g. skin, into a medium with high compressibility, e.g. air, is always connected with relatively high losses, whereas the reverse transmission path would show relatively low losses (compare Eq. (13)).

Analogous to the impedance mismatch within the investigated skin–diaphragm–air–diaphragm interface of the body sounds sensor, the impedance mismatch between the different body tissues can be expected to contribute to the attenuation of the body sounds. For instance, Pasterkamp et al.[16] report that the impedance mismatch between the parenchyma and the chest wall can account for an order of magnitude decrease in the amplitude of $p$. This is because the chest wall is significantly more massive and stiff than the parenchyma, although the chest wall is relatively thin.

## 5. Spatial Distribution of Body Sounds

One would expect from Fig. 13 that the spatial distribution of the hypothetical sound sources inside the body as well as the regional distribution of the surface sounds on the body skin is highly non-uniform. This is because

- sound generation mechanisms lack spatial symmetry with respect to the body axis (Sec. 2) and
- spatial transmission pathways from the sound sources to the skin surface are highly inhomogeneous in terms of acoustic transmission properties (Sec. 4).

The spatial asymmetry of the sound generation mechanisms is primarily given by the massive mediastinum on the left site of the thorax (compare Fig. 13(a)). On the other hand, the inhomogeneous pathways of the sound propagation are caused by the heterogeneous thorax including a mixture of tissue, lung parenchyma, blood, air, and bones (Table 1).

The spatial distribution of the heart sounds was investigated by Kompis et al.[63] The authors demonstrated that the estimated (= hypothetical) sound sources of the first heart sound are spatially constricted at the expected location of the heart itself. In contrast to the first heart sound, the second heart sound gives rise to more complicated patterns of the sound sources which show multiple spatially separated centers close to the heart region.

Indeed, given the generation mechanisms of the heart sounds (Sec. 2.1), the estimated location of the sound sources pertaining to the first heart sound may be expected to remain locally constricted to the heart region. In particular, this could be explained by the location of the sound-generating atrioventricular valves which are situated inside of the heart and thus are relatively isolated from outside (Fig. 2). On the other hand, the reported observation regarding the sources of the second heart sound could be explained by the distal location of the semilunar valves, i.e. their distal location with respect to the heart itself. These valves act as output valves whose closures induce vibrations of the external non-constricted blood and tissues, which, in turn, may result in the multiple scattered sound sources in the immediate vicinity of the heart.

The distribution of the hypothetical sound sources of the vesicular lung sounds is consistent with the origin of these sounds (Sec. 2.2), as proven by many authors.[4,18,19,63,68] Specifically, the estimated distribution supports the concept that the inspiratory sounds are predominantly produced in the periphery of the lung (= distal airways) by distributed sound sources while the expiratory sounds are generated by a more central source in the upper proximal airways.

An important issue is that the transmission of the vesicular lung sounds was shown to be asymmetric, as reported in many papers.[16,19,24,68] In particular, the sound intensity lateralizes with right-over-left dominance at the anterior upper chest and with left-over-right dominance at the posterior upper chest. The lateralization is followed more closely during expiration and for the lower frequencies (below $300\,\mathrm{Hz}$[16] or $600\,\mathrm{Hz}$[26]). In addition, anterior sites show a higher sound intensity than posterior sites. It is likely that the observed asymmetries are related to the effects of

(i)   localization of the cardiovascular structures on the left side of the major airways and

(ii)  unsymmetrical geometry of airways.

The preferential coupling of the vesicular sounds to the right anterior chest, especially at the lower frequencies, could be explained by the massive mediastinum on the left side, for the mediastinum may attenuate the sound coupling to the left anterior lung (and the left anterior chest). The effect of the unsymmetrical airways could be pointed out by the fact that the major left segmental bronchi are directed more posteriorly compared with the right bronchi, because of the anterior position of the heart on the left side. Obviously, this asymmetric setting of the bronchi favors the left-over-right dominance of the sound intensity at the posterior upper chest.

The influence of the frequency on the asymmetric sound propagation should be briefly commented. The strong asymmetry which arises for the lower frequencies only can be explained by the frequency dependant propagation of the body sounds. That is, the low frequency sounds are preferentially bound to the lung parenchyma and inner mediastinum, as discussed in Sec. 4.1.3. As a result, the asymmetrical localization of inner body structures plays an important role only at the lower frequencies. At the higher frequencies, the asymmetry of the sound transmission is weaker because the sound pathway changes to a predominantly airway bound route and is more direct and symmetric, bypassing the effect of the mediastinum.

The regional distribution of the snoring sounds on the skin surface could be approximately derived from the lateralization of passively transmitted sounds introduced at the mouth. These artificially introduced sounds could be roughly equated with the snoring sounds which originate close to the mouth, i.e. in the pharyngeal airway (Sec. 2.3). Given the above assumption and using the data[68] of the passively transmitted sounds, it can be expected that the snoring sounds would lateralize with right-over-left dominance at the anterior upper chest. At the posterior chest, the snoring sounds should be slightly louder on the left side. In addition, anterior sites would be expected to show a higher snoring sound intensity than posterior sites.

The regional distributions of the sound intensities of all three body sound signal $s$ components, i.e. $s_C$, $s_R$, and $s_S$ (simulated snoring), were experimentally investigated by Kaniusas et al.[5] for comparison and for their optimum detection. For this purpose, acoustic sound recordings were carried out with the body sounds sensor (Fig. 1) on two healthy male subjects[ii] in the supine position.

As shown in Fig. 17, the sound intensities were assessed in 10 homologous chest regions (around third, fifth, and seventh intercostal space (IS) anterior left and right, respectively; fifth and seventh IS lateral left and right, respectively) and on the neck (collateral to the trachea). The heart region around the fifth IS on the anterior left was declared as the "standard" detection region. Therefore, all other eleven regions will be referred to as "alternative" regions. In particular, the "standard" region was investigated in comparison with the "alternative" regions.

The assessed sound level $s_{dB}$ was defined as logarithm of $s$ and its components, respectively. Each subfigure in Fig. 17 includes averaged data on $s_{dB}$ pertaining to $s_C$, $s_R$, and $s_S$. The sound levels in the "alternative" regions are given in relation to the "standard" region ($s_{dB} = 0$).

It can be observed that the "standard" heart region is characterized by similar intensities of $s_C$ and $s_S$ which was approximately 5 dB stronger according to Fig. 17(c). This yields a ratio 0 dB : +5 dB between $s_C$ and $s_S$, which favors the simultaneous detection of these two components. Conversely, component $s_R$ is rather weak, its intensity tending to be approximately 30 dB below that of $s_C$ (Fig. 17(b)). The resulting unfavorable ratio 0 dB : −30 dB complicates a synchronous auscultation of respiration, cessation of which represents a key parameter for the detection of apneas (see Footnote b).

---

[ii]It should be noted that healthy males hardly represent typical apnea patients, especially concerning the snoring sounds. In particular, the simulated snoring of healthy males differs markedly from the obstructive snoring of apnea patients (Sec. 2.3).

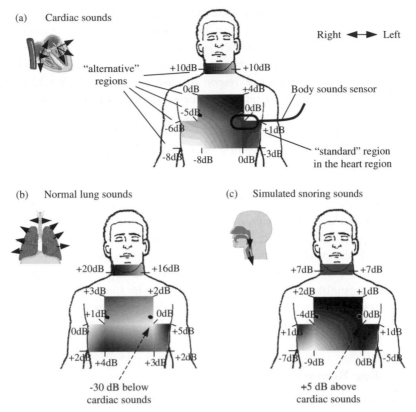

Fig. 17. Local intensity variations of body sounds. Signal amplitudes $s_{dB}$ at "alternative" regions on the chest and neck are given in relation to the "standard" heart region ($s_{dB} = 0$). Values between the measured points are generated using bilinear interpolation and are indicated through the gray tone map. (a) Cardiac sounds $s_C$. (b) Respiratory sounds $s_R$. (c) Simulated snoring sounds $s_S$. The dashed arrows indicate that $s_R$ is 30 dB below $s_C$ at the "standard" region while $s_S$ is 5 dB above $s_C$.

Aiming for comparisons of regional distributions and more balanced intensities, "alternative" regions should be considered. We see the following tendencies:

(i) The intensity of $s_C$ decreases with increasing distance from the heart, i.e. it shows minimum values of about $-8$ dB in the lower right thorax region (Fig. 17(a)). Conversely, it shows a 10 dB maximum at the neck.

(ii) $s_R$ shows only slight local differences at the thorax (Fig. 17(b)), which result from the distributed sources. Strongly enhanced signals arise at the neck (up to $+20$ dB). Contrary to the discussed asymmetric transmission of the vesicular lung sounds, no evident lateralization of $s_R$ can be observed.

(iii) $s_S$ shows a maximum of about $+7$ dB at the neck (Fig. 17(c)), as can be expected in view of the source localization. The intensity decreases with increasing distance, reaching a $-9$ dB minimum in the lower right thorax region.

The experimental results show that optimum auscultation of all three sound components $s_C$, $s_R$, and $s_S$ is not to be expected from the "standard" heart region due to the already mentioned ratio $0\,dB : -30\,dB : +5\,dB$ between the respective components. A more efficient auscultation of $s_R$ or a better balance results for the lower right thorax region around the seventh IS which yields a ratio $-8\,dB : -26\,dB : -4\,dB$, or related to the cardiac region $0\,dB : -18\,dB : +4\,dB$. Another attractive auscultation region would be the neck, the right side yielding a ratio $+10\,dB : -10\,dB : +12\,dB$ or $0\,dB : -20\,dB : +2\,dB$, respectively. As can be seen, the minimum of the intensity of $s_R$ cannot be fully overcome.

All the different components of the body sounds prove to contain spatial information that can be easily assessed using simultaneous sound recordings at different body sites. The use of this spatial information may lead to advanced diagnoses[jj] methods beyond simple single spot sound auscultation, which has already been proposed for both heart sounds[69] and lung sounds.[18] For instance, in the case of the vesicular lung sounds, acoustic images of a pathologically consolidated lung differ substantially from the images of the healthy lung allowing to localize the abnormality.[18] As a practical restriction, the spatial resolution cannot be expected to resolve differences below approximately 2 cm ($\lambda \approx 2.3\,cm$ at $v = 23\,m/s$, Sec. 4.1.1) in the localization of the sound sources.

## 6. Concluding Remarks

Acoustical signals of human biomechanical systems reveal mainly three sound components, namely heart sounds, lung sounds, and snoring sounds. The heart sounds occur predominantly because of the valvular activity of the heart. The generation mechanisms of the lung sounds rely on more complicated biomechanical phenomena. In particular, the tracheobronchial sounds are primarily related to the turbulent airflow and vibrations of the upper airway walls, while the vesicular sounds arise mainly during inspiration, as the air moves from larger airways into smaller ones, hitting the branches of the airways. The snoring sounds are mainly generated by vibrations of the pharyngeal walls and the soft palate.

Given the generation mechanisms of the different body sounds, the hypothetical sources of the heart sounds, tracheobronchial lung sounds, and snoring sounds can be considered, in an approximation, as remaining locally restricted to the heart region, the larger airways, and the upper airways, respectively. Contrary to the latter body sounds, the sources of the vesicular lung sounds are not confined to a certain region but are rather distributed within the whole periphery of the lung.

---

[jj] It is interesting to note that ultrasound methods, i.e. the most prominent spatial imaging methods using acoustic signals of high frequency (MHz range), have not been successfully applied for imaging of the lung parenchyma, primarily because the sound damping of the parenchyma is prohibitively high at the ultrasound frequencies (see frequency dependence of $\alpha$ in Sec. 4.2.1).[63]

In contrast to the heart sounds, the lung and snoring sounds exhibit a high variability from one subject to the other and even from one breath to the next. In addition, the different body sounds cannot be considered as being independent. The arising manifold interrelations in between can be attributed to direct mechanical interrelations between the respective sound sources, neural implications, and indirect effects.

The biomechanical propagation mechanisms of the body sounds reveal that a large percentage of the original sound energy never reaches the surface because of spreading, absorption, scattering, reflection, and refraction losses. In particular, the sound attenuation within the body is highly inhomogeneous due to the heterogeneous thorax composition, and it increases generally with increasing sound frequency. There represents the adipose tissue the strongest sound absorber, whereas the strong lowpass characteristics of the lung should be mentioned as well.

Interestingly, the spatial propagation pathway of the sound waves depends on their frequency; that is, the low frequency sounds are predominantly bound to the inner mediastinum, while the high frequency sounds tend to take an airway bound route. The different pathways have a strong influence on the resulting sound propagation velocity and sound wavelength. In particular, the resulting wavelength determines the type of acoustic field (near or far) on the auscultation site and, on the other hand, the strength of the prevailing scattering, reflection, and refraction effects.

The largest reflection losses arise at the tissue–air passage showing a strong mechanical/acoustical impedance mismatch which impedes an efficient sound auscultation. On the other hand, the concurrent refraction yields a flattened wave front in the air, which favors the auscultation.

The regional distribution of the intensity of the surface sounds (accessible through the auscultation) is highly non-uniform and asymmetric, as well as the spatial distribution of the hypothetical sound sources. This is because the sound generation mechanisms lack spatial symmetry, and the spatial transmission pathways are highly inhomogeneous. As an important property, the strong asymmetry arises only for the lower sound frequencies, which can be explained by the frequency dependant propagation pathways of the body sounds.

The regional mappings of the different body sounds show that the intensity of the heart sounds decreases in the thorax region with increasing distance from the heart, as could be expected from the hypothetical sound sources. However, an absolute maximum is given at the neck, which could be explained by close proximity of the auscultation site to the carotid artery. The intensities of the lung sounds in the different thorax regions yield practically no systematic differences in their amplitude, primarily because the vesicular sounds show distributed sources; however, the intensity increases dramatically at the neck, where the bronchial sounds prevail. Lastly, the snoring sound intensity decreases with increasing distance from the neck, as the relevant sound source is located there. Generally, the regional mappings suggest the right thorax region in the area of the seventh intercostal

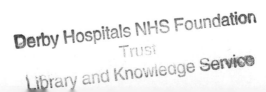

space or the neck to be optimal regions for the simultaneous auscultation of all three types of the body sounds.

Obviously, the relevant sound generation mechanisms in combination with the transmission properties of the body structures and those of the recording system determine the signal properties of the auscultated body sounds. The heart sounds show spectral components in the [0,100] Hz range, the latter components being statistically irrelevant for the lung and snoring sounds. The spectral components of the lung sounds are in the range up to approximately 500 Hz. The snoring sounds exhibit an extremely high variance of their intensity and spectral composition. Normal snoring appears in the range up to approximately 1000 Hz, while obstructive snoring shows amplitudes up to 2000 Hz.

The presented issues pertaining to the biomechanical generation of the body sounds reveal clinically relevant correlations between the physiological phenomena under investigation and the registered biosignals. The analysis of the unique sound transmission from the sound source to the auscultation site offers a solid basis for both proper understanding of the biosignal relevance and optimization of the recording techniques.

## Acknowledgments

This work was supported by the Austrian Federal Ministry of Transport, Innovation and Technology, GZ 140.594/2-V/B/9b/2000. I would like to thank Prof. H. Pfützner and Dipl.-Ing. J. Kosel for valuable comments.

## References

1. M. B. Rappaport and H. B. Sprague, *Am. Heart J.* (1941) 257.
2. M. Abella, J. Formolo and D. G. Penney, *J. Acoust. Soc. Am.* (1992) 2224.
3. P. Y. Ertel, M. Lawrence and W. Song, *J. Audio Eng. Soc.* (1971) 182.
4. R. Loudon and R. L. H. Murphy, *Am. Rev. Respir. Dis.* (1984) 663.
5. E. Kaniusas, H. Pfützner and B. Saletu, *IEEE Trans. Biomed. Eng.* (2005) 1812.
6. B. Saletu and M. Saletu-Zyhlarz, eds., *What You Always Wanted to Know About the Sleep (in German)* (Ueberreuter Publisher, Vienna, 2001).
7. I. Veit, ed., *Technical Acoustics (in German)* (Vogel Publisher, Würzburg, 1996).
8. P. Y. Ertel, M. Lawrence, R. K. Brown and A. M. Stern, *Circulation* (1966) 889.
9. P. Y. Ertel, M. Lawrence, R. K. Brown and A. M. Stern, *Circulation* (1966) 899.
10. P. J. Hollins, *Br. J. Hosp. Med.* (1971) 509.
11. R. M. Rangayyan, ed., *Biomedical Signal Analysis: A Case-Study Approach* (Wiley-IEEE Press, 2002).
12. D. Barschdorff, S. Ester and E. Most, in *Comparative Approaches to Medical Reasoning*, eds. M. E. Cohen and D. L. Hudson (World Scientific Publishing, 1995), p. 271.
13. University of Wales, College of Medicine, *Cardiac Auscultation Site* (http://mentor.uwcm.ac.uk:11280/aspire/cardiac_auscultation/notes/part_2/the_audio_section/,2005).
14. C. Lessard and M. Jones, *Innov. Technol. Biol. Med.* (1988) 116.

15. L. J. Hadjileontiadis and S. M. Panas, *IEEE Trans. Biomed. Eng.* (1997) 642.
16. H. Pasterkamp, S. S. Kraman and G. R. Wodicka, *Am. J. Respir. Crit. Care Med.* (1997) 974.
17. F. Dalmay, M. T. Antonini, P. Marquet and R. Menier, *Eur. Respir. J.* (1995) 1761.
18. M. Kompis, H. Pasterkamp and G. R. Wodicka, *Chest* (2001) 1309.
19. P. Fachinger, *Computer Based Analysis of Lung Sounds in Patients with Pneumonia — Automatic Detection of Bronchial Breathing by Fast-Fourier-Transformation (in German)* (Dissertation, Philipps-University Marburg, 2003).
20. McGill University, Faculty of Medicine, *Molson Medical Informatics Student Projects* (http://sprojects.mmip.mcgill.ca/mvs/, 2005).
21. L. J. Hadjileontiadis and S. M. Panas, in *Proceedings of the 18th Annual EMBS International Conference* (IEEE, 1996), p. 2217.
22. L. J. Hadjileontiadis and S. M. Panas, *IEEE Trans. Biomed. Eng.* (1997) 1269.
23. V. K. Iyer, P. A. Ramamoorthy and Y. Ploysongsang, *IEEE Trans. Biomed. Eng.* (1989) 1133.
24. A. Jones, R. D. Jones, K. Kwong and Y. Burns, *Phys. Ther.* (1999) 682.
25. R. Ferber, R. Millman, M. Coppola, J. Fleetham, C. F. Murray, C. Iber, V. McCall, G. Nino-Murcia, M. Pressman, M. Sanders, K. Strohl, B. Votteri and A. Williams, *Sleep* (1994) 378.
26. G. R. Wodicka, K. N. Stevens, H. L. Golub, E. G. Cravalho and D. C. Shannon, *IEEE Trans. Biomed. Eng.* (1989) 925.
27. G. Liistro, D. Stanescu and C. Veriter, *J. Appl. Physiol.* (1991) 2736.
28. K. Wilson, R. A. Stoohs, T. F. Mulrooney, L. J. Johnson, C. Guilleminault and Z. Huang, *Chest* (1999) 762.
29. R. Beck, M. Odeh, A. Oliven and N. Gavriely, *Eur. Respir. J.* (1995) 2120.
30. F. Cirignota, *Min. Med. Rev.* (2004) 177.
31. J. R. Perez-Padilla, E. Slawinski, L. M. Difrancesco, R. R. Feige, J. E. Remmers and W. A. Whitelaw, *Am. Rev. Respir. Dis.* (1993) 635.
32. F. Series, I. Marc and L. Atton, *Chest* (1993) 1769.
33. B. Truax, ed., *Handbook for Acoustic Ecology* (Cambridge Street Publishing, 1999).
34. J. Schäfer, *Laryngol. Rhinol. Otol.* (1988) 449.
35. J. Schäfer, ed., *Snoring, Sleep Apnea, and Upper Airways (in German)* (Georg Thieme Publisher, 1996).
36. Y. Itasaka, S. Miyazaki, K. Ishikawa and K. Togawa, *Psychiat. Clin. Neurosci.* (1999) 299.
37. M. Moerman, M. De Meyer and D. Pevernagie, *Acta Otorhinolaryngol. Belg.* (2002) 113.
38. J. Cummiskey, T. C. Williams, P. E. Krumpe and C. Guilleminault, *Am. Rev. Respir. Dis.* (1982) 221.
39. K. M. Hartse, V. C. Thessing, G. H. Branham and J. F. Eisenbeis, *Sleep Res.* (1995) 243.
40. P. E. Krumpe and J. M. Cummiskey, *Am. Rev. Respir. Dis.* (1980) 797.
41. D. L. Brunt, K. L. Lichstein, S. L. Noe, R. N. Aguillard and K. W. Lester, *Sleep* (1997) 1151.
42. W. Hida, H. Miki, Y. Kikuchi, C. Miura, N. Iwase, Y. Shimizu and T. Takishima, *Tohoku J. Exp. Med.* (1988) 137.
43. T. N. Liesching, C. Carlisle, A. Marte, A. Bonitati, R. P. Millman, *Chest* (2004) 886.
44. E. Kaniusas, L. Mehnen, H. Pfützner, B. Saletu and R. Popovic, in *Proceedings of International Measurement Confederation*, eds. A. Afjehi-Sadat, M. N. Durakbasa and P. H. Osanna (Austrian Society for Measurement and Automation, 2000), p. 177.

45. A. W. McCombe, V. Kwok and W. M. Hawke, *Clin. Otolaryngol.* (1995) 348.
46. T. Verse, W. Pirsig, B. Junge-Hülsing and B. Kroker, *Chest* (2000) 1613.
47. H. Rauscher, W. Popp and H. Zwick, *Eur. Respir. J.* (1991) 655.
48. T. Penzel, G. Amend, K. Meinzer, J. H. Peter and P. Wichert, *Sleep* (1990) 175.
49. C. A. Kushida, S. Rao, C. Guilleminault, S. Giraudo, J. Hsieh, P. Hyde and W. C. Dement, *Sleep Res. Online* (1999) 7.
50. M. Sergi, M. Rizzi, A. L. Comi, O. Resta, P. Palma, A. De Stefano and D. Comi, *Sleep Breath.* (1999) 47.
51. M. Karam, R. A. Wise, T. K. Natarajan, S. Permutt and H. N. Wagner, *Circulation* (1984) 866.
52. S. Silbernagl and A. Despopoulos, eds., *Pocket-Atlas of Physiology (in German)* (Georg Thieme Publisher, Stuttgart, 1991).
53. C. O. Olsen, G. S. Tyson, G. W. Maier, J. W. Davis and J. S. Rankin, *Circulation* (1985) 668.
54. A. Guz, J. A. Innes and K. Murphy, *J. Physiol.* (1987) 499.
55. M. Elstad, K. Toska, K. H. Chon, E. A. Raeder and R. J. Cohen, *J. Physiol.* (2001) 251.
56. K. Ishikawa and T. Tamura, *Angiology* (1979) 750.
57. W. R. Milnor, ed., *Hemodynamics* (Williams & Wilkins Publisher, Baltimore, 1989).
58. T. J. Pedley, ed., *The Fluid Mechanics of Large Blood Vessels* (Cambridge University Press, Cambridge, 1980).
59. F. Trendelenburg, ed., *Introduction into Acoustic (in German)* (Springer Publisher, Berlin, 1961).
60. D. A. Rice, *J. Appl. Physiol.* (1983) 304.
61. E. Meyer and E. G. Neumann, eds., *Physical and Technical Acoustic (in German)* (Vieweg Publisher, Braunschweig, 1975).
62. A. Bulling, F. Castrop, J. D. Agneskirchner, W. A. Ovtscharoff, L. J. Wurzinger and M. Gratzl, *Body Explorer* (Springer Publisher, CD-ROM, 1997).
63. M. Kompis, H. Pasterkamp, Y. Oh, Y. Motai and G. R. Wodicka, in *Proceedings of the 20th annual EMBS International Conference* (IEEE, 1998), p. 1661.
64. K. R. Erikson, F. J. Fry and J. P. Jones, *IEEE Trans. Son. Ultrason.* (1974) 144.
65. J. B. Calvert, *Sound Waves* (University of Denver, http://www.du.edu/~jcalvert/waves/ soundwav.htm, 2000).
66. P. D. Welsby and J. E. Earis, *Postgrad. Med. J.* (2001) 617.
67. P. D. Welsby, G. Parry and D. Smith, *Postgrad. Med. J.* (2003) 695.
68. H. Pasterkamp, S. Patel and G. R. Wodicka, *Med. Biol. Eng. Comput.* (1997) 103.
69. D. Leong-Kon, L. G. Durand, J. Durand and H. Lee, in *Proceedings of the 20th annual EMBS International Conference* (IEEE, 1998), p. 17.

# CHAPTER 2

# MODELING TECHNIQUES FOR LIVER TISSUE PROPERTIES AND THEIR APPLICATION IN SURGICAL TREATMENT OF LIVER CANCER

JEAN-MARC SCHWARTZ, DENIS LAURENDEAU*, MARC DENNINGER,
DENIS RANCOURT and CLOVIS SIMO

*Department of Electrical and Computer Engineering*
*Laval University, Quebec (Qc) G1K 7P4, Canada*
*\*laurend@gel.ulaval.ca*

This chapter presents a modeling approach for soft tissue properties designed at Laval University as part of the development of a simulation system for liver surgery. Surgery simulation aims at providing physicians with tools allowing extensive training and precise planning of interventions. The design of such simulation systems requires accurate geometrical and mechanical models of the organs of the human body, as well as fast computation algorithms suitable for real-time conditions. Most existing systems use very simple mechanical models, based on the laws of linear elasticity. Numerous biomechanical results yet indicate that biological tissues exhibit much more complex behavior, including important non-linear and viscoelastic effects.

In Sec. 1, we start by reviewing existing methods for the simulation of biological soft tissues. The approach used in our implementation, based on the tensor–mass model, is described in Sec. 2. In Sec. 3, we discuss the implementation issues and show how the efficiency of this model can be improved by an implementation on a distributed computer architecture. Finally, an experimental validation performed on liver tissue and an approach for simulating topological changes are presented in Secs. 4 and 5.

In image-guided cryosurgery, the clinical goal is to provoke a complete destruction of tumoral cells *in situ* through a thermal stress at cryogenic temperatures. Magnetic Resonance Imaging (MRI) guidance allows one to target the tumor site through a percutaneous approach, usually a working channel only a few millimeters in diameter through the skin, as well as to directly monitor the treatment as it takes place. MRI has the advantage of coupling excellent soft-tissue differentiation with high imaging resolution and speed, which results in unmatched visualization of the so-called iceball induced onto the treated tumor.

The SKALPEL-ICT (Simulation Kernel AppLied to the Planning and Evaluation of Image-guided CryoTherapy) project conducted at the Computer Vision and Systems Laboratory at Laval University aims at developing an immersive augmented reality environment for simulating the treatment of liver tumors using image-guided cryotherapy. It is widely recognized that the simulation of surgery through realistic Augmented Reality (AR) environments offers a safe, flexible, and cost-effective solution to the problem of planning the treatment procedures as well as in training surgeons in mastering highly complex manipulations. Augmented Reality attempts to recreate realistic sensory representations through the integration of numerous resources, ranging from high-definition graphics rendering to haptic and auditory feedback.

In the SKALPEL-ICT project, all aspects of the image-guided cryotherapy of liver tumors are being addressed and consists of the development of:

1. image analysis algorithms for the detection of liver tumors in a series of MR slices and the construction of a 3D geometric model of the tumor;
2. a thermal model (and its superimposition on the 3D geometric model) for simulating the growth of the ice ball;
3. a soft tissue model for simulating the mechanical behavior of the liver (and tumor) when submitted to the action of the cryogenic probe;
4. a software simulation framework supporting the above models;
5. a graphical user interface for rendering the different models in 3D as the simulation evolves.

This chapter describes the soft tissue model that has been developed for simulating the mechanical behavior of soft tissue (such as the liver). A review of current techniques for soft tissue modeling is first presented followed by the non-linear viscoelastic model that has been developed in our laboratory. Details on how the model has been implemented in software for real-time performance are also provided. A description of the implementation of the model on a distributed computer architecture is discussed. The procedure that was adopted for calibrating the model on experimental measurements performed on actual soft tissue is described in detail and the validation of the calibrated models is presented. Finally, a description is given on how the model can be exploited for simulating changes in the topology of the tissue during a simulation (e.g. perforation of the liver).

## 1. Soft Tissue Modeling

In this section, we present an overview of methods that have been developed for the modeling and simulation of soft tissue properties. The focus of this chapter being modeling techniques for surgery simulation applications, we do not aim at providing an exhaustive overview of soft tissue models from a biomechanical perspective, but rather focus on fast computational techniques that are suitable for real-time applications.

### 1.1. *Earliest models*

The first deformation models to be introduced in animation and simulation were non-physical models. Some of them, such as the Active Cubes[1] or ChainMail[2,3] models, have been successfully used in medical applications. Although it is possible to represent complex physical properties by purely mathematical or geometric approaches, an important drawback of these approaches is that it is impossible to link the parameters of such models to physically measurable quantities. Non-physical models need to be empirically adjusted to every new situation and are thus very difficult to validate using experimental data.

Terzopoulos[4] first applied mechanical engineering principles to the modeling of deformable objects. His first model used the Lagrangian formulation of the theory of elasticity to simulate deformable objects in one, two, or three dimensions. This pioneering work opened the way to a series of algorithmic developments for the computation of deformations of soft objects.

## 1.2. *Spring-mass models*

With the emergence of medical simulation, the first class of deformation models to gain broad popularity was spring-mass models. The spring-mass approach consists of meshing a surface or volume object into a set of vertices connected by elastic links, assimilated to springs. The mass of the object is entirely lumped at vertices. In most cases, the relation between stress and strain of the elastic links is considered to be linear, but more advanced mechanical models can be implemented. In the linear elastic case, the dynamic properties of such a system are led by the following relation:

$$m_i\ddot{\mathbf{x}}_i + d_i\dot{\mathbf{x}}_i + \sum_{k\in N(i)} c_k\mathbf{e}_k = \mathbf{f}_i, \tag{1}$$

where $\mathbf{x}_i$ is the coordinate vector of vertex $i$, $m_i$ is the mass associated with $i$, $d_i$ is the damping coefficient associated with $i$, $N(i)$ is the set of neighbors of $i$, $c_k$ is the stiffness of the link between $i$ and $k$, $\mathbf{e}_k$ the elongation of the link between $i$ and $k$ with regard to the rest state, and $\mathbf{f}_i$ are external forces applied to vertex $i$.

Numerous applications of this model to soft tissue simulation have been presented. It has been used, among others, in the simulation of bile surgery,[5] for facial surgery and the prediction of facial deformations,[6,7] and in the simulation of the human thigh.[8] It is implemented by the Karlsruhe Endoscopic Surgery Trainer,[9] a virtual reality-based training system for minimally invasive surgery.

Spring-mass models are fast enough to deal with the high-speed requirements of real-time simulation. However, they fail in accurately modeling the mechanical properties of soft tissues, particularly when only two-dimensional meshes are used. An additional drawback of the spring-mass representation is that the obtained properties can depend on the topology of the mesh, i.e. the way vertices are connected by links, which is not unique for a given set of vertices.

### 1.3. *Boundary element methods*

Other methods have been developed with the aim of modeling the physics of linear elasticity in a more rigorous way. Some of these methods are based on the laws of solid mechanics, represented by Navier's equation:

$$(\mathbf{Nu})(\mathbf{x}) + \mathbf{b}(\mathbf{x}) = 0, \tag{2}$$

where $\mathbf{x}$ is the field of points forming an object, $\mathbf{u}$ is the field of displacements, $\mathbf{b}$ is the field of external forces applied to the object, and N is a linear differential operator of second degree.

This equation can be solved by Boundary Element Method, which consists of meshing the boundary of the system into discrete elements. Inside every element, displacement fields are considered to be linear functions of the displacements of vertices. Equation (2) is then integrated on each element, resulting in a linear system of equations with three equations for each vertex.

Despite its apparent complexity, this method can be fast enough to be used in real-time applications for two reasons.[10] First, only the surface of the object needs to be meshed instead of the entire volume, resulting in a significantly smaller number of equations than for Finite Element (FE) Methods. Second, sets of elementary responses (Green functions) can be pre-computed and be later combined in real time due to the linearity property of the system to be solved. This method has been successfully applied to the simulation of liver deformations.[11] However, comparisons with experimental measurements revealed that the linear elastic model is accurate for describing liver properties only in the case of small deformations and low deformation speeds. Adapting boundary element methods to real-time non-linear simulation still remains a challenging task.

### 1.4. *Finite element methods*

The FE method appears as the most promising approach for modeling tissue deformations with good physical accuracy. FE-based methods implement a continuous representation of matter. An object can be meshed into three-dimensional elements, and force and displacement fields are approximated by continuous interpolation functions inside every element. However, such methods are computationally expensive, and, for a long time, were considered as being unsuitable for real-time applications. Bro-Nielsen and Cotin[12,13] first demonstrated the opposite by introducing several innovations.

FM models can be either quasi-static or dynamic. In the first case, the resulting system of equations for a linear elastic deformation model can be written as:

$$\mathbf{K}\,\mathbf{u} = \mathbf{f}, \tag{3}$$

where $\mathbf{u}$ is a vector containing the displacements of all vertices, $\mathbf{f}$ is a vector containing all external forces, and $\mathbf{K}$ is the stiffness matrix of the system.

Solving this system of equations for **u** basically implies computing the inverse of matrix **K**, a task that is too computationally expensive in the general case. Bro-Nielsen and Cotin first introduced a condensation of the stiffness matrix, consisting in transforming Eq. (3) so that surface variables can be isolated:

$$\mathbf{K_{ss}\, u_s = f_s}. \tag{4}$$

The new matrix $\mathbf{K_{ss}}$ has significantly smaller dimensions than the original matrix **K**. This matrix is then inverted directly: although that operation may be time-consuming, it can be performed during an off-line computational step. During runtime simulation, only the following product needs to be computed to obtain the deformations of the object:

$$\mathbf{u_s = K_{ss}^{-1}\, f_s}. \tag{5}$$

In applications related to medical simulations, surface contacts are usually restricted to a small number of points. As a result, $\mathbf{f_s}$ contains a large number of null elements, and computing $\mathbf{u_s}$ is fast.

When the quasi-static hypothesis is too restrictive, Eq. (3) can be transformed into a dynamic equation:

$$\mathbf{M\,\ddot{u} + D\,\dot{u} + K\,u = f}, \tag{6}$$

where **M**, **D**, and **K** are respectively mass, damping, and stiffness matrices. This system can still be solved by condensation and direct inversion of $\mathbf{K_{ss}}$. Although vector $\mathbf{f_s}$ now contains a large number of non-null elements, which are derived from the discretization of speed and acceleration terms, the method is still fast enough for real-time computations.

This approach was applied to the simulation of real-time deformations of liver, and was shown to be efficient for meshes containing as many as 250 vertices for a dynamic model, and 1500 vertices for a quasi-static model.[13,14] However, an important drawback of the approach was that simulating topological changes (i.e. tearing, cutting, or perforation) could not be achieved. If the topology of the mesh changes, the stiffness matrix of the system changes as well and needs to be re-inverted, but this operation is too computationally expensive to be performed in real time.

## 1.5. *Linear elastic tensor-mass model*

To cope with the problem of topological changes, a new FE-based method was later introduced by Cotin *et al.*[15] Instead of solving the FE-based systems of equations globally, a local and iterative approach was introduced. With a linear elastic mechanical model, and assuming a linear interpolation of strain fields on tetrahedral mesh elements, the strain energy of every element can be expressed as a function of the displacements of its four vertices. Then the elastic force $\mathbf{f}_i$ exerted on vertex $i$ as a result of the deformation of a tetrahedron can be computed by derivation of the strain energy. This results in the following expression:

$$\mathbf{f}_i = \frac{1}{36\,V} \sum_{j=0}^{3} (\lambda\,\mathbf{m}_i \otimes \mathbf{m}_j + \mu\,(\mathbf{m}_i \cdot \mathbf{m}_j)\,\mathbf{I}_3 + \mu\,\mathbf{m}_j \otimes \mathbf{m}_i)\,\mathbf{u}_j, \tag{7}$$

where $V$ is the volume of the tetrahedron, $\lambda$ and $\mu$ are the Lamé coefficients of the material, $\mathbf{I}_3$ is the identity matrix of dimension 3, $\mathbf{u}_j$ is the displacement of vertex $j$, and $\mathbf{m}_j$ are vectors defined by the following relations:

$$\mathbf{m}_0 = (\mathbf{P}_2 - \mathbf{P}_1) \wedge (\mathbf{P}_3 - \mathbf{P}_1), \tag{8}$$
$$\mathbf{m}_1 = (\mathbf{P}_2 - \mathbf{P}_3) \wedge (\mathbf{P}_0 - \mathbf{P}_2), \tag{9}$$
$$\mathbf{m}_2 = (\mathbf{P}_0 - \mathbf{P}_3) \wedge (\mathbf{P}_1 - \mathbf{P}_3), \tag{10}$$
$$\mathbf{m}_3 = (\mathbf{P}_0 - \mathbf{P}_1) \wedge (\mathbf{P}_2 - \mathbf{P}_0), \tag{11}$$

where $\mathbf{P}_j$ are the vertices of the tetrahedron. It is important to note that expressions (8)–(11) are valid for a direct orientation of vertex numbers, i.e. the product $(\mathbf{P}_1 - \mathbf{P}_0) \wedge (\mathbf{P}_2 - \mathbf{P}_0)$ should be directed toward vertex $\mathbf{P}_3$. These expressions are not symmetrical with respect to vertex numbers, as all $\mathbf{m}_j$ vectors are directed toward the outside of the tetrahedron.

A series of tensors $\mathbf{K}_{ij}^T$ can then be defined as:

$$\mathbf{K}_{ij}^T = \frac{1}{36\,V} (\lambda\,\mathbf{m}_i \otimes \mathbf{m}_j + \mu\,(\mathbf{m}_i \cdot \mathbf{m}_j)\,\mathbf{I}_3 + \mu\,\mathbf{m}_j \otimes \mathbf{m}_i) \tag{12}$$

enabling expression (7) to be rewritten as:

$$\mathbf{f}_i = \sum_{j=0}^{3} \mathbf{K}_{ij}^T \mathbf{u}_j. \tag{13}$$

Expression (13) is valid for an isolated tetrahedron. However, in an object mesh, elements are not isolated and interactions between neighboring tetrahedrons must be taken into account. Every tetrahedron $T$ has 16 associated $\mathbf{K}_{ij}^T$ tensors. $\mathbf{K}_{ij}^T$ represents the influence of a displacement of vertex $j$ in creating a force exerted onto vertex $i$. Two types of such tensors can therefore be considered: for $i = j$, $\mathbf{K}_{ii}^T$ expresses the influence of vertex $i$ onto itself. All such tensors will be multiplied by the same displacement $\mathbf{u}_i$ in (13), independently from the tetrahedron they belong to. Therefore, computational performance can be optimized by first summing up all $\mathbf{K}_{ii}^T$ tensors, before multiplying the result by $\mathbf{u}_i$. In a similar way, all tensors $\mathbf{K}_{ij}^T$ corresponding to the same edge $(i, j)$ can be summed up, independently of the considered tetrahedron, before being multiplied by $\mathbf{u}_i$. The generalized expression of (13) in a complete mesh thus becomes:

$$\mathbf{f}_i = \mathbf{K}_{ii}\,\mathbf{u}_i + \sum_{j \in \mathrm{N}(i)} \mathbf{K}_{ij}\,\mathbf{u}_j, \tag{14}$$

where $\mathbf{K}_{ii}$ is the sum of all tensors $\mathbf{K}_{ii}^T$ associated with adjacent tetrahedrons of vertex $i$, $\mathbf{K}_{ij}$ is the sum of all tensors $\mathbf{K}_{ij}^T$ associated with adjacent tetrahedrons of edge $(i, j)$, and $\mathrm{N}(i)$ is the set of neighboring nodes of vertex $i$.

Expression (14) makes it possible to compute all internal forces in the mesh in a given deformation state. This relation still needs to be integrated in time for the system to exhibit dynamic behavior. Dynamic motion is derived from Newton's equation:

$$m_i\,\ddot{\mathbf{u}}_i = -\gamma_i\,\dot{\mathbf{u}}_i + \mathbf{f}_i, \tag{15}$$

where $m_i$ is the mass associated with vertex $i$, and $\gamma_i$ is a damping coefficient associated with $i$.

Equation (15) assumes that mass and damping effects are lumped at nodes. This simplifying hypothesis is frequently made in FE applications, as it leads to uncoupling the differential equations corresponding to different nodes, resulting in independent equations for every node. In addition, making this hypothesis is the only way to maintain real time compatibility, and does not significantly affect the precision of the results.[15]

Several methods are available for integrating Eq. (15) numerically. The implementation described in this chapter uses an explicit Euler integration scheme, expressed by:

$$\mathbf{x}(t + \Delta t) = \frac{1}{m_i + \gamma_i\,\Delta t}(\Delta t^2\,\mathbf{f}(t) + (2m_i + \gamma_i\,\Delta t)\,\mathbf{x}(t) - m_i\,\mathbf{x}(t - \Delta t)), \tag{16}$$

where $\Delta t$ is the time interval between two iterations. Explicit schemes are faster than implicit schemes, but they have the drawback of being only conditionally stable. Some authors have preferred Runge–Kutta schemes as they offer a good compromise between computational speed and numerical stability.

## 2. Non-linear Modeling

The previous section presented a number of methods allowing the simulation of linear elastic tissues in real time. Unfortunately, biological soft tissues are usually poorly described by linear elasticity.[16,17] Improved methods need to be developed for describing the behavior of soft tissues accurately with the aim of developing biomedical simulation systems.

It is important to note that *non-linearity* can have two different meanings in the context of continuum mechanics. In the classical theory of linear elasticity, two different assumptions of linearity are made.[18] First, the strain tensor contains quadratic terms in its complete expression, and these terms are discarded in linear models. This approximation relies on the assumption that second-order terms are small compared to linear terms, which is only true when deformations remain small. Force vectors are then proportional to displacements, for that reason this case is sometimes referred to as *geometrical linearity*. A second and independent approximation consists of assuming a linear relation between strain and stress tensors. This case can be referred to as *physical linearity*. Models described in literature as non-linear may discard only one or both of these approximations.

## 2.1. *Non-linear finite element models*

Several FE-based approaches for real time applications involving some type of non-linearity have been presented in recent years. Mahvash and Hayward[19] presented a method for computing the haptic response of non-linear deformable objects from the data obtained by off-line simulation. The haptic response at any point of the object's surface was obtained by interpolation of pre-computed responses for neighboring nodes. This approach is not based on physical modeling of tissue properties, and can therefore be used for simulating a wide range of mechanical properties.

Cotin *et al.*[14] introduced non-linearity into their quasi-static model by adding corrective terms to linear equations. Corrections were derived from experimental measurements and approximated by polynomial functions. In an axial configuration, such corrections can be expressed as a function of axial displacement, and can be added to the results provided by a linear model without much additional computational load.

Zhuang and Canny[20] presented a FE-based method allowing fast computation of geometrically non-linear deformations, thus remaining valid for large deformations. Their approach consisted of constructing a global stiffness matrix while concentrating mass into the vertices of the mesh. Motion equations of individual vertices could then be uncoupled, enabling their individual and explicit integration. This approach appears to be close to the tensor-mass model in its principle, except for the construction of a global stiffness matrix. Wu *et al.*[21] presented a very similar method that furthermore integrates physical non-linearity, by the inclusion of Mooney–Rivlin and Neo-Hookean material models. In addition, an adaptive meshing mechanism was implemented, consisting of increasing the resolution of the mesh in areas that are highly deformed for improved quality.

The earlier methods used global reconstruction of the stiffness matrix, and are therefore not suitable for computing topological changes in real time. Debunne *et al.*[22] developed a local approach that is quite close to the tensor-mass model, but they used adaptive meshing for improved resolution in highly deformed areas. A non-linear strain tensor was used, and the difference between linear and quadratic terms provided a basis for evaluating the intensity of deformations: when this difference exceeded a given threshold, a higher resolution mesh was used. This method should in principle allow the simulation of topological changes, but such an implementation has not been presented.

Picinbono *et al.*[23] presented an extension of the tensor-mass model based on the St Venant–Kirchhoff model of elasticity, thus integrating geometrical non-linearity. The model was derived from a similar process as for the linear tensor-mass model. The general expression of the elastic energy based on the St Venant–Kirchhoff model was discretized, resulting in an extended expression of (7) containing additional second- and third-order terms. This method was reported to require five times as much computational time as the linear method, thus remaining compatible with real-time applications.

Recently the problem of simulating topological changes for non-linear materials has been addressed by Mendoza and Laugier.[24] They presented a methodology to simulate three-dimensional cuts in deformable objects, using a non-linear strain tensor to allow large displacements. Haptic feedback has been implemented with this method, showing that FE approaches can perform well in cases involving both non-linear modeling and topological changes.

## 2.2. *Non-linear extensions of the tensor-mass model*

As previously stated, non-linearity can be understood in different ways. In this section, we describe an extension of the tensor-mass method integrating physical non-linearity, developed by authors at Laval University in the context of the development of a simulation system for liver cryosurgery. We subsequently present an integration of this model[25] with the geometrically non-linear model developed by Picinbono *et al.*[23]

### 2.2.1. *Principle*

The tensor-mass model was chosen as a basis in order to benefit from its advantages, including its high computational performance and its flexibility for simulating topological changes. A first possibility for extending the tensor-mass model could consist in adding higher order terms to expression (7). However, the model would then be constrained to a particular type of mechanical law, with no guarantee that the behavior will correspond to biological tissue. Neither would an iterative addition of higher order terms until satisfying accuracy is reached be an appropriate solution, as it would lead to considerable increase in computational time.

The present model adopts a different approach, consisting of adapting mechanical properties both locally and dynamically: *locally*, as the tensor-mass model relies on local solving of differential equations, allowing mechanical properties to be changed for individual FEs without affecting the entire system; *dynamically*, as deformations change over time and different non-linear effects can be expected depending on the amplitude of deformations.

Mechanical properties are defined for every FE by stiffness tensors $\mathbf{K}_{ij}^T$. The expression of these tensors shows that they can be divided into two parts, so as to extract the Lamé coefficients:

$$\mathbf{K}_{ij}^T = \frac{\lambda}{36\,V}(\mathbf{m}_i \otimes \mathbf{m}_j) + \frac{\mu}{36\,V}(\mathbf{m}_i \cdot \mathbf{m}_j\,\mathbf{I}_3 + \mathbf{m}_j \otimes \mathbf{m}_i). \tag{17}$$

This expression relies on the principle of isotropy of continuous materials. It was shown that, under this assumption and after considering all possible symmetries, only two degrees of freedom remain in a three-dimensional linear relation between stress and strain.[26] These two degrees of freedom correspond to the two Lamé coefficients in linear elasticity theory, $\lambda$ and $\mu$. Therefore, the space spanned by $\lambda$ and $\mu$ in (17) covers all possible deformation behaviors satisfying isotropy constraints for a given tetrahedron. Acting on $\lambda$ and $\mu$ is therefore a convenient way to modify the properties of the element.

Doing so does not add excessive computational overload, as the qualities offered by the tensor-mass model can still be benefited from. By defining two additional tensors $\mathbf{A}_{ij}^T$ and $\mathbf{B}_{ij}^T$:

$$\mathbf{A}_{ij}^T = \frac{1}{36\,V}(\mathbf{m}_i \otimes \mathbf{m}_j), \tag{18}$$

$$\mathbf{B}_{ij}^T = \frac{1}{36\,V}(\mathbf{m}_i \cdot \mathbf{m}_j\,\mathbf{I}_3 + \mathbf{m}_j \otimes \mathbf{m}_i), \tag{19}$$

Eq. (17) can easily be rewritten as:

$$\mathbf{K}_{ij}^T = \lambda\,\mathbf{A}_{ij}^T + \mu\,\mathbf{B}_{ij}^T. \tag{20}$$

The mechanical properties of the element can now be modified by introducing two non-linear functions $\delta\lambda$ and $\delta\mu$:

$$\mathbf{K'}_{ij}^T = (\lambda + \delta\lambda(T))\,\mathbf{A}_{ij}^T + (\mu + \delta\mu(T))\,\mathbf{B}_{ij}^T, \tag{21}$$

that again can be rewritten as:

$$\mathbf{K'}_{ij}^T = \mathbf{K}_{ij}^T + \delta\lambda(T)\,\mathbf{A}_{ij}^T + \delta\mu(T)\,\mathbf{B}_{ij}^T. \tag{22}$$

Finally, forces can be computed using the extended stiffness tensor:

$$\mathbf{f}_i = \sum_{j=0}^{3} \left( \mathbf{K}_{ij}^T + \delta\lambda(T)\,\mathbf{A}_{ij}^T + \delta\mu(T)\,\mathbf{B}_{ij}^T \right) \mathbf{u}_j. \tag{23}$$

Functions $\delta\lambda$ and $\delta\mu$, which can be defined arbitrarily, determine the type of simulated non-linear behavior. Tensors $\mathbf{A}_{ij}^T$ and $\mathbf{B}_{ij}^T$ can still be pre-computed, since, as for $\mathbf{K}_{ij}^T$, they only depend on the geometry of the mesh element at rest. At runtime the computation of forces involves two additional terms. This increase in computational load is still manageable, and computation time remains constant for all types of non-linear functions. Furthermore, all operations remain local thus offering the opportunity of simulating topological changes in real time.

## 2.2.2. *Measure of deformation*

In Eq. (22), $\delta\lambda$ and $\delta\mu$ are two arbitrary functions defining a non-linear behavior. These functions must be expressed with respect to the local deformation of mesh elements. Some parameter quantifying local deformation is therefore needed to serve as an argument for these two functions.

Different approaches are possible for choosing such a parameter. In FE methods, several types of *shape measures* have been defined and are often used for assessing mesh quality. Shape measures can provide the needed assessment of the deformation of individual elements. A detailed study of the properties of three tetrahedron shape measures, including the minimum solid angle, the radius ratio, and the mean ratio, was published by Liu and Joe.[27] Although the notion of mesh quality is subjective to some extent, most of these shape measures have similar properties in that if one measure approaches zero for a poorly-shaped tetrahedron, so does the other, and that each measure attains a maximum value only for a regular tetrahedron.

For that reason, the choice of a particular shape value is not expected to alter the non-linear behavior significantly, and this choice should be mainly directed toward computational efficiency. With this in mind we selected the tetrahedron mean ratio, which can be computed directly from the lengths of a tetrahedron's edges by the following expression:

$$\rho = \frac{12\,(3\,V)^{2/3}}{\sum_{0 \leq i < j \leq 3} l_{ij}^2},\tag{24}$$

where $l_{ij}$ are the lengths of the tetrahedron's edges, and $V$ is the volume of the tetrahedron.

A different possible choice for the measure of deformation consists of using invariants of the strain tensor. They are scalar variables that are independent of the position and orientation of the coordinate referential, and thus depend only on the deformation of an element. A second order tensor $\tau$ possesses three invariants:

$$I_1 = \mathrm{tr}(\tau) = \lambda_1 + \lambda_2 + \lambda_3,\tag{25}$$

$$I_2 = \frac{1}{2}\left(\mathrm{tr}(\tau)^2 - \mathrm{tr}(\tau^2)\right) = \lambda_1\lambda_2 + \lambda_2\lambda_3 + \lambda_3\lambda_1,\tag{26}$$

$$I_3 = \det(\tau) = \lambda_1\lambda_2\lambda_3,\tag{27}$$

where $\lambda_1$, $\lambda_2$, $\lambda_3$ are the eigenvalues of $\tau$. For the strain tensor, $I_1$, $I_2$, and $I_3$ can respectively be interpreted as measures of affine, anisotropic, and volume deformations.

Several combinations of these invariants can be defined. In mechanics, the second invariant $J_2$ of the deviation of the strain tensor is frequently used to determine the elastic limit of materials, by the so-called von Mises criterion.[18] $J_2$ is therefore a good candidate for use as a measure of the intensity of local deformations. Using the notations defined in Sec. 1.5, its expression is

$$J_2 = \frac{1}{844\,V^2} \sum_{i,j=0}^{3} (6\,(\mathbf{u}_i \cdot \mathbf{m}_j)(\mathbf{m}_i \cdot \mathbf{u}_j) + 6\,(\mathbf{u}_i \cdot \mathbf{u}_j)(\mathbf{m}_i \cdot \mathbf{m}_j) - (\mathbf{u}_i \cdot \mathbf{m}_i)(\mathbf{m}_j \cdot \mathbf{u}_j))$$

$$(28)$$

### 2.2.3. Integration of geometrical non-linearity

Picinbono et al.[23] developed an extension of the tensor-mass model using a non-linear Cauchy–Green strain tensor, while keeping physical linearity. The properties and overall structure of the tensor-mass algorithm remain unchanged, but the extension resulted in a number of additional terms in the expression of forces:

$$\mathbf{f}_i = \sum_{j=0}^{3} \mathbf{K}_{ij}^T \mathbf{u}_j + \sum_{j,k=0}^{3} (\mathbf{u}_k \otimes \mathbf{u}_j)\,\mathbf{c}_{jki}^T + \frac{1}{2}(\mathbf{u}_j \cdot \mathbf{u}_k)\,\mathbf{c}_{ijk}^T + 2 \sum_{j,k,l=0}^{3} d_{jkli}^T\,(\mathbf{u}_l \otimes \mathbf{u}_k)\,\mathbf{u}_j,$$

$$(29)$$

where $\mathbf{K}_{ij}^T$ are the stiffness tensors defined by (12), $\mathbf{c}_{jki}^T$ are vectors, and $d_{jkli}^T$ are scalars defined by

$$\mathbf{c}_{ijk} = \frac{1}{216\,V^2}[\lambda\,\mathbf{m}_i(\mathbf{m}_j \cdot \mathbf{m}_k) + \mu\,(\mathbf{m}_k(\mathbf{m}_i \cdot \mathbf{m}_j) + \mathbf{m}_j(\mathbf{m}_i \cdot \mathbf{m}_k))] \qquad (30)$$

$$d_{ijkl} = \frac{1}{1296\,V^3}\left[\frac{\lambda}{4}(\mathbf{m}_i \cdot \mathbf{m}_j)(\mathbf{m}_k \cdot \mathbf{m}_l) + \frac{\mu}{2}(\mathbf{m}_i \cdot \mathbf{m}_l)(\mathbf{m}_j \cdot \mathbf{m}_k)\right]. \qquad (31)$$

Force contributions from different mesh elements are then added together as was done in the linear case. However, this operation is more complex here. In the linear case, only two types of contributions existed: tensors $\mathbf{K}_{ii}^T$ associated with a vertex $i$, and tensors $\mathbf{K}_{ij}^T$ associated with an edge $(i,\,j)$. Now, additional terms include contributions associated with faces $(i,\,j,\,k)$ and with tetrahedrons $(i,\,j,\,k,\,l)$, and the total number of different contributions is 31. The general structure of the algorithm remains unchanged though, as all additional parameters depend only on the rest geometry of tetrahedrons and on their Lamé coefficients.

Physical non-linearity can be integrated into this model following the same principle as described in Sec. 2.2.1. Every stiffness parameter appearing in (29) can be decomposed into two parts, proportional to $\lambda$ and $\mu$, respectively. As the same shape or deformation measure can be used for all terms of (29), no additional parameter needs to be added to the full model.

### 2.2.4. Integration of viscoelasticity

Most experimental characterizations of biological soft tissues revealed that these tissues exhibit viscoelastic behavior in addition to non-linear properties. In its most general form, the theory of viscoelasticity can describe a very wide range of behaviors.[26] However, only the simplest forms of viscoelasticity can reasonably be integrated into a model in a real-time context.

The simplest type of viscoelastic law is described by a linear viscous component, whose stress tensor is proportional to the derivative of the strain tensor:

$$\sigma_{ij}^{(v)} = \eta\,\dot\varepsilon_{ij}, \tag{32}$$

where $\eta$ is the viscosity coefficient. Forces exerted by such an element onto a vertex can be derived in the tensor-mass framework in a similar way as for linear elasticity. A rigorous demonstration must take into account the fact that differential deformations and works have to be considered instead of global elastic works, since viscous forces are not conservative. With the assumption that individual steps be small enough for differential steps to be added together neglecting higher order terms, a similar expression as (13) can be obtained, where displacements are replaced by displacement speeds:

$$\mathbf{f}_i^{(v)} = \sum_{j=0}^{3} \mathbf{K}_{ij}^{(v)T}\,\dot{\mathbf{u}}_j \tag{33}$$

with

$$\mathbf{K}_{ij}^{(v)T} = \frac{\eta}{72\,V}\,(\mathbf{m}_i \cdot \mathbf{m}_j\,\mathbf{I}_3 + \mathbf{m}_j \otimes \mathbf{m}_i). \tag{34}$$

Total forces in an integrated model are obtained by summation of linear, non-linear, and viscous forces:

$$\mathbf{f}_i = \sum_{j=0}^{3}\,(\mathbf{K}_{ij}^{T} + \delta\lambda\,\mathbf{A}_{ij}^{T} + \delta\mu\,\mathbf{B}_{ij}^{T})\,\mathbf{u}_j + \mathbf{K}_{ij}^{(v)T}\,\dot{\mathbf{u}}_j, \tag{35}$$

where $\mathbf{K}_{ij}^{T}$ are the stiffness tensors defined by (12), $\mathbf{A}_{ij}^{T}$ and $\mathbf{B}_{ij}^{T}$ are the non-linearity tensors defined by (18) and (19), and $\mathbf{K}_{ij}^{(v)T}$ are the viscosity tensors defined by (34).

The resulting viscoelastic model is of Voigt–Kelvin type, and only provides approximate modeling of properties of biological soft tissue. The Voigt–Kelvin model is nevertheless considered appropriate for modeling viscoelastic solids, and has been used for describing biological materials and polymers. However, it is not suitable for modeling viscoelastic fluids. When high computational speed is a top priority, this model is the simplest that can be introduced into the tensor-mass framework with limited computational expense, as more advanced models involve differential equations containing coupled stress and strain terms.

## 3. Implementation and Performance

For an efficient implementation of the algorithms described in the previous section, an object-oriented data structure was designed so as to optimize computational speed during the runtime phase. An overview of this structure and of the algorithms exploiting it is presented in the following.

### 3.1. *Data structure*

The following classes were designed to handle FE meshes (Fig. 1):

- SKMesh represents the complete mesh. All other classes are accessible from this class through arrays of pointers. SKMesh additionally contains pre-computed tensors associated with vertices and edges, resulting from summing up individual stiffness tensors associated with tetrahedrons.
- SKVertex represents a vertex in the mesh. It contains the rest position, current and previous positions, speed of displacement, and force applied onto the vertex. Some vertices may be fixed so as to model links with other objects.
- SKEdge represents an edge in the mesh. Edges are linked by pointers to their two vertices.
- SKFace represents a face in the mesh. Faces are linked by pointers to their three vertices and also contain references to their two adjacent tetrahedrons.
- SKTetrahedron represents a tetrahedron in the mesh. It contains all its associated pre-computed tensors, including $\mathbf{K}_{ij}^T$, $\mathbf{A}_{ij}^T$, $\mathbf{B}_{ij}^T$, and $\mathbf{K}_{ij}^{(v)T}$, as defined in Sec. 2. Variables representing the deformation measure used for computing non-linear properties are included. Tetrahedrons are also linked by pointers to their four vertices. Every tetrahedron contains a pointer to an SKTissue

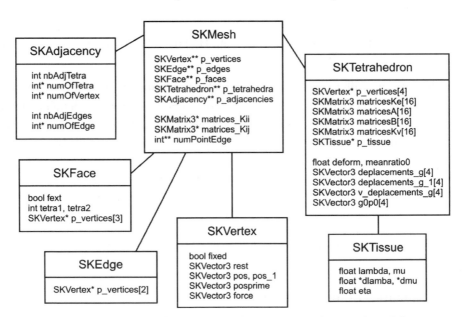

Fig. 1.   Schematic description of the data structure used for implementation of the tensor-mass algorithm.

structure, so that different tissue properties can be assigned to different mesh elements.

- SKAdjacency describes the neighborhood relationship between individual tetrahedrons. It contains data structures giving the lists of neighboring edges and tetrahedrons of each vertex. This structure is essential for real time performance, as the algorithm requires fast access to the neighboring elements of each vertex.

- SKTissue describes the mechanical properties of soft tissue. We chose to describe non-linear tissue properties by two tables containing the values of $\delta\lambda$ and $\delta\mu$ for different values of the deformation measure. This approach has the advantage of not assuming any particular shape for non-linear functions. Furthermore, this description can be refined as wished by adjusting the width of intervals in the table.

## 3.2. *Algorithm*

The main steps of the tensor-mass algorithm are presented in Fig. 2. The most costly steps, including construction of the mesh, of adjacencies, and computation of stiffness tensors, are all performed during an offline computational phase. Once the

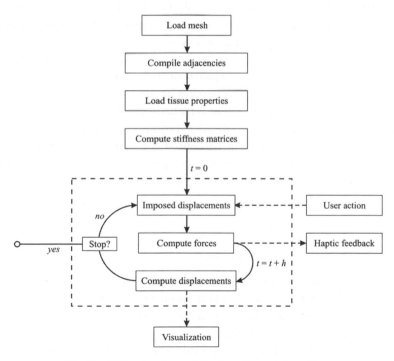

Fig. 2. Main structure of the tensor-mass algorithm.

- For every tetrahedron $T$:
  - Compute the current measure of deformation of $T$
  - Compute current displacements of the vertices of $T$
  - Compute current speeds of the vertices of $T$
- For every vertex $i$:
  - Initialize the force to 0
  - Add the linear contribution of matrix $\mathbf{K}_{ii}$
  - For every edge $(i, j)$ adjacent to vertex $i$:
    - Determine whether $i$ is first or second in edge $(i, j)$
      - If first: add the linear contribution of matrix $\mathbf{K}_{ij}$
      - If second: add the linear contribution of the transposed of matrix $\mathbf{K}_{ij}$
  - For every tetrahedron $T$ adjacent to vertex $i$:
    - For every vertex $k$ of tetrahedron $T$:
      - Add the non-linear contributions of matrices $\mathbf{A}_{ik}^{T}$ and $\mathbf{B}_{ik}^{T}$
      - Add the visco-elastic contributions of matrix $\mathbf{K}_{ik}^{(v)T}$

Fig. 3.   Detail of algorithm for the computation of forces.

algorithm enters the runtime phase, it runs as a loop with alternating computations of forces and displacements. The action of the user (e.g. through the probe) is rendered by imposing displacements to some points of the mesh. Visualization can be rendered following each computation of displacements and haptic feedback after each computation of forces. Higher rendering quality may be achieved by implementing additional response interpolation techniques.[28]

The highest cost of the runtime phase lies in the computation of forces, which is described in detail in Fig. 3. The lists of tetrahedrons and vertices must be scanned entirely. Scanning the list of tetrahedrons is required for updating shape measures after each iteration. Forces are then computed for every vertex in a second loop. Computation of linear elastic, non-linear, and visco-elastic forces are all performed in the same loop.

### 3.3.  Computational speed

#### 3.3.1.  Load of different mechanical models

Computational speed statistics presented in this section were compiled for a 2 GHz Pentium III processor with a test mesh comprising 768 tetrahedrons and 225 vertices. The computational time required for 200 iterations with different mechanical models is shown in Table 1.

The physically non-linear algorithm leads to an approximate fivefold increase in computation time compared to the linear elastic algorithm without viscoelasticity,

Table 1.   Computational speed for different mechanical models.

| Mechanical model | Time for 200 iterations (s) |
| --- | --- |
| Linear elasticity | 0.17 |
| Physical non-linearity | 0.96 |
| Viscoelasticity | 0.6 |
| Physical non-linearity and viscoelasticity | 1.23 |
| Physical and geometrical non-linearity | 6.5 |

and to a sevenfold increase with viscoelasticity. Addition of geometrical non-linearity leads to a significant decrease in performance, due to the large number of additional terms that need to be computed in real time.

### 3.3.2. *Dependence on mesh size*

Simulations of deformations were conducted for different meshes in order to observe the dependence of the computational performance of the algorithm on mesh size (Fig. 4). Speed is not exactly linear with regard to the number of mesh elements; it also depends on the geometry of the object as the algorithm contains different loops proportional to the numbers of tetrahedrons and vertices. An almost linear dependence on the number of mesh elements can nevertheless be observed globally.

In combination with the values from Table 1, these measurements allow us to set limits on the size of meshes that are suitable for real-time applications. When an iteration rate of 50 Hz is set as a target, meshes of up to 17000 tetrahedrons may be used with a linear elastic model, 2500 tetrahedrons with a physically non-linear and

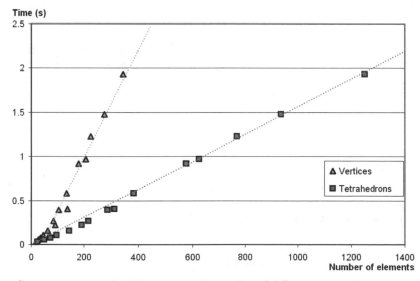

Fig. 4.   Computation time for 200 iterations for meshes of different sizes with a physically non-linear and viscoelastic mechanical model.

viscoelastic model, and 350 tetrahedrons with a complete non-linear model. The first two models are therefore appropriate for typical meshes used in biomedical simulation, while the complete model has more limited performance.

### 3.3.3. *Dynamic adaptation*

Computation of non-linear and viscoelastic forces accounts for a significant part of the computation time of the algorithm. It is therefore judicious to check whether these extensions are relevant at all times and in all parts of the mesh, and to introduce a mechanism for discarding these contributions when they are not essential.

In medical applications, high loads and deformations are usually concentrated in small areas of the modeled object. It is therefore possible to discard non-linear computations in wide areas undergoing small deformations, as a linear elastic model is usually sufficient in such areas. This can be achieved simply by introducing a non-linearity threshold. For mesh elements whose deformation measure does not exceed the defined threshold, only linear elastic terms need to be taken into account, while the full model will be used for mesh elements whose deformation measure exceeds the threshold. The local and dynamic nature of the tensor-mass algorithm is essential here, as the switch between a linear elastic model and a fully non-linear model can be decided for both individual elements and individual iterations.

Figure 5 illustrates the benefit of this adaptation. When the non-linearity threshold is set to a high value, a non-linear model is used throughout the entire mesh. When a low non-linearity threshold is selected, very few elements use a

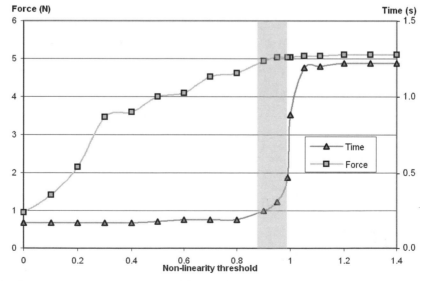

Fig. 5.   Computation time and computed forces after 200 iterations with dynamic adaptation of non-linear modeling. The gray-shaded area indicates the optimal non-linearity threshold range.

non-linear model, leading not only to reduced computation time but also to degraded precision of force values. However, an optimal area can be identified (gray-shaded zone in Fig. 5) where the computation time is significantly reduced while force values are not significantly altered. This area corresponds to the case where a non-linear model is used only for a small number of mesh elements where its contribution is essential.

## 3.4. *Implementation of the model on a distributed computer architecture*

The model presented in the previous sections was implemented as a sequential algorithm running on a standard single processor computer (see Secs. 4 and 5 for a discussion of the results). A distributed implementation of the model was also developed in order to investigate how it would behave with respect to model size and computation speed compared to the sequential implementation.

### 3.4.1. *Principle*

The distributed implementation was developed on a Beowulf cluster architecture. The cluster, which is modest compared to modern high-performance computing devices but can still be used for studying algorithm distribution, is composed of 28 nodes (CPU: AMD Athlon 1.2 Ghz, memory: 768 Mb) running on Linux. All nodes are connected with 100 Mb/s Ethernet links and eight nodes are connected with both 100 Mb/s and 1 Gb/s Ethernet links.

The METIS software package[34] was used for partitioning the FE mesh. The reason for choosing METIS is that it allows for partitioning the mesh with respect to the *elements* or the *nodes*. The Adaptive Communication Environment (ACE) library[35] was used for implementing the network communication between cluster nodes. ACE is an open-source multi-platform object-oriented communication library that is widely used in networking applications.

The data structure that was used for the distributed implementation was the same as for the sequential algorithm (Fig. 1). Figure 6(a) shows the modular structure of the sequential algorithm running on a single computer while Fig. 6(b) shows how this structure was transformed to fit in a distributed architecture using ACE.

The distributed implementation separates user input (which consists of positioning the cryogenic probe or a haptic device mimicking the probe) from the non-linear viscoelastic computation and the graphics rendering the appearance of the mesh as it deforms under the influence of the probe. The three separate modules use the ACE network package for exchanging information.

Figure 7 shows the hardware design of the system while Fig. 8 presents the flowchart of the distributed algorithm with the different steps.

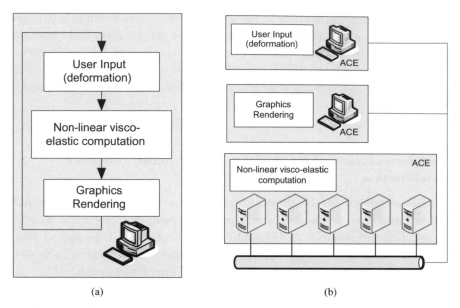

Fig. 6.    Structure of the computing modules for a single computer sequential implementation (a) and a distributed implementation (b). User input consists of sending the position of the cryogenic probe (or any haptic I/O device mimicking the probe) to the non-linear viscoelastic computation module which itself sends the position of the nodes in the mesh to the rendering module.

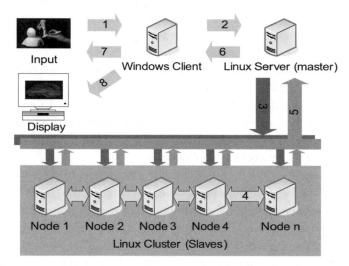

Fig. 7.    Hardware architecture of the distributed implementation of the viscoelastic simulation. The input device is controlled by the Windows Client and the displacement of the cryogenic probe is sent to this computer (1). The Windows Client sends displacement values to the Linux Server (2) which sends this information to the nodes composing the Linux Cluster (3). The nodes in the cluster compute forces and exchange information (4). Force values are sent back to the Linux Server (5) which forward them to the Windows Client (6) which itself forward them to the input device for haptic feedback (7) and to the graphics display for visualization (8).

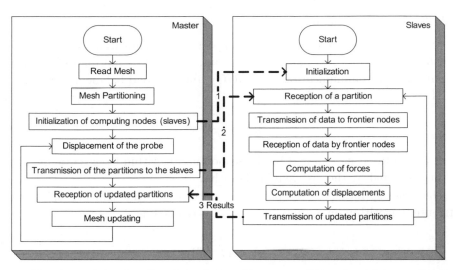

Fig. 8.   Flowchart of the distributed simulation. The master (Linux Server) is responsible for reading and partitioning the mesh used by the simulation. The master then initializes the slave nodes in the cluster and enters the simulation loop which reads the displacement of the probe, sends the information to the slave nodes, receives the updated partitions, and updates the mesh. The slaves, after initialization by the master, receive the partitions of the mesh, send data to frontier nodes (e.g. nodes common to partitions residing on different slaves), receive data from frontier nodes, compute forces resulting from the displacement of the probe, compute the new position of the nodes in the mesh, and transmit the updated partition to the master.

The algorithm is simple and, following initialization of the master and the slaves in the cluster, consists of two loops. The first loop runs on the server and is responsible for collecting user input (e.g. displacement of the probe), sending the partitions to the slaves and waiting until the updated partitions are ready for graphics rendering. The second loop runs on the slaves and is responsible for computing forces and mesh deformation and for sending the updated partitions to the master. Each slave is responsible for computing a subset (partition) of the complete mesh. Frontier nodes are nodes which are located at the limit between partitions and information for these nodes must be shared by slaves responsible for neighboring partitions.[a] Two types of communication occur during a simulation: global communications are concerned with the exchange of information between the master and the slaves while local communications are responsible for exchanging information between slaves managing neighboring partitions in the mesh. Of course, all communications are synchronized in order to maintain consistency of shared data (e.g. the mesh representing the model).

A more elaborate description of the technical details relevant to the distributed simulation can be found in Simo.[36]

---

[a]Assuming that a node-based partition is being implemented.

### 3.4.2. Performance evaluation

Several parameters were used to compare the sequential and distributed implementations of the model: speed up, scale up, normalized efficiency, computation vs. communication ratio (R/C), and the load balancing efficiency.

The *speed up* is defined as:

$$S_{n,P} = \frac{T_{n,1}}{T_{n,P}}, \tag{36}$$

where $T_{n,1}$ is the time required by the sequential algorithm to execute and $T_{n,P}$ is the time required by the distributed algorithm.

The *scale up* measures the potential performance that can be achieved by a distributed algorithm on a given cluster and is defined as:

$$T_m = \frac{G_m}{G_n} T_n, \tag{37}$$

where $G_m$ and $G_n$ are the mesh sizes and $T_m$ and $T_n$ are the theoretical times required for solving the problem for meshes $G_m$ and $G_n$, respectively.

The *normalized efficiency* is defined as the ratio between the increase of computational performance obtained with the distributed algorithm (compared with the sequential implementation) and the number of processors (e.g. the "cost" of distributing the algorithm):

$$E_{n,P} = \frac{S_{n,P}}{P}, \tag{38}$$

where $S_{n,P}$ is the gain in computational performance and $P$ is the number of processing nodes.

The computation vs. communication ratio is defined as:

$$R_{n,P} = \frac{R}{C}. \tag{39}$$

In Eq. (39), $R$ is the time devoted to computations while $C$ is the time devoted to communications (global and local).

Finally, the *load balancing efficiency* defined in Eq. (40) allows the measurement of the effects of code optimization of the sequential algorithm on the overall performance of the distributed algorithm:

$$L_{n,P} = \frac{\sum_{i=1}^{P} T_i}{\max(T_i)}, \tag{40}$$

where $T_i$ is the computation time for node $i$ and $P$ is the number of computing nodes.

The simulation that was used for estimating the performance of the distributed implementation of the non-linear viscoelastic model consisted of applying a deformation with constant speed on the face of a mesh (excluding the initial collision detection between the probe and the mesh) similar to the one shown in Fig. 21

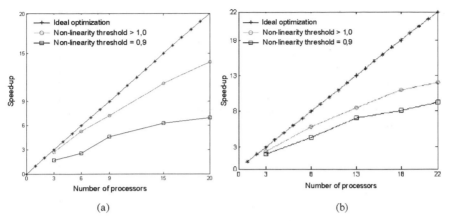

Fig. 9. Speed up values for a 32,256-element mesh (a) and an 18,960-element mesh (b) and for different values of the non-linearity threshold (see Fig. 5).

and measuring the computation time for computing the forces and the new mesh configuration. Figure 9(a) shows the speed up of the distributed algorithm for a mesh made up of 32,256 elements and for a mesh made up of 18,960 elements. A better speed up occurs for a value of the non-linearity threshold greater than 1. The performance decreases for a threshold value of 0.9 because of poor dynamic load balancing. It can also be seen that, for a threshold value greater than 1, the increase in speed up slows down above six processors because of load balancing and communication overhead. Finally, for a given number of processors, the speed up is higher for larger meshes. Although this phenomenon is not fully understood, there is evidence that this behavior results from the coarser granularity of the partition of meshes with a larger number of elements, which implies a larger $R/C$ ratio.

Figure 10 shows the plot of the normalized efficiency versus the number of processors for different values of the non-linearity threshold. These results show that efficiency decreases with the number of processors and this effect is especially true for a value of the non-linearity threshold of 0.9, which means that distributing the algorithm is not efficient. However, for threshold values greater than one, a 70% efficiency can be achieved with 20 processors with increased precision of the computation results. This means that efforts for distributing the computation are best rewarded for experiments where accuracy is important and sequential optimization is not easy to implement.

Figures 11(a) and 11(b) show the scale up that was obtained for five and ten processors, respectively (and a value of the non-linearity threshold greater than 1). In general, the relation between linear scale up and the scale up that was measured on the actual simulation is maintained which means that the simulation time grows linearly with the number of elements in the model. In addition, both plots are identical up to a scale factor. This is a demonstration that the distributed algorithm is efficient and that the simulation time can be extrapolated for a given size of the model.

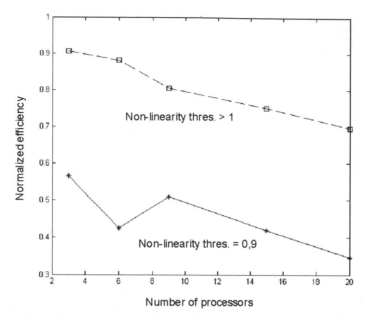

Fig. 10.   Normalized efficiency versus number of processors for different values of the non-linearity threshold. 32,256 elements, 900 iterations.

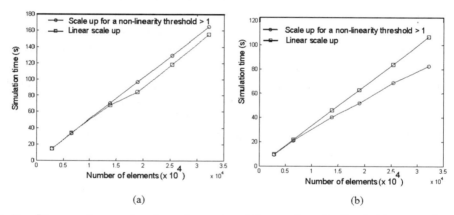

(a)                                                        (b)

Fig. 11.   Linear scale up and scale up for a value of the non-linearity threshold greater than 1.5 processors — 900 iterations (a) 10 processors — 900 iterations (b).

### 3.4.3. *Implementation strategies*

Two strategies can be adopted for partitioning the model for distributed simulation: (i) node-based and (ii) element-based. For a node-based partition, only the nodes located at frontiers between partitions need to be duplicated on two (or more) processors while the complete element needs to be duplicated for an element-based partition.

Before comparing the two different approaches, three definitions must be introduced.

The "waiting time" $T_w$ is defined as the time that flows between the moment a slave node starts sending data at the frontier of its partition and the moment it has received all the data at the frontier of other partitions. This time includes the time spent for local communications between slave nodes. During $T_w$, slave nodes are idle and do not perform useful computation. The "computation time" $T_c$ is the time spent computing forces and displacements. Finally, the global communication time $T_g$ is the time spent at global communications between the master and the slaves (including synchronization). Based on the previous definitions, the simulation time $T_s$ is defined as

$$T_s = T_w + T_c + T_g. \tag{41}$$

Since it is difficult to measure $T_g$, it is rather estimated with Eq. (41) as

$$T_g = T_s - (T_c + T_w). \tag{42}$$

Figure 12 shows the speed up that is obtained for a node-based partitioning strategy compared to an element-based strategy (for both an average simulation time and maximum simulation time). The performance of the node-based strategy is clearly the best. In addition, a "superlinearity" behavior is observed for the node-based average when the speed up is computed for the average computation time (instead of with the maximum computation time). This is explained by the fact that the average time smooths the effect caused by non-optimal load balancing between the processors in the cluster. It is important to note that the average time reflects

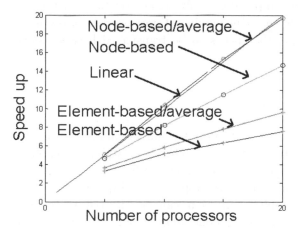

Fig. 12. Speed up of the distributed algorithm for node-based partitioning and element-based partitioning.

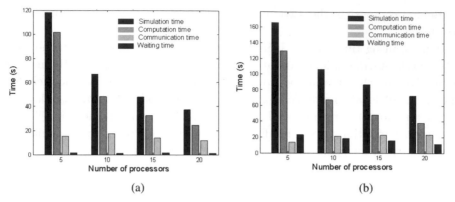

Fig. 13.    Plots of different time parameters for a 25,344-element mesh (900 iterations, non-linearity threshold > 1). (a) Node-based partition. (b) Element-based partition.

the overall performance of the distributed algorithm while the maximum time is the one that sets the refresh cycle time of the mesh.

Finally, Fig. 13 compares the different time values for node-based and element-based partitions. For a node-based partition (Fig. 13(a)), the proportion between the simulation time and the computation time is maintained as the number of processors increases. It can also be observed that the waiting time is small compared to the computation time. This is explained by the fact that the amount of data (16 bytes per node) that is exchanged between partitions (e.g. slaves in the cluster) is very small.

For an element-based partition (Fig. 13(b)), the proportion between the simulation time and the computation time is also maintained as the number of processors increases. The waiting time tends to decrease with the number of processors while the communication time increases. In addition, the waiting time for the element-based partition is always greater than the waiting time for the node-based partition for the same number of processors because the amount of data (192 bytes per element) that needs to be transferred between slaves in the cluster is greater.

### 3.5. Numerical stability

Stability is a recurrent problem in the numerical integration of dynamic equations. Unconditionally stable integration schemes exist, but the explicit Euler scheme used in our implementation is only conditionally stable. The key parameter affecting stability is the time interval $\Delta t$ appearing in Eq. (16).

A rigorous stability criterion can be derived mathematically in the one-dimensional case. Assuming a one-dimensional dynamic equation of the form

$$m\,\ddot{u} = -\gamma\,\dot{u} - k\,u \tag{43}$$

discretized by the following explicit Euler scheme:

$$(m + \gamma \Delta t)\, x(t + \Delta t) + (k\, \Delta t^2 - 2m - \gamma \Delta t)\, x(t) + m\, x(t - \Delta t) = 0, \tag{44}$$

it can be shown that integration will be stable if

$$\Delta t \leq \frac{1}{k}(\gamma + \sqrt{\gamma^2 + 4km}). \tag{45}$$

No rigorous stability criterion could be derived in the three-dimensional case, but an approximate criterion can be obtained by drawing an analogy between a one-dimensional model and a three-dimensional cylinder. The previous criterion then becomes:

$$\Delta t \leq \frac{h}{SE}\left(\gamma + \sqrt{\gamma^2 + 4\frac{SEm}{h}}\right), \tag{46}$$

where $S$ and $h$ are respectively the characteristic section and height of the modeled object, and $E$ is Young's modulus. When $SEm \ll h\gamma^2$, Eq. (46) reduces to

$$\Delta t \leq \frac{2\gamma h}{SE}. \tag{47}$$

Equations (46) and (47) indicate that the stability limit decreases linearly with Young's modulus. Deformations of soft tissues are easier to model than deformations of more rigid objects for that reason. Although relying on a broad approximation, the stability criterion predicted by Eqs. (46) and (47) was verified in simulation tests (Fig. 14).

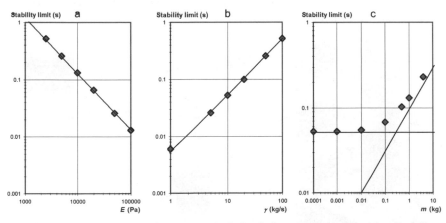

Fig. 14.  Stability limits derived from numerical simulations of three-dimensional meshes as a function of different model parameters. (a) $E$ Variable, $\gamma = 100$, $m = 0.0006$. (b) $E = 2500$, $\gamma$ Variable, $m = 0.0006$. (c) $E = 2500$, $\gamma = 10$, $m$ variable. All three graphs use logarithmic scales.

## 4. Experimental Measurements and Validation

### 4.1. *Mechanical setup*

We performed experimental measurements on animal liver in order to assess the suitability of the presented approach to the simulation of biological soft tissue. The experimental setup is shown in Fig. 15. A 2.4 mm diameter biopsy needle was mounted on a 5 lbs Totalcomp TMB-5 load cell. Vertical movement was controlled by a step-motor whose velocity ranged from 2 to 10 mm/s. The needle perforated a sample of deer liver placed in a container. The force modulus exerted onto the needle was acquired together with the position of the needle at the rate of 500 Hz by an A/D sampling board and plotted.

Measurements were repeated several times for different positions and various contact angles between the needle and the sample, to avoid biases due to a particular geometrical configuration or local non-homogeneity of liver tissue. The liver membrane was conserved in all experiments, as it is present in the case of a real surgical intervention.

### 4.2. *Experimental results*

Several series of measurements were conducted using three different perforation speeds, i.e. 2, 6, and 10 mm/s (Fig. 16). Results showed good reproducibility, as force curves obtained at different positions and for different orientations of the sample were very similar. The properties of liver tissue therefore appear to be quite homogeneous. Membrane rupture occurred at variable times though, for force values between 2 and 4 N, without showing any correlation to the perforation speed.

Force curves show as expected that liver behavior is highly non-linear and that a linear model is not suitable. An overlay of curves obtained at different speeds shows that forces grow faster with higher perforation speeds, thus confirming the viscoelastic nature of liver tissue.

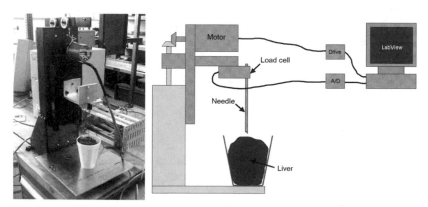

Fig. 15. Experimental setup for the characterization of mechanical properties of liver tissue and validation of the simulation model.

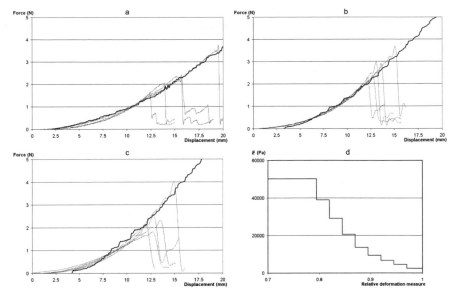

Fig. 16.   Five independent experimental force curves (light gray) and simulated forces (black) for three different perforation speeds: (a) 2 mm/s; (b) 6 mm/s; (c) 10 mm/s; (d) Relation between Young's modulus and the local deformation measure used in the simulation model.

## 4.3.  Comparisons with simulation models

### 4.3.1.  Physically non-linear model

These experimental results were used to fit parameters of a physically non-linear and viscoelastic tensor-mass model. The number of parameters being quite important, fitting had to be conducted by iteratively comparing simulation results to the experimental data. No automatic procedure has been developed for this task yet. Parameter values obtained by fitting are given in Table 2, and simulated forces are displayed on Fig. 16 over experimental curves.

High values of non-linear corrections, as compared to linear Lamé coefficients, had to be used to fit experimental curves. Non-linear corrections were kept constant for deformation measures under 0.795, as higher corrections below that value did not produce any noticeable effect on simulation results (low deformation measures correspond to high deformations in compression, the deformation measure of an undeformed element being one). Because of the axial symmetry of the experimental setup, the Poisson coefficient could not be derived from the experimental results. It was therefore kept constant at 0.4 throughout our model, leading to fixed proportions between $\lambda$ and $\mu$.

### 4.3.2.  Full non-linear model

As stated in Sec. 2, using a linear strain tensor can no longer be considered a valid approximation when large deformations occur. This property becomes clearly

Table 2.  Parameter values of the mechanical model used in the simulations displayed in Fig. 16. The tetrahedron mean ratio $\rho$ (24) was used as a deformation measure.

| Parameters | Values |
|---|---|
| Lamé coefficients $\lambda$ and $\mu$ | 3600; 900 |
| Viscosity coefficient $\eta$ | 600 |
| Non-linear corrections $\delta\lambda$ and $\delta\mu$ by intervals of deformation measure: | |
| $> 0.97$ | 0; 0 |
| 0.945–0.97 | 3000; 750 |
| 0.92–0.945 | 6000; 1500 |
| 0.895–0.92 | 10,000; 2500 |
| 0.87–0.895 | 16,000; 4000 |
| 0.845–0.87 | 26,000; 6500 |
| 0.82–0.845 | 38,000; 9500 |
| 0.795–0.82 | 52,000; 13,000 |
| $< 0.795$ | 68,000; 17,000 |

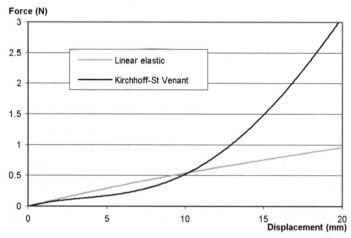

Fig. 17.   Simulations of compression of liver tissue for physically linear mechanical models: the gray curve was obtained by using a linear strain tensor, while the black curve was obtained using the non-linear Cauchy–Green strain tensor.

visible when simulations using linear and non-linear strain tensors are compared for a physically linear model (Fig. 17). Forces computed using the Kirchhoff–St Venant elasticity model remain very close to linear elastic forces for deformation lower than approximately 10 mm, but the two models significantly diverge from each other at higher deformations. Although most mesh elements undergo small deformations in a needle compression simulation, elements that are very close to the needle are likely to undergo large deformations, and such elements are important contributors to the forces exerted onto the needle.

Simulation results using a physically and geometrically non-linear model are displayed in Fig. 18. As stated in Sec. 3.3.1, this model lacks the computational performance to be suitable for real time simulation of large meshes. It nevertheless achieves very good modeling of experimental results. Of particular interest is that the values required for non-linear corrections are significantly lower than for the physically only non-linear model (Table 3). As highly deformed mesh elements are poorly modeled by a linear strain tensor, lower forces indeed need to be compensated by increasing the values of non-linear corrections. The full non-linear model is therefore expected to describe more accurately the physical properties of tissues. On the other hand, both models are able to reproduce the measured properties with good precision, and choosing a physically only non-linear model remains justified from an empirical point of view.

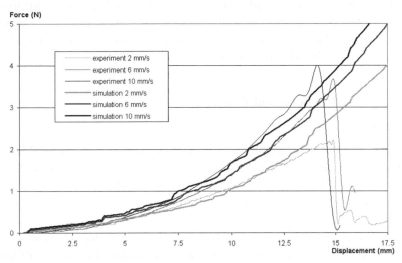

Fig. 18. Simulations of liver tissue compression using a full non-linear model and comparisons with experimental data.

Table 3. Parameter values of the mechanical model used in the simulations displayed in Fig. 17. The strain tensor invariant $J_2$ (28) was used as a deformation measure.

| Parameters | Values |
|---|---|
| Lamé coefficients $\lambda$ and $\mu$ | 4000; 1000 |
| Viscosity coefficient $\eta$ | 500 |
| Non-linear corrections $\delta\lambda$ and $\delta\mu$ | |
|    by intervals of deformation measure: | |
| $< 8.10^{-9}$ | 0; 0 |
| $8.10^{-9}$–$28.10^{-9}$ | 4000; 1000 |
| $28.10^{-9}$–$48.10^{-9}$ | 8000; 2000 |
| $> 48.10^{-9}$ | 12,000; 3000 |

### 4.3.3. *Limitations*

There are two main limitations to the previous experimental characterizations. First, forces were only measured at a single point and in one dimension. While this is sufficient for evaluating the haptic response in a needle insertion experiment, additional measurement points would be required for fully assessing the mechanical model and characterizing the three-dimensional behavior of liver tissue. Such validation poses important experimental challenges, and the development of new methods to validate real time soft tissue deformation models has been the object of further research.[29]

The second limitation arises from the fact that properties of *ex vivo* tissues differ from those of living tissue, mostly because of the absence of perfusion. It has nevertheless been observed on the brain tissue that a model developed from *in vitro* data could accurately reproduce *in vivo* soft tissue behavior by appropriately increasing material parameters describing instantaneous stiffness.[30] The effect of perfusion remains important though and may be assessed by newly developed setups, thus eliminating the need to resort to *in vivo* experiments.[31]

## 5. Simulation of Topological Changes

### 5.1. *Overview*

This section is aimed at presenting an approach for coping with the problem of real-time topological changes in the modeling of needle insertion in soft tissue. Simulation of needle insertion has become particularly important with the development of brachytherapy, a therapy consisting of the percutaneous insertion of radioactive sources into malignant tissue.

Simulation of needle insertion differs from the simulation of other medical tasks in several ways. First, the needle does not only manipulate the surface of the organ and friction plays a significant role during insertion. Second, biopsy needles are flexible and their deformation should be taken into account. Alterovitz *et al.*[32] developed a simulation approach of needle insertion in soft tissue for the planning of prostate brachytherapy, based on a two-dimensional dynamic FE model. Goksel *et al.*[33] presented a three-dimensional needle–tissue interaction model applied to the same context and achieved computational rates faster than 1 kHz. These approaches were taking friction into account, but relied on linear elastic mechanical modeling. In the following, we present an overview of how the tensor-mass framework may be adapted to the simulation of needle insertion, and more generally to tasks involving topological changes in three-dimensional models.

### 5.2. *Algorithm*

As described in Sec. 3, our tensor-mass implementation has been designed to allow simulation of topological changes in real time. Of crucial importance in this context is the SKAdjacency class, storing lists of adjacent tetrahedrons and edges for every vertex in the mesh. The main requirement when a topological change occurs consists of updating this information.

An algorithm for removing a tetrahedron from a mesh is presented in Fig. 19. It is possible to simulate a tear in a tissue using the same approach, except that no tetrahedron has to be removed in this case and only adjacency links need to be broken. This algorithm relies on information about mesh faces being external or internal. If the tetrahedron to be removed possesses one or more external faces, these faces will disappear completely from the mesh after removal of the tetrahedron. However, an internal face is shared by two different tetrahedrons and will remain present in the mesh. Similarly, a vertex or an edge belonging only to external faces of the tetrahedron to be removed will disappear from the mesh. Elements to be deleted from the model can be easily identified that way, and adjacency information can then be updated.

During the process of tetrahedron removal, stiffness tensors associated with the vertices and edges of the deleted tetrahedron have to be updated. These tensors need not be recomputed from scratch though, as the only required operation is a summing up of $\mathbf{K}_{ij}^{T}$ tensors associated with individual tetrahedrons (Sec. 1.5) and not a new computation of these tensors. The computational overload due to tetrahedron removal

- For every vertex $i$ of tetrahedron $T_0$:
  - Set matrices $\mathbf{K}_{ii}$ to zero
  - If all faces of $T_0$ containing $i$ are external:
    - Delete vertex $i$
    - Delete matrix $\mathbf{K}_{ii}$
- For every edge $(i, j)$ of tetrahedron $T_0$:
  - Set matrices $\mathbf{K}_{ij}$ to zero
  - If all faces of $T_0$ containing $(i, j)$ are external:
    - Delete edge $(i, j)$
    - Delete matrix $\mathbf{K}_{ij}$
    - Delete adjacency links to $(i, j)$ from vertices $i$ and $j$
- For every face $F$ of tetrahedron $T_0$:
  - If $F$ is external: delete $F$
- Delete tetrahedron $T_0$
- Delete adjacency links to $T_0$ from remaining vertices and faces of $T_0$
- Recompute matrices $\mathbf{K}_{ii}$ and $\mathbf{K}_{ij}$ that were set to zero but not deleted

Fig. 19.   Algorithm for removing a tetrahedron $T_0$ from a tensor-mass model.

therefore remains limited. In trials conducted on meshes of about 4000 elements, additional time due to tetrahedron removal did not exceed 0.01 s.

## 5.3. *Simulation approach*

Experimental force measurements in needle perforation revealed that forces exhibit a highly unpredictable pattern after perforation of the liver membrane (Fig. 20). A succession of peaks of variable height and variable frequency was observed. This behavior may be due to both friction between the needle and liver tissue and heterogeneity of the tissue itself. Accurate simulation of this behavior will therefore require the development of new approaches for modeling these properties.

The relevance of the tensor-mass framework for simulating the perforation of non-linear tissue in real time can nevertheless be demonstrated (Fig. 21). The approach followed in this example consisted of removing a tetrahedron every time the force intensity exerted onto the needle exceeded a defined threshold.

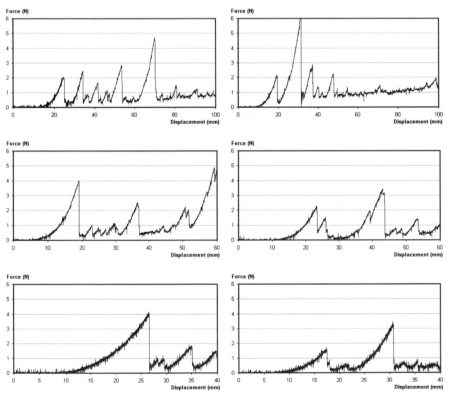

Fig. 20. Examples of experimental force measurements in liver perforation by a biopsy needle. Perforation speed was 10 mm/s for the curves in the top row, 6 mm/s in the middle row, and 2 mm/s in the bottom row.

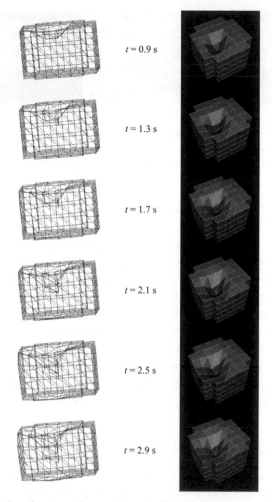

Fig. 21.   Simulation of perforation of a model mesh. One tetrahedron was removed every time the force intensity exerted onto the needle exceeded a defined threshold. Soft tissue properties were modeled by a physically non-linear tensor-mass model whose parameters are given in Table 2.

## 6. Conclusion

As mentioned in the Introduction, the non-linear viscoelastic model presented in this chapter was developed as a component of a Magnetic Resonance Imaging guided simulator for cryotherapy. Figure 22(a) shows the graphics rendering of the simulation environment with the open-field magnetic resonance imager and the patient (a 3D rendering of the Visible Human[37]). Figure 22(b) shows a close-up of the tumor and an avatar for the probe. The 3D model of the tumor was built from the analysis of a stack of MR images of a real patient. Figure 22(c) shows a close-up of the liver being deformed by a probe (not shown). The non-linear viscoelastic

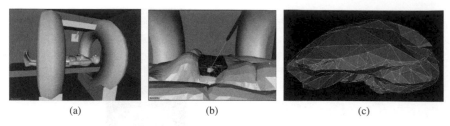

(a)                         (b)                         (c)

Fig. 22.  Virtual environment recreating the operating room with the open-field Magnetic Resonance Imaging device (a); Close-up of a tumor (green) being perforated by a probe (b); Three-dimensional model of a tumor being deformed (c), following the viscoelastic non-linear model described in Sec. 3 and validated experimentally by the experiments described in Sec. 4.

model is computed in real time and generates the forces and displacements that come into play in a simulation.

In this chapter, we presented a model allowing the simulation of biological soft tissue properties that combines computational efficiency and physical accuracy. Although this model was developed in the context of liver surgery simulation, it is expected to be generic enough for allowing its usage in different contexts and for different types of deformable materials. Experimental data are crucial to the presented approach, as it relies on empirical functions for modeling non-linear tissue behavior. In the future, the development of improved experimental setups and methodologies for better characterization of the complex properties of living tissues will be crucial for further improving the accuracy of deformation models and surgery simulation systems.

## Acknowledgments

The authors acknowledge the financial support of the Natural Sciences and Engineering Council of Canada (NSERC) through the Strategic Grant Program. Thanks go to Drs Christian Moisan and Amidou Traoré from Centre Hospitalier Universitaire de Québec (CHUQ) for providing technical and scientific advice on cryotherapy and to Dr Annette Schwerdtfeger for proofreading the manuscript. Constructive comments on the mass-tensor model presented in this chapter were provided by Dr Hervé Delingette from INRIA Sophia-Antipolis.

## References

1. M. Bro-Nielsen, *Proc. CVRMed '95* (1995) 535–541.
2. S. F. Gibson, *IEEE Trans. Vis. Comput. Graph.* **5**(4) (1999) 333–348.
3. Y. Li and K. Brodlie, *Comput. Graph. Forum* **22**(4) (2003) 717–728.
4. D. Terzopoulos, J. Platt, A. Barr and K. Fleischer, *Proc. SIGGRAPH'87* (1987) 269–279.
5. S. A. Cover, N. F. Ezquerra, J. F. O'Brien, R. Rowe, T. Gadacz and E. Palm, *IEEE Comput. Graph. Appl.* **13**(6) (1993) 68–75.

6. Y. Lee, D. Terzopoulos and K. Waters, *Proc. SIGGRAPH '95* (1995) 55–62.
7. R. M. Koch, M. H. Gross, F. R. Carls, D. F. von Büren, G. Fankhauser and Y. I. H. Parish, *Proc. SIGGRAPH '96* (1996) 421–428.
8. D. d'Aulignac, R. Balaniuk and C. Laugier, *Proc. ICRA 2000* **3** (2000) 2452–2457.
9. U. Kühnapfel and H. K. Çakmak and H. Maaß, *Comput. Graph.* **24**(5) (2000) 671–682.
10. D. L. James and D. K. Pai, *Proc. SIGGRAPH '99* (1999) 65–72.
11. C. Monserrat, U. Meier, M. Alcañiz, F. Chinesta and M. C. Juan, *Comput. Meth. Prog. Biomed.* **64**(2) (2001) 77–85.
12. M. Bro-Nielsen and S. Cotin, *Proc. EUROGRAPHICS '96* (1996) 57–66.
13. M. Bro-Nielsen, *Proc. IEEE* **86**(3) (1998) 490–503.
14. S. Cotin, H. Delingette and N. Ayache, *IEEE Trans. Vis. Comput. Graph.* **5**(1) (1999) 62–73.
15. S. Cotin, H. Delingette and N. Ayache, *Vis. Comput.* **16**(8) (2000) 437–452.
16. J. D. Humphrey, *Proc. R. Soc. Lond. A* **459**(2029) (2003) 3–46.
17. Y. C. Fung, *Biomechanics: Mechanical Properties of Living Tissues*, 2nd edn. (Springer-Verlag, New York, 1993), pp. 1–22.
18. Y. C. Fung, *Foundations of Solid Mechanics* (Prentice-Hall, Englewood Cliffs, 1965).
19. M. Mahvash and V. Hayward, *IEEE Comput. Graph. Appl.* **24**(2) (2004) 48–55.
20. Y. Zhuang and J. Canny, *Proc. ICRA 2000* **3** (2000) 2428–2433.
21. X. L. Wu, M. S. Downes, T. Goktekin and F. Tendick, *Comput. Graph. Forum* **20**(3) (2001) c349–c358.
22. G. Debunne, M. Desbrun, M.-P. Cani and A. H. Barr, *Proc. SIGGRAPH 2001* (2001) 31–36.
23. G. Picinbono, H. Delingette and N. Ayache, *Graph. Models* **65**(5) (2003) 305–321.
24. C. Mendoza and C. Laugier, *Lec. Notes Comput. Sci.* **2673** (2003) 175–182.
25. J.-M. Schwartz, M. Denninger, D. Rancourt, C. Moisan and D. Laurendeau, *Med. Image Anal.* **9**(2) (2005) 103–112.
26. P. C. Chou and N. J. Pagano, *Elasticity: Tensor, Dyadic, and Engineering Approaches* (Van Nostrand, Princeton, 1967), pp. 204–224.
27. A. Liu and B. Joe, *BIT* **34**(2) (1994) 268–287.
28. M. Mahvash and V. Hayward, *IEEE Trans. Robot.* **21**(1) (2005) 38–46.
29. A. E. Kerdok, S. M. Cotin, M. P. Ottensmeyer, A. M. Galea, R. D. Howe and S. L. Dawson, *Med. Image Anal.* **7**(3) (2003) 283–291.
30. K. Miller, K. Chinzei, G. Orssengo and P. Bednarz, *J. Biomech.* **33**(11) (2000) 1369–1376.
31. A. E. Kerdok, M. P. Ottensmeyer and R. D. Howe, *J. Biomech.* in press (2006).
32. R. Alterovitz, J. Pouliot, R. Taschereau, I.-C. J. Hsu and K. Goldberg, *Proc. MMVR 11* (2003) 19–25.
33. O. Goksel, S. E. Salcudean, S. P. DiMaio, R. Rohling and J. Morris, *Lect. Notes Comput. Sci.* **3749** (2005) 827–834.
34. Family of Multilevel Partitioning Algorithms, http://www-users.cs.umn.edu/˜karypis/metis/.
35. The Adaptive Communication Environment, http://www.cs.wustl.edu/s̆chmidt/ACE.html.
36. C. Simo, Parallélisation d'un simulateur pour déformation de tissus mous, Master's thesis, Laval University, 2005
37. http://www.nlm.nih.gov/research/visible/visible_gallery.html.

# CHAPTER 3

# A SURVEY OF BIOMECHANICAL MODELING OF THE BRAIN FOR INTRA-SURGICAL DISPLACEMENT ESTIMATION AND MEDICAL SIMULATION

M. A. AUDETTE

*Innovation Center Computer Assisted Surgery — ICCAS, Leipzig*
*michel.audette@medizin.uni-leipzig.de*

M. MIGA

*Dept. Biomedical Engineering, Vanderbilt University*

J. NEMES

*Dept. Mechanical Engineering, McGill University*

K. CHINZEI

*Advanced Inst. for Science & Technology — AIST, Japan*

T. M. PETERS

*Imaging Research Laboratories*
*Robarts Research Inst., Univ. of Western Ontario*

Biomechanical modeling of human and animal brain tissue is a growing field of research, whose applications currently include simulating, with a view to minimizing, head injuries in car impacts, generically modeling dynamic behavior in the surgical theater, such as brain shift, and increasingly, providing medical experts with clinical tools such as surgical simulators and predictive models for tumour growth. This chapter provides an overview of the literature on the biomechanics of the brain, with a particular emphasis on applications to intrasurgical brain shift estimation and to surgical simulation. Included is a discussion of the underlying continua, of numerical estimation techniques, and of related cutting and resection models.

*Keywords*: Surgical simulation; image-guided neurosurgery; rheology; mass-spring systems; finite elements; viscoelasticity; poroelasticity; mixture models; cutting; haptics; meshing.

## 1. Introduction

Biomechanical modeling of human and animal brain tissue is a growing field of research, the applications of which currently include simulating, with a view to minimizing head injuries in car impacts,[85] generically modeling dynamic behavior in the surgical theater, such as brain shift,[73] and increasingly, providing medical experts with clinical tools such as surgical simulators[29] and predictive models for tumour growth.[38,81] Another clinical application currently being investigated is the compensation of a 3D patient-specific graphical model, used in image guidance, for intrasurgical brain shift,[22,50] in a manner that integrates quantitative displacement information provided in the OR by a range sensor or by a hand-held locating device.

The requirements of surgical simulation and intrasurgical deformation estimation for image guidance are a trade-off between computational efficiency and realism, due to the need of the former to provide a response to a virtual surgical intervention that is representative of human tissue in terms of continuity and motion amplitude, and of the latter to give the surgeon precise volumetric displacement information on demand, within a short time frame deemed tolerable in a surgical context. However, in the case of simulation, this trade-off favors efficient computation, i.e. update rates in excess of 100 Hz, possibly reaching 1000 Hz,[14] particularly if haptic feedback is involved. In contrast, image guidance will tolerate somewhat larger computation times if a high degree of realism, such as quantitatively predicting material behavior to sub-mm resolution, can be achieved.

The focus of this chapter is to review the important contributions to biomechanical modeling of healthy and pathological brain tissue, as well as general techniques applicable to simulation and accurate image guidance of brain surgery, such as numerical efficiencies and the modeling of surgical cutting and resection.

## 2. Preliminaries

### 2.1. *Biomechanics*

Biomechanics[23] is the study of the mechanics of living tissue, particularly from a continuum mechanics[43] perspective. The latter is the branch of mechanics concerned with external loading forces in solids and liquids, with the resulting deformation or flow of these materials, and the state of internal traction, or *stress*, inherent in these materials. The deformation of a solid is referred to as *strain*.[43]

The dynamic behavior of an individual material or tissue is characterized in a manner relating stress to strain by its constitutive equations. These are relevant to characterizing the dynamics of the brain because the latter's equations of motion involve both stress and strain, but cannot be solved without expressing the unknown stress tensor field as a function of the strain tensor field, which can be estimated from known displacements. Generally, the relation between stress and strain is not closed-form, and its analysis benefits from some formulations of idealized material response.

Furthermore, biomechanical modeling of the brain is often approached by finding a numerical solution for the displacements, deformations, stresses, and forces, as well as possibly other states, such as hydrostatic pressure, in relation to a history of "loading." The approaches for estimating or simulating biomechanical deformations are characterized by a trade-off between computational efficiency and material fidelity, and the nature of this trade-off can be viewed as a spectrum

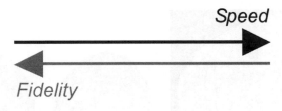

Fig. 1. Illustration of trade-off between computational efficiency and material fidelity.

between two poles, as illustrated by Fig. 1. At the fast but materially approximative end of the spectrum lies mass-spring systems. At the other end of the spectrum, computationally slow but more descriptive, we have classical finite elements (FEs), which can characterize even large (finite) deformations and non-linear elasticity. As shall be seen, there are intermediate solutions between the latter model and classical FEs, which lie between these two poles in the speed/fidelity spectrum.

A mass-spring system[83] is an approximation of a biomechanical system as a collection of point masses connected by elastic springs, and is derived from the field of computer animation. The parameters available to determine the biomechanical behavior are the mass values and the visco-elastic spring characteristics.

FE modeling[8,88] has become the standard method for quantitatively analyzing a wide variety of engineering problems, typically of a mechanical or electromagnetic nature, and in particular for material deformation. The analysis of material deformation is based on expressing equations that characterize the mechanical equilibrium and that must be satisfied everywhere in the system under investigation. An exact solution would require force and momentum equilibrium at all times everywhere in the body, but the FE method replaces this requirement with the weaker one that equilibrium must be maintained in an average sense over a finite number of divisions, elements, of the volume of the body.

The actual division of complex geometries into simple shapes, such as tetrahedra and hexahedra, corresponds to the *meshing* problem.[64] It is illustrated in Fig. 2 that features meshes developed by Zhou[86] and Kleiven,[37] and is still an active research area. Interested readers can refer to some useful web pages.[46,64]

### 2.1.1. *Elastic solid models*

The simplest idealized solid is the Hookean solid, which is characterized by a linear elastic response. For a cylindrical bar subject to a tensile or compressive stress $\sigma$ in its axial direction, the resulting strain $\epsilon$ is given by $\sigma = E\epsilon$, where $E$ is Young's modulus and is a characteristic of the material. This relationship can also be stated in terms of a compliance $J$: $\epsilon = J\sigma$. Furthermore, intuitively one would

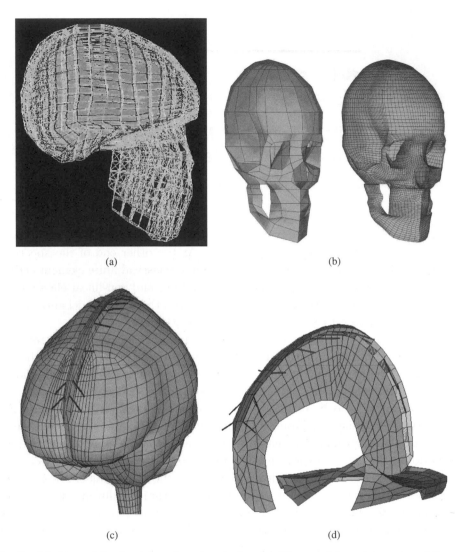

Fig. 2. Meshing of the head based on hexahedra: (a) Zhou model used in automobile crash studies; (b)–(d) recent model developed by Kleiven, featuring meshing of (b) cranial bone (at two resolutions), (c) brain tissue, and (d) falx tentorium.

expect this cylinder to undergo a decrease or increase in its diameter, respectively. Indeed, the ratio of radial strain $\epsilon_d$ to axial strain $\epsilon_a$ is given by Poisson's ratio: $\nu = -\frac{\epsilon_d}{\epsilon_a}$ and is also a characteristic of the material. In 3D, an elastic material is characterized by the stress tensor $\boldsymbol{\sigma}$ that is linearly proportional to the strain tensor $\boldsymbol{\epsilon}$:

$$\boldsymbol{\sigma} = \mathcal{C}\boldsymbol{\epsilon} \text{ or } \sigma_{ij} = C_{ijkl}\epsilon_{kl} \quad \text{and} \quad \boldsymbol{\epsilon} = \mathcal{S}\boldsymbol{\sigma} \text{ or } \epsilon_{ij} = S_{ijkl}\sigma_{kl}, \tag{1}$$

where $\mathcal{C} = [C_{ijkl}]$ and $\mathcal{S} = [S_{ijkl}]$ are fourth order tensors ($3^4 = 81$ components) of elastic moduli and compliance, respectively, and where the Einstein summation convention is used.[a]

If we assume small displacement gradients and neglect rigid motion, $\epsilon$ and $\sigma$ can be referred to *current* coordinates $x_i$, $i = 1, 2, 3$, and are *Cauchy stress* and *small strain*, respectively. Expression (1) simplifies considerably under assumptions of elastic and symmetry and isotropy, namely:

$$C_{ijkl} = \lambda \delta_{ij} \delta_{kl} + \mu \left( \delta_{ik} \delta_{jl} + \delta_{il} \delta_{jk} \right) , \tag{2}$$

where $\lambda$ and $\mu$ are Lamé's elastic constants and $\delta$ is the Kronecker delta.[b,43] These are related to Young's and Shear moduli $E$ and $G$, and to Poisson's ratio $\nu$ as follows:

$$\mu = G = \frac{E}{2(1+\nu)} \quad \text{and} \quad \lambda = \frac{\nu E}{(1+\nu)(1-2\nu)}, \tag{3}$$

whereby the isotropic Hookes law is a system of six equations of the stress components $\sigma_x\, \sigma_y\, \sigma_z\, \tau_{xy}\, \tau_{yz}\, \tau_{zx}$ expressed as follows:

$$
\begin{aligned}
\epsilon_x &= \frac{1}{E}[\sigma_x - \nu(\sigma_y + \sigma_z)] & \gamma_{yz} &= \frac{1}{G_{yz}}\tau_{yz} \\
\epsilon_y &= \frac{1}{E}[\sigma_y - \nu(\sigma_z + \sigma_x)] & \gamma_{zx} &= \frac{1}{G_{zx}}\tau_{zx} . \\
\epsilon_z &= \frac{1}{E}[\sigma_z - \nu(\sigma_x + \sigma_y)] & \gamma_{xy} &= \frac{1}{G_{xy}}\tau_{xy}
\end{aligned}
\tag{4}
$$

For a large, or *finite*, deformation assumption, the generalized Hookes law is expressed as

$$\tilde{\boldsymbol{T}} = \boldsymbol{C}\boldsymbol{E} \quad \text{or} \quad \tilde{T}_{IJ} = C_{IJKL}E_{KL} , \tag{5}$$

where $\tilde{\boldsymbol{T}}$ and $\boldsymbol{E}$ are referred to as *material* coordinates $X_I$, $I = 1, 2, 3$, associated with the initial (natural) state of the material, and are the *second Piola–Kirchoff stress* and *Lagrangian finite strain* tensors, respectively.[43] An illustration of these coordinates appears in Fig. 3. Here $\boldsymbol{C}$ is the Right Cauchy–Green strain tensor defined as $\boldsymbol{C} = \boldsymbol{F}^T\boldsymbol{F}$, where $\boldsymbol{F}$ is the *deformation gradient* tensor. In turn, we define

$$d\boldsymbol{x} = \boldsymbol{F} \cdot d\boldsymbol{X} \quad \text{or} F_{kM} = \frac{\partial x_k}{\partial X_M} . \tag{6}$$

It is important to note that stress and strain must be defined with respect to the same configuration, initial or current; i.e. that they are *work-conjugate*.

---

[a]Indices that are repeated on either side of the equal sign, in this case $k$ and $l$, indicate summations over these indices. This convention is maintained throughout the text.
[b]$\delta_{pq} = 1$ if $p = q$, and 0 if $p \neq q$.

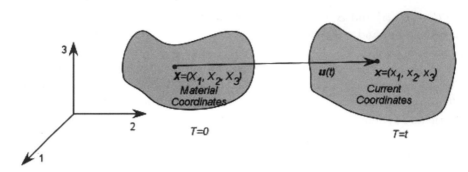

Fig. 3. Illustration of an evolving body, with material and current (or spatial) coordinates associated with it.

Motivation for adopting large deformation and non-linearly elastic assumptions can be seen in the work of Miller[57] and Tendick[84] with their respective collaborators. First, deformations involved in surgery can exceed the small scale assumed in linear elasticity. Second, the motion involved may feature a rigid-body component that may be indistinguishable from the deformation, unless the continuum mechanics preserve material frame-indifference. However, in contrast with the small-strain case, where the displacement gradient $\frac{\partial u_i}{\partial x_j}$ decomposes additively into a sum of a pure strain and a pure rotation,[43] for a large deformation the deformation gradient decomposes into a product of two tensors, according to the *Polar Decomposition Theorem*. The first tensor represents *rigid body rotation* $\boldsymbol{R}$ while the other represents right or left *stretch* $\boldsymbol{U}$ or $\boldsymbol{V}$:

$$\boldsymbol{F} = \boldsymbol{R} \cdot \boldsymbol{U} = \boldsymbol{V} \cdot \boldsymbol{R} \ . \tag{7}$$

The Polar Decomposition Theorem is generally exploited in large deformation FE modeling, by numerically implementing frame-indifferent tensor analysis based on quantities invariant to rigid-body motion. Moreover, research has also emphasized material non-linearity, and these models are described in Sec. 3.1.

### 2.1.2. *Fluid models*

A simple fluid idealization that is relevant to modeling the fluid constituent of brain tissue is the Newtonian fluid. Fluid at rest or in uniform flow cannot sustain a shear stress, so that the shear (off-diagonal) components of stress are null. Moreover, stress in this case is assumed hydrostatic (its principal stresses are equal): $\sigma_{ij} = -p\delta_{ij}$. In a deforming fluid, the total stress includes a viscosity component that is a function of the rate-of-deformation tensor $\mathbf{D}$: $\boldsymbol{\sigma} = -p\mathbf{I} + \mathcal{F}(\mathbf{D})$. If $\mathcal{F}$ is assumed linear, i.e.

$$\sigma_{ij} = -p\delta_{ij} + C_{ijkl} D_{kl} \ , \tag{8}$$

the fluid is called Newtonian. Under assumptions of symmetry and isotropy, the viscosity tensor $[C_{ijkl}]$ also simplifies in the same manner as Eq. (2), where this time $\lambda$ and $\mu$ are two independent parameters of viscosity. Also, if the shear terms are deemed negligible, the deforming fluid is called inviscid.

## 2.2. *Numerical estimation*

### 2.2.1. *Finite element modeling*

The displacement FE method numerically solves for unknown displacements, deformations, stresses, forces, and possibly other variables of a solid body. An exact solution would require force and momentum equilibrium at all times everywhere in the body,

$$\int_S \mathbf{t}dS + \int_V \mathbf{f}dV = 0 \int_S (\mathbf{x} \times \mathbf{t})\,dS + \int_V (\mathbf{x} \times \mathbf{f})\,dV = 0, \tag{9}$$

but the FE method replaces this requirement with a weaker one that equilibrium must be maintained in an average sense over a finite number of divisions of the volume of the body. These divisions, or *elements*, are simple shapes such as triangles and rectangles for surfaces, and tetrahedra and hexahedra for volumes, and the method relies on estimating the displacement at their vertices, or *nodes*. The application of the equilibrium equations to numerical analysis is based on using Gauss' theorem to restate the equilibrium conditions as a single integral, called the *Principle of Virtual Work*.

The volume that is modeled is defined as $\Omega$ and is subject to boundary conditions. Assuming Cartesian coordinates, and adopting the nomenclature of Ref. 88, the displacement at the node $i$ of a given element is labeled $\mathbf{a}_i = [u_i \ v_i \ w_i]^T$, while the displacement at any point in $\Omega$ is expressed $\mathbf{u} = [u(x, y, z) \ v(x, y, z) \ w(x, y, z)]^T$. The latter is fully determined by the nodal displacements and by the *shape functions* that govern the interpolation between them. For a tetrahedral element, we have:

$$\mathbf{u} = [(\mathbf{I}N_i)\ (\mathbf{I}N_j)\ (\mathbf{I}N_m)\ (\mathbf{I}N_p)]\mathbf{a}^e \equiv \mathbf{N}\mathbf{a}^e, \tag{10}$$

where $N_i = 1$ at node $(x_i, y_i, z_i)$ but zero elsewhere, and so on, and where $\mathbf{a}^e_{12 \times 1} = [\mathbf{a}_i \ \mathbf{a}_j \ \mathbf{a}_p \ \mathbf{a}_p]^T$ is comprised of all nodal displacements within a given tetrahedral element. For a small strain assumption, the relationship between strain and nodal displacement is a simple one:

$$\epsilon = \begin{bmatrix} \epsilon_x \\ \epsilon_y \\ \epsilon_z \\ \gamma_{xy} \\ \gamma_{yz} \\ \gamma_{xz} \end{bmatrix} \equiv \begin{bmatrix} \frac{\partial u}{\partial x} \\ \frac{\partial v}{\partial y} \\ \frac{\partial w}{\partial z} \\ \frac{\partial u}{\partial y} + \frac{\partial v}{\partial x} \\ \frac{\partial v}{\partial z} + \frac{\partial w}{\partial y} \\ \frac{\partial w}{\partial x} + \frac{\partial u}{\partial z} \end{bmatrix} = \mathbf{B}\mathbf{a}^e \equiv [\mathbf{B}_i \ \mathbf{B}_j \ \mathbf{B}_m \ \mathbf{B}_p]\mathbf{a}^e, \tag{11}$$

where for example $\mathbf{B}_i$ is obtained by deriving $\mathbf{I}N_i$ appropriately. The Virtual Work Principle states that for a virtual displacement $\delta\mathbf{a}^e$ applied to the system, static equilibrium requires that the external virtual work must equal the internal work done within the element. Defining *nodal forces* $\mathbf{q}^e$ that are statically equivalent to boundary stresses and body forces comprising boundary conditions, and $\mathbf{b}$ the concentrated loads acting on the body, the Virtual Work Principle is expressed for an infinitesimal volume:

$$\delta\mathbf{a}^{eT}\mathbf{q}^e = \delta\boldsymbol{\epsilon} : \boldsymbol{\sigma} - \delta\mathbf{u}^T\mathbf{b}. \tag{12}$$

This expression is integrated with respect to volume, while also substituting for $\delta\boldsymbol{\epsilon}$ and $\delta\mathbf{u}$:

$$\delta\mathbf{a}^{eT}\mathbf{q}^e = \delta\mathbf{a}^{eT}\left(\int_{V^e}\mathbf{B}^T\boldsymbol{\sigma} - \mathbf{N}^T\mathbf{b}\right)dV. \tag{13}$$

Finally, $\boldsymbol{\sigma}(\mathbf{a}^e, \mathbf{B}, \boldsymbol{\sigma}_0)$ is estimated according to the constitutive properties of the assumed continuum. For a linearly and isotropically elastic solid,[43] whose constitutive properties $\mathcal{C}$ simplify to a matrix $\mathbf{D}(\lambda, \mu)$, and after some manipulation,[88] we have

$$\mathbf{q}^e = \mathbf{K}^e\mathbf{a}^e + \mathbf{f}^e, \text{ where } \mathbf{K}^e = \int_{V^e}\mathbf{B}^T\mathbf{D}\mathbf{B}dV \text{ and}$$

$$\mathbf{f}^e = -\int_{V^e}\mathbf{N}^T\mathbf{b}dV - \int_{V^e}\mathbf{B}^T\mathbf{D}\boldsymbol{\epsilon}_0 dV + \int_{V^e}\mathbf{B}^T\boldsymbol{\sigma}_0 dV. \tag{14}$$

Summing the elemental stiffness matrices and forces we obtain:

$$\mathbf{K}\mathbf{a} = \mathbf{f}. \tag{15}$$

The matrix $\mathbf{K}$ is called the *stiffness matrix*, and has a sparse structure. The unique solution of expression (15) requires one or more boundary conditions, which modify the stiffness matrix and make it non-singular. For some dynamic systems, this equation may be modified to further include *mass* ($\mathbf{M}$) and *damping* ($\mathbf{C}$) effects:

$$\mathbf{M}\ddot{\mathbf{a}} + \mathbf{C}\dot{\mathbf{a}} + \mathbf{K}\mathbf{a} = \mathbf{f}. \tag{16}$$

The Principle of Virtual Work can be seen as equating internal deformation energy with external energy generated by external forces over a domain $\Omega$[84,88]:

$$\int_{\Omega^e}\delta U d\Omega = \int_{\Omega^e}\mathbf{f}^T\delta\mathbf{u}d\Omega, \tag{17}$$

where $\delta$ indicates the *variation* of a quantity. For material non-linearity and large geometric deformation, it is natural to solve FEs expressed in terms of a *Strain Energy Density* (SED) function $U$, which is a material-related function of *invariants* of the Cauchy–Green deformation tensor $\mathbf{C}$. Various SED functions are reviewed in more detail in Sec. 3.1.

### 2.2.2. Toward constitutively realistic surgical simulation: Multi-rate FE and other efficiencies

In a brain shift estimation context, we are interested in the collection of nodal displacements $a_i$ that solve expression (15). The application of FE methods to intrasurgical deformation estimation is discussed in Sec. 3, within a broader survey of FE modeling of the brain. In a surgical simulation context, the concentrated loads term also accounts for user-controlled virtual cutting forces, and the corresponding set of nodal displacements is then found. Haptic feedback to the user can be computed from the surface tractions and body forces on the elements in contact with the surgical tool.

A volumetric, dynamically deformable FE approach was long thought to be too slow for implementing haptic feedback in the context of surgical simulation.[c] Recently however, some researchers have demonstrated practical computational efficiencies for accelerating FE numerical schemes, designed with haptic rate force feedback in mind.

As illustrated in Fig. 4, Astley[3] has demonstrated a multi-scale multi-rate FE software architecture based on a hierarchy of meshes, featuring a *parent* and one or more *child* meshes, which can be updated independently and at different rates. This decoupling is accomplished by representing each system as a simple equivalent, inspired from the Norton and Thevenin equivalents of electronic circuit analysis, within each other's stiffness matrix. Each child mesh can be dense and in theory non-linearly elastic (although the concept was demonstrated only with

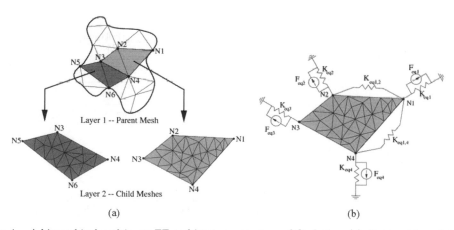

(a)                                             (b)

Fig. 4.   A hierarchical multi-rate FE architecture, courtesy of O. Astley: (a) division of mesh into parent and child elastic subsystems; (b) use of Thevenin-like equivalents to model parent and child 1 subsystems, as seen by child mesh 2.

[c]In contrast to FE methods reliant on extensive precomputation,[9,13] which may preclude changes in volumetric topology.

linear elasticity) and is restricted to a small volume relevant to haptic and visual interaction, while maintaining the parent mesh linearly elastic and relatively sparse.

Çavuşoğlu and Tendick[15] also proposed a method for multi-rate FE computation, capable of different update rates for the physical model and for haptic feedback. The haptic-rate force command is achieved by *model reduction* based on systems theory. The haptic rendering problem is analogous to interpolating a simple one-dimensional 10 Hz signal at 1000 Hz, illustrated in Figs. 5 and 6. In an ideal case, it would be possible to update the physical model at the haptic rate, coinciding with Fig. 5(a) and the solid line in Fig. 6: $force_1(n) = f(x[n])$. However, current computing capabalities preclude this possibility. In the simplest force model, seen in Fig. 5(b) and the dash-dot line in Fig. 6, 1000 Hz force can be generated from the 10 Hz model by maintaining the former constant between samples of the latter: $force_2(n) = f(x[N])$. The next model applies a force that is a low-pass filtered version of the piecewise constant one, whose output is sampled at 1000 Hz: $force_3(n) = f(x[N]) * lpf[n]$. In the last model, force at every time sample $n$ is computed from a *linearization* of the non-linear physical model, based on its tangent

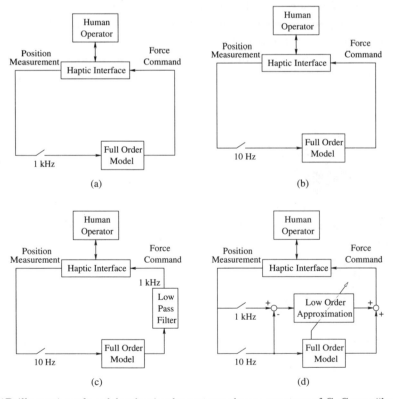

Fig. 5.   1D illustration of model reduction by systems theory, courtesy of C. Çavuşoğlu: (a) ideal case; (b) constant force model; (c) low-pass filtered model; (d) tangent model based on linearization of physical model.

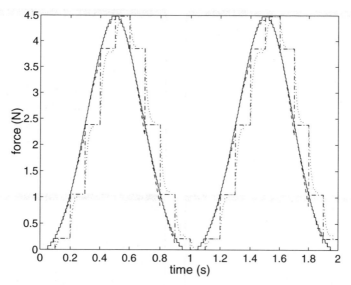

Fig. 6.  1D time samples of four models, courtesy of C. Çavuşoğlu. Solid line: ideal case; dash-dot line: constant force model; dotted line: low-pass model; dashed line: tangent model.

value at its last update: $force_4(n) = f(x[N]) + f'(x[N])[x(n) - x(N)]$. This model coincides with the situation in Fig. 5(d) and the dashed line in Fig. 6, which is almost indistinguishable from the solid line. The authors then describe how to achieve a *low-order linear model*, for haptic rendering, from non-linear FE mesh systems, as well as analyze the stability of their method.

Wu and Tendick propose *multigrid* (MG) FE approach for efficiently and stably resolving geometrically and materially non-linear model,[85] in conjunction with non-linear FE model of Ref. 84, and as illustrated in Figs. 7 and 8. They argue for using a MG framework to divide-and-conquer to efficiently resolve large displacements and non-linear material models, propagating a solution from coarse to progressively finer meshes. Moreover, the MG framework is seen as applying divide-and-conquer in the frequency domain, where the residual error at a given resolution influences processes at nearby frequencies. MG methods use three operators in solving for $X$ a problem of the type $T(X) = b$. The smoothing operator $G()$ takes a problem and its approximated solution $X(i)$, where $i$ is an index indicating the grid level, and computes an improved $X(i)$ using a one-level iterative solver. This smoothing is performed on all but the coarsest mesh. The restriction operator $R()$ takes the residual of $T(X(i)) - b(i)$, and maps it to $b(i + 1)$ on coarser level $i + 1$. The interpolation operator $P()$ projects the correction to an approximate solution $X(i)$ on the next finer mesh. One of the important implementation issues with this method is determining the spatial correspondence between grids of different resolutions. The multigrid algorithm is described as advantageous in stability and convergence over single level explicit integration, and provides real-time performance.

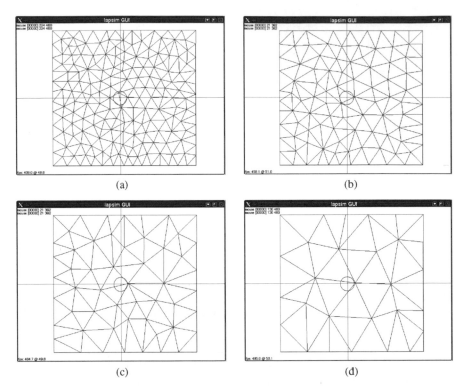

Fig. 7.    Illustration of Wu multi-grid implementation, from finest (a) to coarsest (d).

Basdogan[7] has proposed two efficiencies for the dynamic FE equilibrium
equations contained in expression (16): first, a *modal transformation and reduction*,
as suggested by Pentland[67] in the context of active surface models, and last,
a new technique called the *Spectral Lanczos Decomposition* method, based on the
re-arrangement and the Laplace transformation of expression (16). Berkley[9] has
investigated the effects of permuting the stiffness matrix to make it narrowly banded
and prioritizing the rows of expression (15), according to the importance of the node:
boundary condition, visible, interior, or contact node. Bro-Nielsen and Cotin[13] have
also considered a new partition of the FE system equation, on the basis of surface
and interior nodes, and have proposed a method that inverts the stiffness matrix in a
precomputated manner. However, the complexity of stiffness matrix processing may
limit the applicability of these techniques, given that surgically induced changes in
topology would impose a sequence of new stiffness matrices over time.

### 2.2.3. *Mass-spring and mass-tensor systems*

A mass-spring system is characterized by each node $i$, having a mass $m_i$ and position
$\mathbf{x}_i$, and being imbedded in a mesh where each edge coincides with a spring $k$. Each

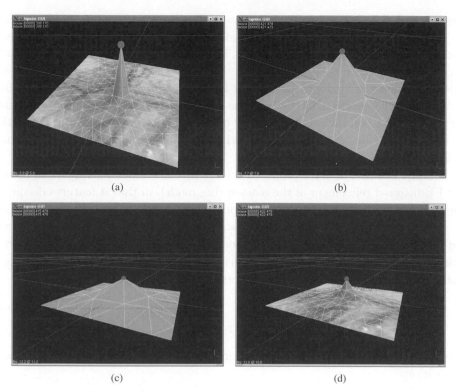

Fig. 8.  Interactive non-linearly elastic modeling through multi-grid methods. (a) Initial lifting of node in dense mesh, in response to grabbing node, with neighboring elements undergoing very large deformation. (b) Displacement restricted onto coarse mesh, with distortion distributed over a larger region due to larger elements. (c) Redistribution of stress over coarse mesh. (d) Spreading of deformation from coarse to fine mesh.

node is subject to an equation of the form[83]:

$$m_i \frac{d^2\mathbf{x}_i}{dt^2} + \gamma_i \frac{d\mathbf{x}_i}{dt} + \mathbf{g}_i = \mathbf{f}_i \quad i = 1, \ldots, N, \text{ where} \tag{18}$$

$$\mathbf{g}_i(t) = \sum_{j \varepsilon \mathcal{N}_i} \mathbf{s}_k, \quad \text{where } \mathbf{s}_k = \frac{c_k e_k}{\|\mathbf{r}_k\|} \mathbf{r}_k. \tag{19}$$

In this equation, $\mathbf{s}_k$ represents the force on the $k$th spring linking the node $i$ to a neighboring node $j$. This force is a function of the vector separation of the nodes $\mathbf{r}_k = \mathbf{x}_j - \mathbf{x}_i$, of the deformation of the spring $e_k = \|\mathbf{r}_k\| - l_k$, and of the characteristics of the spring: its natural length $l_k$, its stiffness $c_k$, and its velocity-dependent damping $\gamma_i$. The quantity $\mathbf{f}_i$ is the net external force acting on node $i$, which may include a surgical tool or the effect of gravity.

In general, mass-spring systems are used mainly for surgical simulation,[17,60] and somewhat less for estimating brain shift, with the possible exceptions of Edwards[20] and of Škrinjar,[75] because of the difficulty in making spring constants conform to the measured properties of elastic anatomical tissues and the criticality of accurate constitutive modeling in the OR. Their use in surgical simulation involves modeling the effect of surgical forces $\mathbf{f}_i$ in expression (18) by integrating the equations of motion forward through simulated time. The sum of spring forces $\mathbf{g}_i$ on the nodes in contact with the virtual tool, can then provide the user with a sense of tissue resistance. Škrinjar[75] adopted a method based on the Kelvin viscoelastic spring–dashpot model (see Sec. 3.1.1.), where the spring force expression (19) also features a term dependent on the relative velocity between nodes $i$ and $j$. Edwards[20] further incorporated terms that promote material incompressibility and inhibit surface folding in the deformation computation.

Finally, Cotin et al. have proposed the mass-tensor model,[17] which can be seen as a FE-inspired refinement of the mass-spring model, in that it features decoupled computation for individual tetrahedra comprising a mesh, but estimates the force on each vertex from a linear *tetrahedral stiffness* matrix $\mathbf{K}$, as well as from current and initial vertex positions $\mathbf{p}_i$ and $\mathbf{p}_i^0$. For a given vertex at $\mathbf{p}_i$, the elastic force $\mathbf{f}_i$ acting on it is the sum of contributions from adjacent tetrahedra, where adjacency is stored in a data structure and can be updated as the topology evolves:

$$\mathbf{f}_i = \mathbf{K}_{ii}\mathbf{p}_i^0\mathbf{p}_i + \sum_{j\varepsilon N(\mathbf{p}_i)} \mathbf{K}_{ij}\mathbf{p}_j^0\mathbf{p}_j. \qquad (20)$$

This method has been extended by Picinbono et al.[68] for anisotropically elastic applications.

## 2.3. Cutting models

An important complement to biomechanical tissue modeling for surgical simulation applications is a model that formally represents the effect of cutting forces, as they relate to changes in tissue shape and to haptic feedback to the user. The application of cutting models to intrasurgical brain motion estimation is perhaps less obvious, given the difficulty of estimating the amount and distribution of resected tissue.[73] However, were such quantitative information available, the consideration of cutting forces would clearly complement intrasurgical body forces (gravity, intrasurgically administered drugs, etc.[32,44]) currently accounted for in published brain models.

Contributions to the modeling of surgical resection are mostly qualitative, emphasizing topological changes to meshes as well as heuristics for synthesizing forces to the user, rather than based on formal *fracture mechanics* analysis.[2] Neumann[60] proposed a simple, highly efficient implementation of several types of tools used in ophthalmic surgery, in conjunction with a mass-spring representation of an eye. These tools included a pick for elevating tissue, a cutting blade, a drainage needle, a laser used to seal tissues, and a suction instrument. Basdogan et al.[6] modeled the collision detection of a cutting tool as a line segment indenting a polygon, and simulated a spring damping force proportional to the velocity of the tool. Bielser and Gross[10] performed a thorough investigation of the topological effect of a cutting tool on a tetrahedral volume element. They proposed five subdivision patterns for their cutting algorithm, corresponding to completely or partially split tetrahedra, and suggested collision detection strategies. They also offered a haptic scalpel model, interacting with mass-springs system and featuring a cutting force that is decomposed into components in the plane of the blade and normal to this plane.

Clearly, research of this kind is invaluable for the accurate simulation and haptic rendering of surgical tools, and will have an important impact on the realism of surgical simulation in the future, particularly as quantitative *fracture mechanics* analysis is incorporated. In that vein, Greenish and Hayward[27] investigated with animal experiments the cutting forces of surgical instruments, the work which was subsequently refined in Ref. 16. Also, as illustrated in Fig. 9, Malvash and Hayward[41,42] proposed a fracture mechanics model that expressed cutting as a sequence of three modes of interaction between the surgical tool and the body: *deformation, cutting,* and *rupture.* Deformation states 1 and 2, in the absence and in the presence of a crack, respectively, feature a curve with reversible work done *fracture toughness* of a material. The cutting mode curve illustrates a tool applying a load initially beyond $J_c$, undergoing a displacement, and doing irreversible work. Finally, the rupture mode is characterized by a load large enough to cause fracture, prior to any displacement beyond the rupture point $\delta_r$ and may serve as a transition between deformation and cutting. Finally, O'Brien *et al.* have proposed efficient fracture mechanics models of both *brittle*[61] and *ductile*[62] materials for computer graphics applications, which could also be transposed to surgery simulation. In

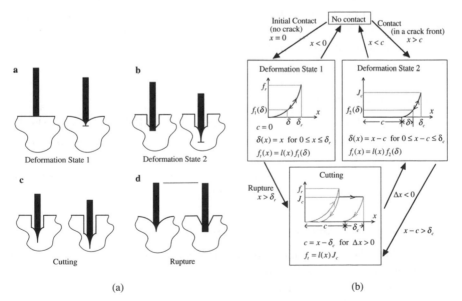

Fig. 9. Cutting model proposed by Mahvash and Hayward. (a) Illustration of tool–body interaction modes; (b) Possible sequences of interaction modes. Reproduced with permission.

brittle fracture, no plastic deformation occurs prior to fracture, so that if the fractured pieces are glued back together, the original shape can be reconstituted. In contrast, ductile fracture is characterized by substantial plastic deformation taking place. How to best apply these abstractions to biological materials still remains an open question.

## 3. Finite Element Modeling of the Brain

There exist three categories of brain FE models, in terms of the types of loads simulated:

- those that view the brain under *impacts*, typically caused by auto collisions[35,70,81,85];
- those that model the effect of *pathologies*[38,60,82];
- and recently, those that model *surgical loads*.[51,57,75]

Brain models can also be classified according to the nature of their underlying idealized material or *continuum*, which may consider brain tissue either as

- a strictly *visco- or hyper-elastic solid*, or
- as a *hybrid of elastic solid and inviscid fluid constituents* (poro-elastic or biphasic).

There is a correlation between these categorizations: most impact collision models view brain matter as a simple elastic solid, whereas tumor growth models account not only for solid and fluid constituents, but possibly for biological and biochemical factors as well, modeled as pseudo-forces,[82] and finally surgical models of both solid[56,74,84] and solid–liquid hybrid[1,50,76] types exist.

### 3.1. *Solid brain models*

This section provides an overview of solid continua and FE models of the brain, tracing their history from early impact response research, through *rheological* studies characterizing constitutive properties by experiments featuring the compression and stretching of animal brain tissue, to recent physical models better adapted for resolving surgically induced displacements.

#### 3.1.1. *Non-linear solid continua: Hyper-elastic and Viscoelastic solids*

Beyond the *linearly elastic* solid, two other idealized solids are commonly found in the literature: *hyper-elastic* and *viscoelastic* solids. Elasticity theory posits that a deformation is thermodynamically *reversible* provided that it occurs at an infinitesimal speed, where thermodynamic equilibrium is maintained at every instant.[40] At finite velocities, the body is not always in equilibrium, processes will take place that return it to equilibrium, and these processes imply that the motion is irreversible and that mechanical energy is dissipated into heat. Hyper-elasticity ignores these thermal effects: work done in hyper-elastic deformation is assumed stored and available for reversing the deformation, while viscoelasticity makes no such assumption.

A hyper-elastic material is also characterized by a *strain-energy function U* (or *elastic potential function*, also denoted $W$), which is a scalar function of one of the strain or deformation tensors, whose derivative with respect to deformation determines the corresponding stress component:

$$\sigma_{ij} = \frac{\partial U(\epsilon)}{\partial \epsilon_{ij}}, \tag{21}$$

where $[\sigma_{ij}]$ and $[\epsilon_{ij}]$ are work-conjugate stress and strain measures. Hyper-elasticity is based on the assumption that the elastic potential always exists as a function of strains alone.[43] One special case of this strain energy function is the Mooney–Rivlin expression for isotropic incompressible material[26]:

$$U = \sum_{i=0}^{N} \sum_{j=0}^{N} C_{ij}(I_1 - 3)^i (I_2 - 3)^j \text{ that, taking } N = 1, \text{ reduces to}$$

$$U = C_{10}(I_1 - 3) + C_{01}(I_2 - 3), \tag{22}$$

where $I_1$ and $I_2$ are the first two of the three *invariants* of the strain tensor:

$$I_1 = \lambda_1^2 + \lambda_2^2 + \lambda_3^2, I_2 = \lambda_1^2 \lambda_2^2 + \lambda_2^2 \lambda_3^2 + \lambda_1^2 \lambda_3^2, \quad \text{and} \quad I_3 = \lambda_1^2 \lambda_2^2 \lambda_3^2, \text{ where} \tag{23}$$

$\lambda_i$ represent the principal stretch ratios of a deformed material (note that $I_3 = 1$ for an incompressible material).

Viscoelasticity is characterized by a relationship between stress and strain that depends on time, and constitutive relations are typically expressed as an integral, i.e.

$$\boldsymbol{\sigma}(t) = \int_0^t C(t - \tau) \frac{d\boldsymbol{\epsilon}(\tau)}{d\tau} d\tau \quad \text{or} \quad \boldsymbol{\epsilon}(t) = \int_0^t S(t - \tau) \frac{d\boldsymbol{\sigma}(\tau)}{d\tau} d\tau. \tag{24}$$

Some phenomena associated with viscoelastic materials include *creep*, whereby strain increases with time under constant stress; *relaxation*, where stress decreases with time under constant strain; and finally, a dependency of the effective stiffness on the rate of application of the load.[39]

Finally, transient creep and relaxation responses can be modeled as exponentials, for example, $J(t) = J_0(1 - e^{-t/\tau_c})$ and $E(t) = E_0 e^{-t/\tau_r}$, respectively. Exponential response functions arise in simple discrete models composed of *springs*, which are perfectly elastic ($\sigma_s = E\epsilon_s$), and *dashpots*, which are perfectly viscous ($\sigma_d = \eta d\epsilon_d/dt$; we can envision a piston whose motion causes a viscous fluid to move through an aperture). Consequently, spring–dashpot models are considered useful idealizations for viscoelastic behavior. The two simplest such models are the

*Maxwell* model, consisting of a spring and a dashpot in *series*, and the *Voigt/Kelvin* model, with the spring and dashpot arranged in *parallel*.[39]

### 3.1.2. *Impact response FE models*

Early (1960s and early 1970s) studies of impact response were formulated as *analytical* continuum models based on spherical, elliptical, and cylindrical idealizations[36]), but this approach was limited in its applicability by the complex shape of the brain.[81] With the advent of the FE method in the 1970s, the skull, brain, and CSF could be divided into small elements, typically hexahedra, tetrahedra, and shells, and complex geometries could be modeled as the sum of simple shapes.

A comparison of early impact FE models in terms of geometry, material characterization, and boundary conditions is featured by Khalil and Viano.[35] Early FE models relied on simple material and kinetic idealizations, viewing the head as an elastic shell, approximating the skull, filled with fluid. These models assume homogeneous, isotropic, and linearly (visco)-elastic material subject to small deformations. Moreover, many of the earliest models were 2D approximations of coronal[34] and mid-sagittal[71] sections, by virtue of the resolution achievable in comparison with a 3D model. Progressively, more descriptive 3D models, most assuming some form of symmetry, appeared in the late 1970s.[33,72,80] Impact models were characterized by a dynamic equation, typically neglecting damping, i.e. $\mathbf{M\ddot{a} + Ka = f}$ that was numerically integrated.

Research in the 1980s and early 1990s was reviewed by Sauren and Claessens.[70] Material properties were still assumed homogeneous and isotropic; linearly elastic constitutive models were used in general, in combination with small-deformation theory. Notable exceptions include Ueno and Mendis,[45] who employed large-deformation theory. Mendis' characterization based on a large deformation assumption first appeared in his PhD thesis, and was later published (Ref. 45). Subsequently, King and his collaborators, in particular Ruan *et al.*[70] and Zhou *et al.*,[86] described a comprehensive 3D approach that was highly detailed anatomically. The Zhou model, illustrated in Fig. 2, emphasized details of gray and white matter and ventricles to match regions of high shear stress to locations of diffuse axonal injury.

### 3.1.3. *Early rheological studies and strain models*

Early investigations into the constitutive properties of brain tissue are attributed to McElhaney and his collaborators.[21,24] Advani[45,65] introduced more descriptive physical models based on a Mooney–Rivlin strain energy function. More recently, Miller and Chinzei[53] have published studies characterizing brain constitutive properties under conditions approximating surgical loads.

Early reviews of rheological studies of animal and human brain tissue appear in Ommaya[63] and in Galford and McElhaney.[24] McElhaney and his collaborators[21,24] did extensive analyses of the stress–strain relation in human and monkey brain tissue, assuming a viscoelastic model. In Ref. 21, Estes and McElhaney noted that under compressive loading at rates $v$ varying between 0.02 ips and 10 ips, the stress–strain curves were concave upward, suggesting that there was no linear portion where a meaningful Young's modulus might be determined. A model of the form

$$ln(\sigma/\dot{\epsilon}) = a + b \ ln(t), \quad \text{where } t = \frac{h - h_0}{v}, \tag{25}$$

where $h$ and $h_0$ were the instantaneous and original height of a given cylindrical sample, better accounted for the strain rate dependency. Galford and McElhaney[24] performed creep compliance tests with human and monkey brains, in order to characterize a four-parameter model featuring Maxwell and Kelvin idealizations in series. The authors also performed tensile creep studies on scalp and dura samples.

Pamidi and Advani[65] modeled the viscoelastic behavior of human brain tissue under a *large-deformation* assumption, by viewing the constitutive properties in terms of a power function $H$ encompassing inertial, restoring, and dissipative forces:

$$\sigma_{ij} = \partial H / \partial \dot{\epsilon}_{ij}, \quad \text{where } H = \dot{U} + D, \tag{26}$$

where $U$ is the familiar Mooney–Rivlin strain energy function in expression (22), $D$ is the Rayleigh dissipation function of the material, and $\dot{\epsilon}_{ij}$ is a component of the *strain rate* tensor $\dot{\epsilon}$. This formulation led to two discrete spring-and-dashpot non-linear characterizations, as well as a continuum model for an *isochoric* (volume-preserving) deformation.

Mendis *et al.*[45] first adopted a purely hyper-elastic model, again characterized by a first order Mooney–Rivlin strain energy function, and proposed a procedure for estimating the coefficients $C_{01}$ and $C_{10}$ in expression (22) for brain tissue, based on the uniaxial compression data of Estes and McElhaney.[21] Mendis then described a large-deformation FE representation of the uniaxial soft tissue specimens used by Estes, and showed a comparison of the empirical stress values in the latter's compression experiment with the stress predicted by the hyper-elastic FE model. Mendis also proposed a viscoelastic characterization of Estes' brain tissue samples based on a strain energy function *dependent on the time history* of the strain invariants, provided in expression (23):

$$U(t) = \int_0^t C_{10}(t - \zeta)\frac{d}{d\zeta}I_1(\zeta) + C_{01}(t - \zeta)\frac{d}{d\zeta}I_2(\zeta)d\zeta, \tag{27}$$

in order to simulate experimental stress responses at four different strain rates.

### 3.1.4. *Rheological studies and FE models for medical applications*

Both Ferrant[22] and Hagemann[28] have proposed small-strain linearly elastic
FE models in research that dealt specifically with non-rigid registration of the
human brain. Ferrant developed automatic image-based meshing algorithms for
tomographic data, and has applied his model to registering pre- and intraoperative
MR volumes. He has indicated that his registration method does not preclude
the use of non-linear constitutive properties. Hagemann validated his model by
registering 2D pre- and postoperative images of the head of a patient.

Miller and Chinzei conducted similar compression studies as Estes and
McElhaney, but with much reduced loading velocities, appropriate for surgery.[54]
The former pointed out that the strain rates investigated by McElhaney and
his collaborators are relevant to injury modeling, but not as appropriate for
characterizing the effects of surgical loads, particularly given the strong rate
dependency of brain constitutive properties that appeared in their own findings.
They presented results of unconfined uniaxial compression tests of cylindrical
brain tissue samples, based on the apparatus illustrated in Fig. 10. This test was
carried out under three different loading velocities: 500 mm/min, 5 mm/min, and
0.005 mm/min, corresponding to strain rates of about $0.64\,\mathrm{s}^{-1}$, $0.64 \times 10^{-2}\,\mathrm{s}^{-1}$, and
$0.64 \times 10^{-5}\,\mathrm{s}^{-1}$, respectively, and Fig. 11 illustrates the rate dependency of brain
constitutive properties.

Miller proposed a "hyper-viscoelastic" model, based on a generalization of the
Mooney–Rivlin strain energy function expressed as an integral, in the same vein as
Mendis',

$$U(t) = \int_0^t \left\{ \sum_{i+j=1}^N C_{ij}(t-\zeta)\frac{d}{d\zeta}\left[(I_1-3)^i(I_2-3)^j\right] \right\} d\zeta, \qquad (28)$$

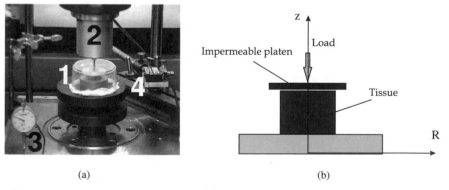

(a)                                                                          (b)

Fig. 10.   Brain tissue rheological studies: (a) illustration of uniaxial compression apparatus;
(b) layout with coordinate axes. Components: 1 — specimen and loading platens; 2 — load cell
to measure axial force; 3 — micrometer to measure axial displacement, and 4 — laser to measure
radial displacement. Courtesy: Karol Miller and Kiyoyuki Chinzei.

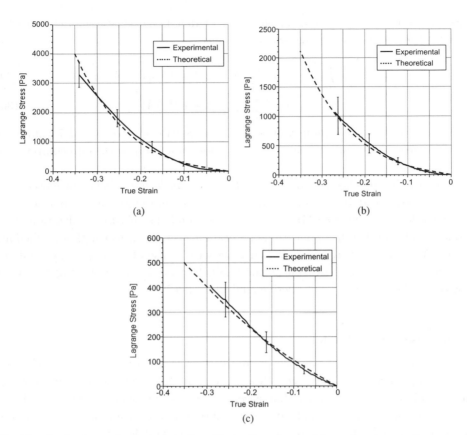

Fig. 11. Brain tissue rheological studies: illustration of uniaxial compression results vs. under three different loading velocities — (a) 500 mm/min; (b) 5 mm/min; (c) 0.005 mm/min. Courtesy: Karol Miller and Kiyoyuki Chinzei.

but he emphasized that a second order characterization was necessary to fully capture the rate-dependent behavior (i.e. $N = 2$). Moreover, their strain-energy function is based on invariants of the left Cauchy–Green deformation tensor. This continuum was subsequently used in a FE implementation[56] using ABAQUS commercial software.[31] In other publications,[52,55] they argued in favor of a purely solid continuum for modeling brain tissue, rather than a hybrid of solid and liquid, on the grounds that the latter does not account for stress–strain rate dependence as well as solid models.

Miller and Chinzei also investigated the material properties of the brain *in extension*,[57] whereby an apparatus similar to that in Fig. 10, but affixed to a tissue cylinder using surgical glue. They came to the conclusion that elastic behavior in extension is significantly different from that in compression, which was not accounted for by any rheological model developed until then. Specifically, energy functions in polynomial form result from the application of even powers of principal stretches $\lambda_1^2$, $\lambda_2^2$, $\lambda_3^2$, etc., which makes no distinction between a positive or negative value. By adopting a generalization of an Ogden hyper-elastic model featuring *unrestricted* (i.e. fractional) powers of stretches,

$$U = \frac{2}{\alpha^2} \int_0^t \left[ \mu(t - \tau) \frac{d}{d\tau} \left( \lambda_1^\alpha + \lambda_1^\alpha + \lambda_1^\alpha \right) d\tau \right], \text{ where} \tag{29}$$

$$\mu = \mu_0 \left[ 1 - \sum_{k=1}^n g_k \left( 1 - e^{-t/\tau_k} \right) \right]. \tag{30}$$

They were able to determine values of $\mu_o = 842\,\text{Pa}$ and $\alpha = -4.7$ that best characterize rate-dependent behavior in a manner consistent with both compression and extension.

Finally, linear elastic models for *tumor growth* have been proposed.[38,82] Kyriacou and Davatzikos[38] simulated the uniform contraction and expansion of a tumor model obtained from MR image data, with a hyper-elastic idealization. This application facilitates the application of a brain atlas to a subject with an imbedded lesion. Wasserman *et al.* incorporated a variety of pseudo-forces to account for biological and chemical, as well as mechanical processes, contributing to tumor growth, in the context of a predictive clinical model.[82]

## 4. Biphasic Brain Models

This section provides an overview of brain models consisting of both solid and liquid components. We first review literature that characterizes the physiology of the cranial cavity in a manner that accounts for its fluid component.[18,30] This is followed by an overview of publications that integrate both components in a hybrid continuum, namely the *poro-elastic*[11,50] and *mixture* models.[1,12,58]

### 4.1. *Biomechanics of the cranial cavity featuring solid and fluid components*

Hakim *et al.*[30] proposed a detailed mechanical interpretation of intracranial anatomy, in a manner that accounted for both solid and fluid components, with an emphasis on describing the phenomenon of hydrocephalus. In particular, the brain parenchyma was described as *submicroscopic sponge of viscoelastic material.* They completed the mechanical picture with a description of the linkage between brain and skull:

> The brain does not rest directly on the inner surfaces of the skull, but is floating within the CSF (that is approximately the same density) and moored in position by the arachnoidal strands that tether the arachnoid membrane to the pia mater.

Hakim also evoked two parallel fluid compartments consisting of the CSF and extracellular spaces of the parenchyma, supplied by separate sources of blood (to the choroid plexuses and directly to the parenchymal tissue), and drained by the intracranial venous system. The CSF is secreted by the choroid plexuses, flows from the lateral ventricles, through the foramens, aqueduct, and subarachnoid spaces, and discharges into the venous system by way of the arachnoidal villi of the superior sagittal sinus. The interaction between the open venous system and the closed CSF system, in particular as it relates to CSF pressure, subdural stress, and ventricular size, was described by rectilinear and spherical models.

Dóczi[18] provided a recent survey of medical literature on volume regulation of brain tissue, in a manner that emphasized fluid distribution as well. In particular, starting from the assumption of incompressibility of the constituents of the skull (blood, CSF, and brain tissue), which implied that their total volume must remain constant, he investigated the enlargement (four- to eight-fold) of hydrocephalic ventricles. Given that the cerebral blood volume and CSF correspond to 50 ml and 100 ml of the available space, he concluded that the brain itself must change in size and described the factors involved in this process.

### 4.2. *Solid–liquid continua: Poro-elastic and mixture continua, with related FE models*

Biot[11] was the first to describe a three-dimensional continuum consisting of porous solid, assumed linearly and isotropically elastic and under small strain, and containing water, assumed incompressible, in its pores. He suggested that such a *consolidation* model, whereby a poro-elastic medium containing an incompressible fluid gradually settling under load, could describe a wet sponge or water-saturated soil. The water in the pores is characterized by $q$ and $p$. The parameter $q$ is the increment of fluid volume per unit of continuum volume. It reflects how saturated the medium is, i.e. if it were unity, the media would be fluid. The parameter $p$ represents the pressure associated with the fluid. Biot modified the 3D Hookean solid model, as appears in expression (4), to account for the fluid pressure term $p$, which after some manipulation[11,50] can be stated simply as the following expression:

$$G\nabla^2\mathbf{u} + \frac{G}{1-2\nu}\nabla\epsilon - \alpha\nabla p = 0 \tag{31}$$

and $\epsilon = \epsilon_x + \epsilon_y + \epsilon_z$ represents the volume increase of the continuum per unit initial volume. This expression represents a system of three equations in four unknowns, $u_1$, $u_2$, $u_3$, and $p$, which requires a fourth equation for its solution. The last equation is derived from the conservation of interstitial fluid mass which, for a constant density incompressible fluid continuum, can be written as,

$$\nabla \cdot \mathbf{v} = 0 \tag{32}$$

where $\mathbf{v}$ is the interstitial fluid flow velocity. Using *Darcy's law*, which governs the flow of fluid in a porous medium, the relationship between flow velocity and interstitial pressure is stated as,

$$\mathbf{v} = -k\nabla p \tag{33}$$

where $k$ is the coefficient of permeability of the porous solid. Substitution (33) into (32), yields the first term in the following expression, and speaks to conservation of interstitial fluid mass,

$$\nabla \cdot (-k\nabla p) = \alpha \frac{\partial \varepsilon}{\partial t} \frac{1}{Q} \frac{\partial p}{\partial t} \tag{34}$$

In (34), the terms on the right-hand-side refer to interaction between fluid and solid matrix. When a porous media is compressed, there is an interaction between the dynamics of interstitial fluid transport and the forces acting on the supportive solid matrix. The transient relationship reflecting the transferal of load between these phases is reflected in the first two terms of (34). Extending further, according to Biot's original theory, while the fluid is assumed incompressible, it is possible to have an unsaturated media, i.e. small gaseous content within pores. While in soft-tissue modeling this term is often neglected, it translates to a net compressibility in the continuum that acts to delay the distribution of pressure. Here, the term $Q$ is a measure of the amount of fluid that can be forced into the porous solid under pressure while the solid matrix is kept constant.

Miga and collaborators solved expression (31) and (33) using the Galerkin Method of Weighted Residuals on spatial domains reflecting porcine and human brains.[47,50] Furthermore, Miga also rigorously investigated the stability of a finite element implementation of the consolidation model and demonstrated a need for fully implicit calculations if using a traditional two-level time stepping scheme.[48] Finally, he has also applied his FE model to characterizing brain shift, on the basis of sparse displacement information,[49] and recently of dense laser-based range data.[51] Figure 12c is an example of a series of brain shift model calculations simulating the effects of gravity-induced deformation. In this case, gravity was acting along the anteroposterior axis and the exposed cortical surface was located at the superior extent. The solutions compare three techniques to use sparse displacement data measured from cortical surface to predict brain shift: (1) modeling changes in buoyancy forces due to cerebrospinal fluid drainage, (2) direct application of cortical shift as displacement boundary conditions, and (3) direct application of cortical shift displacements and subsurface lateral ventricle movement. With each calculation, the cortical surface at the superior extent moved exactly the same but the subsurface displacement field was significantly different. This indicates the importance of understanding how to integrate sparse information appropriately less different subsurface deformation fields may ensue. In more recent reports, Miga and colleagues have developed an integration platform that uses sparse data as acquired by a laser range scanner, pre-computation strategies to improve speed, and linear optimization techniques to correct for brain shift.[19] It should also be noted that this same model has been used to simulate the effects of brain edema and the biomechanics of hydrocephalus.[76,77]

A related but more general continuum, the mixture model, has been developed by Mow et al.[58] and by Bowen et al.,[12] and applied to hydrated soft tissues by

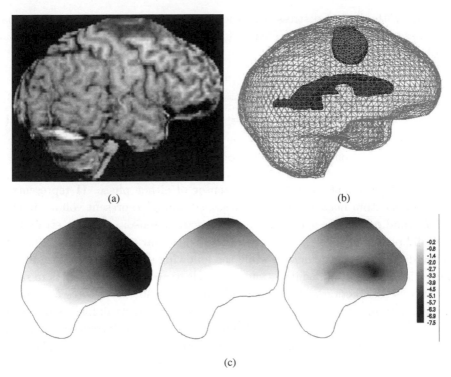

Fig. 12. Poro-elastic model, featuring imbedded tumor, applied to deformation estimation: (a) MR surface rendering of brain and (b) corresponding volumetric mesh; (c) downward displacement map of brain sagittal section, arising from (left) gravity-induced shift, (center) applied surface deformation, and (right) applied surface/ventricle deformations.

Spilker.[76] This model is characterized by each spatial point being simultaneously occupied to some degree by all the constituents comprising the mixture, where the $a$th body is assigned a *reference configuration* $\mathbf{x} = \chi_a(\mathbf{X}_a, t)$. The $a$th constituent is characterized by its *bulk density* $\rho_a(\mathbf{x}, t)$, where $\rho(\mathbf{x}, t) = \sum_{a=1}^{N} \rho_a(\mathbf{x}, t)$, representing the mass of $a$ per unit volume of mixture, and by its *true density* $\gamma_a(\mathbf{x}, t)$ representing the mass of $a$ per unit volume of $a$. The *volume fraction* of the $a$th constituent is given by:

$$\phi_a(\mathbf{x}, t) = \rho_a(\mathbf{x}, t)/\gamma_a(\mathbf{x}, t), \quad \text{where} \quad \sum_{a=1}^{N} \phi_a(\mathbf{x}, t) = 1. \tag{35}$$

Bowen derived equations of balance of linear momentum, moment of momentum and energy for the mixture, in a manner that accounts for their diffusion and on the basis of equations characterizing individual constituents. He then described the special case of an incompressible elastic solid and $N - 1$ incompressible fluids. At the same time, Mow[58] developed the governing equations for a mixture consisting of a solid and a liquid phase, and applied them to characterizing cartilage tissue in accordance with creep and stress relaxation tests. For a system idealized as quasi-static, these equations are expressed as follows, where $s$ and $f$ indicate solid and fluid phases, respectively:

$$\begin{aligned}
&\text{momentum:} && \nabla \cdot \boldsymbol{\sigma}^{\alpha} + \boldsymbol{\Pi}^{\alpha} = 0, \quad \alpha = s, f \\
&\text{constitutive } (s): && \boldsymbol{\sigma}^s = -\phi^s p\mathbf{I} + \lambda_s e^s \mathbf{I} + 2\mu^s \boldsymbol{\epsilon}^s \\
&\text{constitutive } (f): && \boldsymbol{\sigma}^f = -\phi^f p\mathbf{I} \\
&\text{diffusive drag:} && \boldsymbol{\Pi}^s = -\boldsymbol{\Pi}^f = K(\mathbf{v}^f - \mathbf{v}^s) \\
&\text{continuity:} && \nabla \cdot (\phi^f \mathbf{v}^f + \phi^s \mathbf{v}^s) = 0.
\end{aligned} \tag{36}$$

Here, $\nabla$ is the gradient, $\boldsymbol{\sigma}$ is the stress tensor of either phase, $\boldsymbol{\Pi}$ represents the diffusive momentum between the two phases, $\phi^s$ and $\phi^f$ represent volume fractions or *solidity* and *porosity*, respectively, $\mathbf{I}$ is the identity tensor, $\boldsymbol{\epsilon}^s$ is the strain tensor of the solid phase, and $\mathbf{v}$ is the velocity vector. The scalar $p$ is the apparent pressure, $K$ is the diffusive drag coefficient, while the following scalars characterize the solid phase: $e^s$ is the dilatation, while $\lambda_s$ and $\mu_s$ are elastic constants. Needless to say, the simultaneous satisfaction of the system of equations (36) constitutes a formidable challenge, in terms of the expression of their corresponding weak form and their FE-based numerical solution.[1,76] Zhu and Suh[87] have recently formulated a dynamic variant of this model for the subsequent application to brain impact studies.

## 5. Summary

This paper proposed a literature review of the physical modeling of the brain, particularly as these publications relate to estimating its volumetric displacement field during surgery and simulating biomechanical response to virtual surgical tools. We reviewed relevant biomechanical concepts, in particular solid and liquid continua that are common in the literature, as well as leading approaches for numerical simulation. FE models of the brain were categorized foremost on the basis of the underlying continuum: solid and solid–liquid hybrid. The history of solid brain modeling was traced from impact models to models simulating surgical loads. The anatomical basis for a model accounting for solid and liquid components was presented, along with a discussion of the consolidation and mixture models.

## References

1. E. S. Almeida and R. L. Spilker, Mixed and penalty finite element models for the non-linear behavior of biphasic soft tissues in finite deformations: Part I — Alternate formulations, *Int. J. Comp. Meth. Biomech. Biomed. Eng.* **1** (1997) 25–46.
2. T. L. Anderson, *Fracture Mechanics*, 3rd edn. (Taylor & Francis, 2005).
3. O. Astley and V. Hayward, Real-time finite-elements simulation of general viscoelastic materials for haptic presentation, *IROS '97, IEEE/RJS Int. Conf. Intelligent Robots and Systems*, September 1997.

4. O. Astley, A software architecture for surgical simulation using haptics, PhD thesis, McGill University (1999).

5. M. A. Audette, K. Siddiqi and T. M. Peters, Level-set surface segmentation and fast cortical range image tracking for computing intrasurgical deformations, *Med. Image Comput. Comput.-Assist. Interv. (MICCAI99)* 19–22 September 1999, Cambridge, England.

6. C. Basdogan, Simulation of tissue cutting and bleeding for laparoscopic surgery using auxiliary surfaces, in *Conf. Medicine Meets Virtual Reality — MMVR*, eds. J. D. Westwood *et al.* (IOS Press, 1999), pp. 39–44.

7. C. Basdogan, Real-time simulation of dynamically deformable finite element models using modal analysis and spectral lanczos decomposition methods, in *Proc. Medicine Meets Virtual Reality* (2001).

8. K.-J. Bathe, *Finite Element Procedures in Engineering Analysis* (Prentice-Hall, 1982).

9. J. Berkley *et al.*, Banded matrix approach to finite element modeling for soft tissue simulation, *Virt. Real.: Res. Devel. Appl.* **4** (1999) 203–212.

10. D. Bielser and M. H. Gross, Interactive simulation of surgical cuts, in *Pacific Graphics 2000* (IEEE Computer Society Press), pp. 116–125.

11. M. A. Biot, General theory of three-dimensional consolidation, *J. Appl. Phys.* **12** (1941) 155–164.

12. R. M. Bowen, Incompressible porous media models by use of the theory of mixtures, *Int. J. Eng. Sci.* **18** (1980) 1129–1148.

13. M. Bro-Nielsen and S. Cotin, Real-time volumetric deformable models for surgery simulation using finite elements and condensation, *EUROGRAPHICS'96* **15**(3) (1996) 57–66.

14. G. C. Burdea, *Force and Touch Feedback for Virtual Reality* (John Wiley & Sons, 1996).

15. M. C. Çavuşoğlu and F. Tendick, Multirate simulation for high fidelity haptic interaction with deformable objects in virtual environments, in *Proc. IEEE Int. Conf. Rob. Auto. (ICRA)* (2000), pp. 2458–2465.

16. V. B. Chial, S. Greenish and A. M. Okamura, On the display of haptic recordings for cutting biological tissues, *Haptics 2002 — IEEE Virt. Real. Conf.* (2002).

17. S. Cotin, H. Delingette and N. Ayache, Efficient linear elastic models of soft tissues for real-time surgery simulation, *IEEE Trans. Vis. Comput. Graph.* **5**(1) (1999) 62–73.

18. T. Dóczi, Volume regulation of the brain tissue — A survey, *Acta Neurochirurgica* **121** 1–8.

19. P. Dumpuri, R. C. Thompson, B. M. Dawant, A. Cao, M. I. Miga, An atlas-based method to compensate for brain shift. Preliminary results, *Medical Image Analysis*, **11**(2) (2007) 128–145.

20. P. J. Edwards *et al.*, Deformation for image guided interventions using a three component tissue model, in *Proc. Inform. Proc. Med. Imag. — IPMI* (1997), pp. 218–231.

21. M. S. Estes and J. H. McElhaney, Response of brain tissue of compressive loading, *ASME Report 70-BHF-13* (1970).

22. M. Ferrant *et al.*, Registration of 3D intraoperative MR images of the brain using a finite element biomechanical model, *Med. Image Comput. Comput.-Assist. Interv. — MICCAI* (2000) 19–27.

23. Y. C. Fung, *Biomechanics: Mechanical Properties of Living Tissues*, 2nd edn. (Springer-Verlag, 1993).

24. J. E. Galford and J. H. McElhaney, A viscoelastic study of scalp, brain, and dura, *J. Biomech.* **3** (1970) 211–221.

25. S. F. F. Gibson, 3D Chainmail: A fast algorithm for deforming volumetric objects, in *Proc. Symp. Interactive 3D Graphics — ACM SIGGRAPH* (1997), pp. 149–154.

26. A. E. Green and W. Zerna, *Theoretical Elasticity*, 2nd edn. (Clarendon Press, 1968).

27. S. Greenish, Acquisition and analysis of cutting forces of surgical instruments for haptic simulation, Master's thesis, Dept. Electrical and Computer Engineering, McGill University (1998).

28. A. Hagemann *et al.*, Non-rigid matching of tomographic images based on a biomechanical model of the human head, in *Proc. SPIE — Med. Imag.: Image Proc.* (1999).

29. K. V. Hansen and O. V. Larsen, Using region-of-interest based finite element modeling for brain surgery simulation, *Med. Image Comput. Comput-Assist. Interv.— MICCAI'98* (1998) 305–316.

30. S. Hakim, J. G. Venegas and J. D. Burton, The physics of the cranial cavity, hydrocephalus and normal pressure hydrocephalus: mechanical interpretation and mathematical model, *Surg. Neurol.* **5** (1976).

31. Hibbitt, Karlsson and Sorensen, Inc., *ABAQUS Theory Manual* (1995).

32. D. L. G. Hill *et al.*, Estimation of intraoperative brain surface movement, in *Proc. CVRMed-MRCAS* (1997), pp. 449–458.

33. R. R. Hosey and Y. K. Liu, A homeomorphic finite element model of impact head and neck injury, in *Int. Conf. Proc. Finite Elements in Biomechanics*, Vol. 2, ed. B. R. Simon (1980), pp. 851–871.

34. T. T. Khalil and R. P. Hubbard, Parametric study of head response by finite element modeling, *J. Biomech.* **10** (1977) 119–132.

35. T. B. Khalil and D. C. Viano, Critical issues in finite element modeling of head impact, in *Proc. 26th Stapp Car Crash Conf.*, SAE Paper 821150 (1982), pp. 87–101.

36. A. I. King and C. C. Chou, Mathematical modeling, simulation and experimental testing of biomechanical system crash response, *J. Biomech.* (9) (1976) 301–317.

37. S. Kleiven, Finite element modeling of the human head, PhD thesis, Department of Aeronautics, Royal Institute of Technology, Stockholm, Sweden (2002).

38. S. K. Kyriacou and C. Davatzikos, A biomechanical model of soft tissue deformation with applications to non-rigid registration of brain images with tumor pathology, *Med. Image Comput. Comput.-Assist. Interv. — MICCAI'98* (1998) 531–538.

39. R. S. Lakes, *Viscoelastic Solids* (CRC Press, 1999).

40. L. D. Landau and E. M. Lifshitz, *Theory of Elasticity*, 3rd edn., Course of Theoretical Physics, Vol. 7 (Pergamon Press, 1986).

41. M. Mahvash and V. Hayward, Haptics rendering of cutting: A fracture mechanics approach, *Haptics-e — Electron. J. Haptics Res.* **2**(3) (2001).

42. M. Mahvash, Haptic rendering of tool contact and cutting, PhD Thesis, McGill University (2002).

43. L. E. Malvern, *Introduction to the Mechanics of a Continuous Medium* (Prentice-Hall, 1969).

44. C. R. Maurer *et al.*, Measurement of intraoperative brain deformation using a 1.5 Tesla interventional MR system: preliminary results, *IEEE Trans. Med. Imag.* **17**(5) (1998) 817–825.

45. K. K. Mendis, R. L. Stalnaker and S. H. Advani, A constitutive relationship for large deformation finite element modeling of brain tissue, *J. Biomech. Eng.* **117** pp. 279–285.

46. Mesh Generation and Grid Generation on the Web, http://www-users.informatik.rwth-aachen.de/ roberts/meshgeneration.html, maintained by Robert Schneiders.

47. M. I. Miga, K. D. Paulsen, F. E. Kennedy, P. J. Hoopes, A. Hartov and D. W. Roberts, In vivo quantification of a homogeneous brain deformation model

for updating preoperative images during surgery, *IEEE Trans. Biomed. Eng.* **47**(2) (2000) 266–273.

48. M. I. Miga, K. D. Paulsen, J. M. Lemery, S. Eisner, A. Hartov, F. E. Kennedy and D. W. Roberts, Model-updated image guidance: Initial clinical experience with gravity-induced brain deformation, *IEEE Trans. Med. Imag.* **18**(10) (1999) 866–874.

49. M. I. Miga *et al.*, Updated neuroimaging using intraoperative brain modeling and sparse data, *Stereotac. Func. Neurosurg.* **72** (1999) 103–106.

50. M. I. Miga, Development and quantification of a 3D brain deformation model for model-updated image-guided stereotactic neurosurgery, PhD thesis, Dartmouth College, Hanover, NH (1999).

51. M. I. Miga *et al.*, Incorporation of surface-based deformations for updating images intraoperatively, *SPIE Med. Imag. 2001* **2**(24) (2001) 169–178.

52. K. Miller and K. Chinzei, Modeling of brain tissue mechanical properties: biphasic versus single-phase approach, *Comp. Meth. Biomech. Biomed. Eng. — 2*, ed. J. Middleton, M. L. Jones and G. N. Pande, Gordon and Breach Science Publishers (1998), pp. 535–542.

53. K. Miller and K. Chinzei, Simple validation of biomechanical models of brain tissue, *J. Biomech.* **31**(1) (1998).

54. K. Miller and K. Chinzei, Constitutive modeling of brain tissue: experiment and theory, *J. Biomech.* **30**(11/12) (1997) 1115–1121.

55. K. Miller, Modeling soft tissue using biphasic theory — A word of caution, *Comp. Meth. Biomech. Biomed. Eng.* **1** (1998) 261–263.

56. K. Miller, Constitutive model of brain tissue suitable for finite element analysis of surgical procedures, *J. Biomech.* (32) 531–537.

57. K. Miller, *Biomechanics of Brain for Computer Integrated Surgery* (Warsaw University of Technology Publishing House, 2002).

58. V. C. Mow *et al.*, Biphasic creep and stress relaxation of articular cartilage in compression: theory and experiments, *Trans. ASME — J. Biomech. Eng.* **102** (1980) 73–84.

59. T. Nagashima *et al.*, The finite element analysis of brain oedema associated with intracranial meningiomas, *Acta Neurochirurgica*, (Suppl. 51) (1990) 155–157.

60. P. F. Neumann, L. L. Sadler and J. Gieser, Virtual reality vitrectomy simulator, *Med. Image Comput. Comput.-Assist. Interv. — MICCAI'98* (1998) 910–917.

61. J. F. O'Brien and J. K. Hodgins, Graphical modeling and animation of brittle fracture, in *Proc. ACM SIGGRAPH 99, Comput. Graph. Proc.* (1999) 137–146.

62. J. F. O'Brien, A. W. Bargteil and J. K. Hodgins, Graphical modeling and animation of ductile fracture, in *Int. Conf. Comput. Graph. Interact. Tech.* (2002), pp. 291–294.

63. A. K. Ommaya, Mechanical properties of tissues of the nervous system, *J. Biomech.* **1**(2) (1968), pp. 127–138.

64. S. Owen, A Survey of unstructured mesh generation technology, available online at www.andrew.cmu.edu/user/sowen/survey/index.html (1999).

65. M. R. Pamidi and S. H. Advani, Non-linear constitutive relations for human brain tissue, *Trans. ASME* **100** (1978) 44–48.

66. A. Peña *et al.*, Effects of brain ventricular shape on periventricular biomechanics: A finite-element analysis, *Neurosurg.* **45**(1) (1999).

67. A. Pentland and S. Sclaroff, Closed-form solutions for physically based shape modeling and recognition, *IEEE Trans. Pattern Anal. Mach. Intell.* **13**(7) (1991) 715–729.

68. G. Picinbono, H. Delingette and N. Ayache, Real-time large displacement elasticity for surgery simulation: non-linear tensor-mass model. *Med. Imag. Comput. Comput.-Assist. Interv. — MICCAI* (2000) 643–652.

69. J. S. Ruan, T. B. Khalil and A. I. King, Dynamic response of the human head to impact by three-dimensional finite element analysis, *ASME J. Biomech. Eng.* **116** (1994) 44–50.

70. A. A. H. J. Sauren and M. H. A. Claessens, Finite element modeling of head impact: The second decade, in *Proc. 1993 Int. IRCOBI Conf. Biomechanics of Impacts* (1993), pp. 241–254.

71. T. A. Shugar and M. G. Katona, Development of finite element head injury model, *J. Amer. Soc. Civil Engineers*, **101**(E173) (1975) 223–239.

72. T. A. Shugar, A finite element head injury model, Report No. DOT HS 289-3-550-TA, Vol. 1 (1977).

73. M. Sinasac, Master's thesis, McGill University (1999).

74. O. Škrinjar, D. Spencer and J. Duncan, Brain shift modeling for use in neurosurgery, *Med. Image Comput. Comput-Assist. Interv. — MICCAI'98* (1998) 641–649.

75. O. Škrinjar and J. Duncan, Real time 3D brain shift compensation, in *Proc. Inform. Proc. Med. Imag. IPMI* (1999) pp. 42–55.

76. R. L. Spilker and J.-K. Suh, Formulation and evaluation of a finite element model for the biphasic model of hydrated soft tissues, *Comput. Struct.* **35**(4) (1990) 425–439.

77. Y. Tada and T. Nagashima, Modeling and simulation of brain lesions by the finite-element method, *IEEE Eng. Med. Biol.* (1994) 497–503.

78. C. Truesdell and W. Noll, *The Non-linear Field Theories of Mechanics*, 2nd edn (Springer-Verlag, 1992).

79. L. Voo *et al.*, Finite-element models of the human head, *Med. Biol. Eng. Comput.* (1996) 375–381.

80. C. C. Ward and R. B. Thompson, The development of a detailed finite element brain model, in *Proc. 19th Stapp Car Crash Conf.* (1975), pp. 641–674.

81. C. C. Ward, Finite element models of the head and their use in brain injury research, in *Proc. 26th Stapp Car Crash Conf.* SAE Paper 821154 (1982), pp. 71–85.

82. R. Wasserman *et al.*, A patient specific *in vivo* tumor model, *Math. Biosci.* **136**(2) (1996) 111–140.

83. K. Waters, A physical model of facial tissue and muscle articulation derived from computer tomography data, in *Proc. Visual. Biomed. Comput. — SPIE* **1808** (1992) 574–583.

84. X. Wu, M. S. Downes, T. Goktekin and F. Tendick, Adaptive non-linear finite elements for deformable body simulation using dynamic progressive meshes, *EuroGraphics 2001*, appearing in Computer Graphics Forum, **20**(3) (2001) 349–358.

85. X. Wu and F. Tendick, Multi-Grid integration for interactive deformable body simulation, *Int. Symp. Med. Simul.* (2004) 92–104.

86. C. Zhou, T. B. Khalil and A. I. King, A new model comparing impact responses of the homogeneous and inhomogeneous human brain, *Soc. Automot. Eng. Inc. Report #952714* (1995).

87. Q. Zhu and J. K. F. Suh, Dynamic biphasic poroviscoelastic model simulation of hydrated soft tissues and its potential application for brain impact study, in *BED-Vol. 50, Bioeng. Conf. ASME* (2001), pp. 835–836.

88. O. C. Zienkiewicz and R. L. Taylor, *The Finite Element Method*, 4th edn. Vols. 1 and 2 (McGraw-Hill, 1991).

# CHAPTER 4

# TECHNIQUES AND APPLICATIONS OF ROBUST NONRIGID BRAIN REGISTRATION

OLIVIER CLATZ*,†,‡, HERVÉ DELINGETTE*, NECULAI ARCHIP†, ION-FLORIN
TALOS†, ALEXANDRA J. GOLBY†, PETER BLACK†, RON KIKINIS†,
FERENC A. JOLESZ†, NICHOLAS AYACHE* and SIMON K. WARFIELD†

*Asclepios Research Project, INRIA Sophia Antipolis, France
†Surgical Planning Laboratory
Computational Radiology Laboratory
Harvard Medical School, Boston, USA
‡oclatz@bwh.harvard.edu

Intraoperative magnetic resonance (MR) imaging systems allow neurosurgeons to acquire images of the brain during the course of neurosurgical procedures. During surgery, these systems help following the deformation of the brain. However, even if they provide significantly more information than any other intraoperative imaging system, it is not possible to acquire full diffusion tensor, functional MR or high resolution MR images (MRI) in a reasonable time compatible with the procedure.

The intraoperative image can be used to measure the brain deformation during surgery. Applying this deformation to the advanced imaging modalities acquired preoperatively makes them virtually available during surgery. This chapter describes a new algorithm to register 3D preoperative MRI to intraoperative MRI of the brain which has undergone brain shift. This algorithm relies on a robust estimation of the deformation from a sparse noisy set of measured displacements. We propose a new framework to compute the displacement field in an iterative process, allowing the solution to gradually move from an approximation formulation (minimizing the sum of a regularization term and a data error term) to an interpolation formulation (least square minimization of the data error term). An outlier rejection step is introduced in this gradual registration process using a weighted least trimmed squares approach, aiming at improving the robustness of the algorithm. We use a patient-specific model discretized with the finite element method (FEM) in order to ensure a realistic mechanical behavior of the brain tissue.

The slowest step of the algorithm has been parallelized, so that we can perform a full 3D image registration in 35 s (including the image update time) on a heterogeneous cluster of 15 PCs. The algorithm has been tested on six retrospective cases of brain tumor resection, presenting a brain shift of up to 14 mm. The results show a good ability to recover large displacements, and a limited decrease of accuracy near the tumor resection cavity.

## 1. Introduction

### 1.1. *Image-guided neurosurgery*

The development of intraoperative imaging systems has contributed to improving the course of intracranial neurosurgical procedures. Among these systems, the 0.5 T

---

‡Corresponding author.

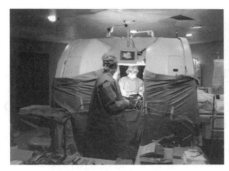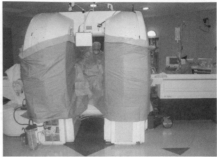

Fig. 1.   The 0.5 T open magnet system (Signa SP, GE Medical Systems) of Brigham and Women's Hospital.

intraoperative magnetic resonance scanner of Brigham and Women's Hospital (Signa SP, GE Medical Systems, Fig. 1) offers the possibility to acquire $256 \times 256 \times 58$ (0.86, 0.86, 2.5 mm) T1 weighted images with the fast spin echo protocol (TR = 400, TE = 16 ms, FOV = $220 \times 220$ mm) in 3 min and 40 s. The quality of every $256 \times 256$ slice acquired intraoperatively is fairly similar to images acquired with a 1.5 T conventional scanner, but the major drawback of the intraoperative image remains the slice thickness (2.5 mm). Images do not show significant distortion but can suffer from artifacts due to different factors (surgical instruments, hand movement, radio-frequency noise from bipolar coagulation). Recent advances in acquisition protocol[1] however make it possible to acquire images with very limited artifacts during the course of a neurosurgical procedure.

The intraoperative MR scanner enhances the surgeon's view and enables the visualization of the brain deformation during the procedure.[2,3] This deformation is a consequence of various combined factors: cerebro spinal fluid (CSF) leakage, gravity, edema, tumor mass effect, brain parenchyma resection or retraction, and administration of osmotic diuretics.[4-6] Intraoperative measurements show that this deformation is an important source of error that needs to be considered.[7] Indeed, imaging the brain during the procedure makes the tumor resection more effective,[8] and facilitates complete resections in critical brain areas. However, even if the intraoperative MR scanner provides significantly more information than any other intraoperative imaging system, it is not clinically possible to acquire image modalities like diffusion tensor MR, functional MR, or high resolution MR images in a reasonable time during the procedure. Illustrated examples of image-guided neurosurgical procedures can be found on the SPL website.[a]

Nonrigid registration algorithms provide a way to overcome the intraoperative acquisition problem: instead of time-consuming image acquisitions during the procedure, the intraoperative deformation is measured on fast acquisitions of intraoperative images. This transformation is then used to match the preoperative

[a]http://splweb.bwh.harvard.edu:8000/pages/projects/mrt/mrt.html.

images on the intraoperative data. To be used in a clinical environment, the registration algorithm must hence satisfy different constraints:

- Speed. The registration process should be sufficiently fast such that it does not compromise the workflow during the surgery; for example, a process time less than or equal to the intraoperative acquisition time is satisfactory.
- Robustness. The registration results should not be altered by image intensity inhomogeneities, artifacts, or by the presence of resection in the intraoperative image.
- Accuracy. The displacement field measured with the registration alorithm should reflect the physical deformation of the underlying organ.

The choice of the number and the frequency of image acquisitions during the procedure remains an open problem. Indeed, there is a trade-off between acquiring more images for accurate guidance and not increasing the time for imaging. The optimal number of imaging sessions may depend on the procedure type, physiological parameters, and the current amount of deformation. Other imaging devices (stereovision, laser range scanner, ultrasound, etc.) could be additionally ·used to assist the surgeon in his/her decision. These perspectives are currently under investigation in our group.[9]

In this chapter, we introduce a new registration algorithm designed for image-guided neurosurgery. We rely on a biomechanical finite element model to enforce a realistic deformation of the brain. With this physics-based approach, *a priori* knowledge in the relative stiffness of the intracranial structures (brain parenchyma, ventricles,etc.) can be introduced.

The algorithm relies on a sparse displacement field estimated with a block matching approach. We propose to compute the deformation from these displacements using an iterative method that gradually shifts from an approximation problem (minimizing the sum of a regularization term and a data error term) toward an interpolation problem (least square minimization of the data error term). To our knowledge, this is the first attempt to take advantage of the two classical formulations of the registration problem (approximation and interpolation) to increase both robustness and accuracy of the algorithm.

In addition, we address the problem of information distribution in the images (known as the aperture problem[10] in computer vision) to make the registration process depend on the spatial distribution of the information given by the structure tensor (see Sec. 2.1.5. for definition).

We tested our algorithm on six cases of brain tumor resection performed at Brigham and Women's Hospital using the 0.5 T open magnet system. The preoperative images were usually acquired the day before the surgery. The intraoperative dataset is composed of six anatomical $256 \times 256 \times 58$ T1 weighted MR images acquired with the fast spin echo protocol previously described. Usually, an initial intraoperative MR image is acquired at the very beginning of the procedure, before opening of the dura-mater. This image, which does not yet show any deformation, is used to compute the rigid transformation between the two positions of the patient in any preoperative image and the image from the intraoperative scanner.

## 1.2. *Nonrigid registration for image-guided surgery*

### 1.2.1. *Modeling the intraoperative deformation*

Because of the lower resolution of the intraoperative imaging devices, modeling the behavior of the brain remains a key issue to introduce *a priori* knowledge in the image-guided surgery process. The rheological experiments of Miller significantly contributed in the understanding of the physics of the brain tissue.[11] His extensive investigation in brain tissue engineering showed very good concordance of the hyperviscoelastic constitutive equation with *in vivo* and *in vitro* experiments. Miga *et al.* demonstrated that a patient-specific model can accurately simulate both the intraoperative gravity and the resection-induced brain deformation.[12,13] A practical difficulty associated with these models is the extensive time necessary to mesh the brain and solve the problem. Castellano-Smith *et al.*[14] addressed the meshing time problem by warping a template mesh to the patient geometry. Davatzikos *et al.*[15] proposed a statistical framework consisting of precomputing the main mode of deformation of the brain using a biomechanical model. Recent extensions of this framework showed promising results for intraoperative surgical guidance based on sparse data.[16]

### 1.2.2. *Displacement-based nonrigid registration*

We propose a displacement-based nonrigid registration method consisting of optimizing a parametric transformation from a sparse set of estimated displacements.

Alternative methods include intensity-based methods, where the parametric transformation is estimated by minimizing a global voxel-based functional defined on the whole image. It should be noted that although these algorithms are by nature computationally expensive, the work of Hastreiter *et al.*[17] based on an openGL acceleration, or the work of Rohlfing and Maurer[18] using shared-memory multiprocessor environments to speed up the free form deformation-based registration[19] recently demonstrated that such algorithms could be adapted to the intraoperative registration problem.

The following review of the literature is purposely restricted to registration algorithms based on approximation and interpolation problems in the context of matching corresponding points using an elastic model constraint.

**Interpolation.** Simple biomechanical models have been used to interpolate the full brain deformation based on sparse measured displacements. Audette[20] and Miga *et al.*[21] measured the visible intraoperative cortex shift using a laser range scanner.

The displacement of deep brain structures was then obtained by applying these displacements as boundary conditions to the brain mesh. A similar surface based approach was proposed by Skrinjar *et al.*[22] and Sun *et al.*,[23] imaging the brain surface with a stereovision system. Ferrant *et al.*[24] extracted the full cortex and ventricles surfaces from intraoperative MR images to constrain the displacement of the surface of a linear finite element model. These surface-based methods showed very good accuracy near the boundary conditions, but suffered inside the brain due to lack of data.[6] Rexilius *et al.*[25] followed Ferrant's efforts by incorporating block-matching estimated displacements as internal boundary condition to the FEM model (leading to the solution presented in Sec. 2.3.2.). However, the method proposed by Rexilius was not robust to outliers. Ruiz-Alzola *et al.*[26] proposed through the Kriging interpolator a probabilistic framework to manage the noise distribution in the sparse displacement field computed with the block-matching algorithm. Although first results show qualitative good matching, it is difficult to assess the realism of the deformation since the Kriging estimator does not rely on a physical model.

**Approximation.** The approximation-based registration consists of formulating the problem as a functional minimization decomposed into a similarity energy and a regularization energy. Because its formulation leads to well-posed problems, the similarity energy often relies on a block- (or feature) matching algorithm. In 1998, Yeung *et al.*[27] showed that impressive registration results on a phantom using an approximation formulation combining ultrasound speckle tracking with a mechanical finite element model. Hata *et al.*[28] registered preoperative with intraoperative MR images using a mutual information based similarity criterion (see Wells *et al.* for details about mutual information[29]) and a mechanical finite element model to get plausible displacements. They could perform a full image registration using a stochastic gradient descent search in less than 10 min, for an average error of 40% of true displacement. Rohr *et al.*[30] improved the basic block-matching algorithm by selecting relevant anatomical landmarks in the image and by taking into account the anisotropic matching error in the global functional. Shen and Davatzikos[31] investigated this idea of anatomical landmarks and proposed an attribute vector for each voxel reflecting the underlying anatomy at different scales. In addition to the Laplacian smoothness energy, their energy minimization involves two different data similarity functions for pushing and pulling the displacement to the minimum of the functional energy.

## 2. Method

We have developed a registration algorithm to measure the brain deformation based on two images acquired before and during the surgery. The algorithm can be decomposed into three main parts, presented in Fig. 2. The first part consists of building a patient-specific model corresponding to the patient position in the

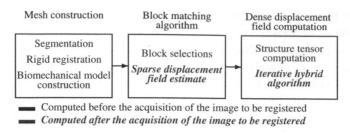

Fig. 2.   Overview of the steps involved in the registration process.

open-magnet scanner. Patient-specific in this algorithm's context refers to having a coarse finite element model that approximately matches the outer curvature of the patient's cortical surface and lateral ventricular surfaces. The second part is the block-matching computation for selected blocks. The third part is the iterative hybrid solver from approximation to interpolation.

As suggested in Fig. 2, a large part of the computation can be done before acquiring the intraoperative MR image. In the following section, we propose a description of the algorithm sequence, making a distinction between preoperative and intraoperative computations. Indeed, since the preoperative image is available hours before surgery, we can use preprocessing algorithms to

- segment the brain, the ventricles, and the tumor.
- Build the patient-specific biomechanical model of the brain based on the previous segmentation.
- Select blocks in the preoperative image with relevant information.
- Compute the structure tensor in the selected blocks.

Note that the rigid registration between the preoperative image and the intraoperative image is computed before the acquisition of the image is registered, after the beginning of the procedure. Indeed, the rigid motion between the two positions of the patient is estimated on the first intraoperative image acquired at the very beginning of the surgical procedure, before opening the skull and the dura.

After the first intraoperative acquisition showing deformations, it is important to minimize the computation time. As soon as this image is acquired, we compute for each selected block in the preoperative image the displacement that minimizes a similarity measure. We choose the coefficient of correlation as the similarity measure, also providing a confidence in the measured displacement for every block.

The registration problem, combining a finite element model with a sparse displacement field, can then be posed in terms of approximation and interpolation. The two formulations, however, come with weaknesses, further detailed in Sec. 2.3.1. We thus propose a new gradual hybrid approach from the approximation to the interpolation problem, coupled with an outlier rejection algorithm to take advantage of both classical formulations.

## 2.1. *Preoperative MR image treatment*

### 2.1.1. *Segmentation*

We use the method proposed by Mangin *et al.*[32] and implemented in Brainvisa[b] to segment the brain in the preoperative images (see Fig. 3). The tumor segmentation is extracted from the preoperative manual delineation created by the physician for the preoperative planning.

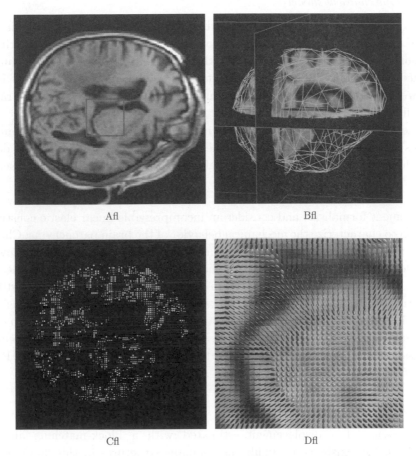

Fig. 3.  Illustration of the preoperative processes. (A) Preoperative image. (B) Segmentation of the brain and 3D mesh generation (we only represent the surface mesh for visualization convenience). (C) Example of block selection, choosing 5% of the total brain voxels as blocks centers. Only the central voxel of the selected blocks is displayed. (D) Structure tensor visualization as ellipsoids (zoom on the red square); the color of the tensors demonstrates the fractional anisotropy.

[b]http://www.brainvisa.info/.

### 2.1.2. Rigid registration

We match our initial segmentation to the first intraoperative image (actually acquired before the dura-mater opening) using the rigid registration software developed at INRIA by Ourselin et al.[33,34] This software, also relying on block-matching, computes the rigid motion that minimizes the transformation error with respect to the measured displacements. Detailed accuracy and robustness measures can be found in Ref. 35.

### 2.1.3. Biomechanical model

The full meshing procedure is decomposed into three steps: we generate a triangular surface mesh from the brain segmentation with the marching cubes algorithm.[36] This surface mesh is then decimated with the YAMS software.[37] The volumetric tetrahedral mesh is finally built from the triangular one with another INRIA software: GHS3D.[38] This software optimizes the shape quality of all tetrahedra in the final mesh.

The mesh generated has an average number of 10,000 tetrahedra (about 1700 vertices), which proved to be a reasonable trade-off between the number of degrees of freedom and the number of matches (about 1–15, see Sec. 2.3.2. for a discussion of the influence of this ratio).

We rely on the finite element theory (see Fung[39] for a complete review of the finite element formalism) and consider an incompressible linear elastic constitutive equation to characterize the mechanical behavior of the brain parenchyma. Choosing the Young modulus for the brain tissue $E = 694\,\mathrm{Pa}$ and assuming slow and small deformations ($\leq 10\%$), we have shown that the maximum error measured on the Young modulus with respect to the state of the art brain constitutive equation[11] is less than 7%.[40] We chose a Poisson's ratio $\nu = 0.45$, modeling an almost incompressible brain tissue. Because the ventricles and the subarachnoid space are connected to each other, the CSF is free to flow between them. We thus assume very soft and compressible tissue for the ventricles ($E = 10\,\mathrm{Pa}$ and $\nu = 0.05$).

### 2.1.4. Block selection

The relevance of a displacement estimated with a block-matching algorithm depends on the existence of highly discriminant structures in this block. Indeed, a homogeneous block lying in the white matter of the preoperative image might be similar to many blocks in the intraoperative image so that its discriminant ability is lower than a block centered on a sulcus. We use the block variance to measure its relevance and only select a fraction of all potential blocks based on this criterion (an example of 5% block selection is given in Fig. 3).

The drawback of this method is a selection of blocks in clusters, where overlapping blocks share most of their voxels. We thus introduce the notion of prohibited connectivity between two block centers to prevent two selected blocks to be too close to each other. We implemented a variety of connectivity criteria and obtained best results using the 26 connectivity (with respect to the central voxel), preventing two distinct blocks of $7 \times 7 \times 7$ voxels to share more than 42% overlapping voxels. Note that this prohibited connectivity criterion leads to a maximum of 30,000 blocks selected in an average adult brain ($\approx 1300 \, \text{cm}^3$) imaged with a resolution of $0.86 \, \text{mm} \times 0.86 \, \text{mm} \times 2.5 \, \text{mm}$. Note also that the $7 \times 7 \times 7$ blocks used are about three times longer in the $Z$ direction because of the anisotropic voxel size.

In addition, to anticipate the ill-posed nature of finding correspondences in the tumor resection cavity, we performed the block selection inside a mask corresponding to the brain without the tumor.

### 2.1.5. *Computation of the structure tensor*

It has been proposed in the literature to use the information distribution around a voxel as a means of selecting blocks[26] or as an attribute considered for the matching of two voxels.[31] Recent works assess the problem of ambiguity raised by the anisotropic character of the intensity distribution around a voxel in landmark matching-based algorithms: edges and lines lead, respectively, to first and second order ambiguities, meaning that a block correlation method can only recover displacements in their orthogonal directions. Rohr *et al.*, account for this ambiguity by weighting the error functional related to each landmark displacement with a covariance matrix.[30]

We consider the normalized structure tensor $T_k$ defined in the preoperative image $I$ at position $O_k$ by

$$T_k = \frac{G * (\nabla I(O_k))(\nabla I(O_k))^T}{\text{trace} \left[ G * (\nabla I(O_k))(\nabla I(O_k))^T \right]}, \tag{1}$$

where $\nabla I(O_k)$ is the Sobel gradient computed at voxel position $O_k$, and $G$ defines a convolution kernel. A Gaussian kernel is usually chosen to compute the structure tensor. In our case, since all voxels in a block have the same influence, we use a constant convolution kernel $G$ in a block so that each $(\nabla I(O_k))(\nabla I(O_k))^T$ has the same weight in the computation of $T_k$.

This positive definite second order tensor represents the structure of the edges in the image. If we consider the classical ellipsoid representation, the more the underlying image resembles a sharp edge, the more the tensor elongates in the direction orthogonal to this edge (see image D of Fig. 3). The structure tensor provides a 3D measure of the smoothness of the intensity distribution in a block and thus a confidence in the measured displacement for this block. In Sec. 2.3., we will see how to introduce this confidence in the registration problem formulation.

## 2.2. *Block-matching algorithm*

Also known as template or window matching, the block-matching algorithm is a simple method used for decades in computer vision.[41,42] It makes the assumption that a global deformation results in translation for small parts of the image. Then the global complex optimization problem can be decomposed into many simple ones: considering a block $B(O_k)$ in the reference image centered in $O_k$, and a similarity metric between two blocks $M(B(O_a), B(O_b))$, the block-matching algorithm consists of finding positions $O'_k$ that maximize the similarity:

$$\arg\max_{O'}[M(B(O_k), B(O'_k))].  \tag{2}$$

Performing this operation on every selected block in the preoperative image produces a sparse estimation of the displacement between the two images (see Fig. 4). In our algorithm, the block-matching is an exhaustive search performed once, and limited to integral voxel translation. It is limited to the brain segmentation, thus restricting the displacements to the intracranial region.

The choice of the similarity function has largely been debated in the literature, we will refer the reader to the article of Roche *et al.*[13] for a detailed comparison of them. In our case, the mono-modal (MR-T1 weighted) nature of the registration problem allows us to make the strong assumption of an affine relationship between the two image intensity distributions. The correlation coefficient thus appears as a natural choice adapted to our problem:

$$c = \frac{\sum_{X \in B}(B_F(X) - \overline{B}_F)(B_T(X) - \overline{B}_T)}{\sum_{X \in B} B_F(X)B_T(X) - \overline{B}_F\overline{B}_T},  \tag{3}$$

where $B_F$ and $B_T$ denote, respectively, the block in the floating and in the reference image, and $\overline{B}$ denotes the average intensity in block $B$. In addition, the value of the correlation coefficient for two matching blocks is normalized between 0 and 1 and reflects the quality of the matching: a value close to 1 indicates two blocks very similar, while a value close to 0 for two blocks very different. We use this value as a confidence in the displacement measured by the block-matching algorithm.

## 2.3. *Formulation of the problem: approximation versus interpolation*

As we have seen in Sec. 1.2., the registration problem can be either formulated as an approximation, or as an interpolation problem. In this section, we will show how to formulate our problem in both terms and describe the associated advantages and disadvantages.

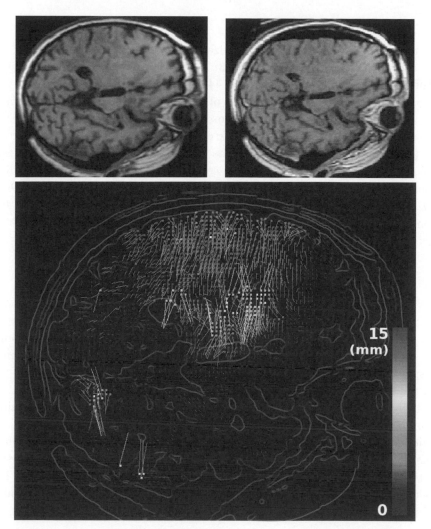

Fig. 4. Block-matching-based displacements estimation. Top left: slice of the preoperative MR image. Top right: intraoperative MR image. Bottom: the sparse displacement field estimated with the block-matching algorithm and superposed to the gradient of the preoperative image (5% block selection, using the coefficient of correlation). The color scale encodes the norm of the displacement, in millimeters.

### 2.3.1. *Approximation*

The approximation problem can be formulated as an energy minimization. This energy is composed of a mechanical and a matching (or error) energy:

$$W = \underbrace{U^T K U}_{\text{Mechanical energy}} + \underbrace{(HU - D)^T S (HU - D)}_{\text{Matching energy}} \tag{4}$$

with

- $U$, the mesh displacement vector of size $3n$, with $n$ number of vertices.
- $K$, the mesh stiffness matrix of size $3n \times 3n$. Details about the building of the stiffness matrix can be found in Ref. 44
- $H$ is the linear interpolation matrix of size $3p \times 3n$. One mesh vertex $v_i$, $i \in [1 : n]$, corresponds to three columns of $H$ (columns $[3*i+1 : 3*i+3]$). One matching point k (i.e. one block center $O_k$) corresponds to three rows of $H$ (rows $[3*k+1 : 3*k+3]$). The $3 \times 3$ submatrices $[H]_{ki}$ are defined as $[H]_{kc_j} = diag(h_j, h_j, h_j)$ for the four columns $c_j$, $j \in [1 : 4]$, corresponding to the four points $v_{c_j}$ of the tetrahedron containing the center of the block $O_k$, and $[H]_{ki} = 0$ everywhere else. The linear interpolation factors $h_j$, $j \in [1 : 4]$, are computed for the block center $O_k$ inside the tetrahedron with

$$\begin{bmatrix} h_1 \\ h_2 \\ h_3 \\ h_4 \end{bmatrix} = \begin{bmatrix} v_{c_1}^x & v_{c_2}^x & v_{c_3}^x & v_{c_4}^x \\ v_{c_1}^y & v_{c_2}^y & v_{c_3}^y & v_{c_4}^y \\ v_{c_1}^z & v_{c_2}^z & v_{c_3}^z & v_{c_4}^z \\ 1 & 1 & 1 & 1 \end{bmatrix}^{-1} \begin{bmatrix} O_k{}^x \\ O_k{}^y \\ O_k{}^z \\ 1 \end{bmatrix}. \tag{5}$$

- $D$, the block-matching computed displacement vector of size $3p$, with $p$ number of matched points. Note that $HU - D$ defines the error on estimated displacements.
- $S$, the matching stiffness of size $3p \times 3p$.
  Usually, a diagonal matrix is considered in the matching energy aiming at minimizing the sum of squared errors. In our case, this would lead to $S = \frac{\alpha}{p}I$. $I$ defines the identity matrix, and, $\alpha$ defines the trade-off between the mechanical energy and the matching energy, it can also be interpreted as the stiffness of a spring toward each block-matching target (the unit of $\alpha$ is N m$^{-1}$). The $\frac{1}{p}$ factor is used to make the global matching energy independent of the number of selected blocks.

We propose an extension to the classical diagonal stiffness matrix $S$ case, taking into account the matching confidence from the correlation coefficient (Eq. 3) and the local structure distribution from the structure tensor (Eq. 1) in the matching stiffness. These measures are introduced through matrix $S$, which becomes a block-diagonal matrix whose $3 \times 3$ submatrices $S_k$ are defined for each block $k$ as

$$S_k = \frac{\alpha}{p} c_k T_k. \tag{6}$$

The influence of a block thus depends on two factors:

- the value of the coefficient of correlation: the better the correlation is (coefficient of correlation closer to 1), the higher the influence of the block on the registration will be;

- the direction of matching with respect to the tensor of structure: we only consider the matching direction colinear to the orientation of the intensity gradient in the block.

The minimization of Eq. 4 is classically obtained by solving $\frac{\partial W}{\partial U} = 0$:

$$\frac{\partial W}{\partial U} = [K + H^T S H]U - H^T S D = 0, \tag{7}$$

leading to the linear system

$$[K + H^T S H]U = H^T S D. \tag{8}$$

Solving Eq. 8 for $U$ leads to the solution of the approximation problem. As shown in Fig. 5, the main advantage of this formulation lies in its ability to smooth the initial displacement field using strong mechanical assumptions. The approximation formulation, however, suffers from a systematic error: whatever the value chosen for $E$ and $\alpha$, the final displacement of the brain mesh is a trade-off between the preoperative rest position and the measured positions so that the deformed structures never reach the measured displacements (visible in Fig. 5 for the ventricles and the cortical displacement).

### 2.3.2. *Interpolation*

The interpolation formulation consists of finding the optimal mesh displacements $U$ that minimize the data error criterion:

$$\arg\min_U (HU - D)^T (HU - D). \tag{9}$$

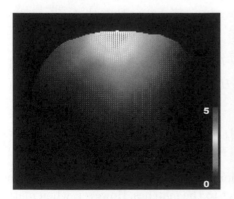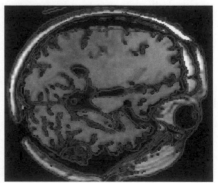

Fig. 5.   Solving the registration problem using the approximation formulation (shown on the same slice as Fig. 4). Left: dense displacement computed as the solution of Eq. 8. Right: gradient of the target image superimposed on the preoperative deformed image using the computed displacement field. We can observe a systematic error on large displacements.

The vertex displacement vector $U$ satisfying Eq. 9 is then given by

$$U = (H^T H)^{-1} H^T D. \tag{10}$$

The possible values for $D$ are restricted to integral voxel translations. However, the displacement of a single vertex depends on all the matches included in the surrounding tetrahedra so that its displacement is a weighted combination of all these matches. The mesh thus also serves the function of regularization on the estimated displacements. Therefore, if the ratio of the number of degrees of freedom ($U$) to the number of block displacement ($D$) is small enough (typically $< 0.1$), subvoxel accuracy (with respect to the "true" transformation) can be expected, even with integral displacements. Conversely, if the previous ratio is greater than or close to 1, the regularization due to the limited number of degrees of freedom is lost, and the transformation can be discontinuous because of the sampling effect. Using a refined mesh could thus induce an additional displacement error (up to half a voxel size), and makes this method inappropriate to estimate brain tissue stress. The ratio we used is about 15 matches per vertex.

Solving Eq. 10 without matches in a vertex cell leads to an undetermined displacement for this vertex. The sparseness of the estimated displacements could thus prevent some areas of the brain from moving because they are not related to any blocks. One way of assessing this problem is to take into account the mechanical behavior of the tissue. The problem is turned into a mechanical energy minimization under the constraint of minimum data error imposed by Eq. 10. The minimization under constraint is formalized through the Lagrange multipliers stored in a vector $\tilde{F}$:

$$\tilde{W} = U^T K U + \tilde{F}^T H^T (HU - D). \tag{11}$$

The Lagrange multiplier vector $\tilde{F}$ of size $3n$ can be interpreted as the set of forces applied at each vertex $U$ in order to impose the displacement constraints. Note that the second term $\tilde{F}^T H^T (HU - D)$ is homogeneous to an elastic energy. Once again, the optimal displacements and forces are obtained by writing that $\frac{\partial \tilde{W}}{\partial U} = 0$ and $\frac{\partial \tilde{W}}{\partial \tilde{F}} = 0$. One then obtains:

$$KU + H^T H \tilde{F} = 0, \tag{12}$$
$$H^T HU - H^T D = 0. \tag{13}$$

A classic method is then to solve

$$\begin{bmatrix} K & H^T H \\ H^T H & 0 \end{bmatrix} \begin{bmatrix} U \\ \tilde{F} \end{bmatrix} = \begin{bmatrix} 0 \\ H^T D \end{bmatrix}. \tag{14}$$

The main advantage of the interpolation formulation is an optimal displacement field (that minimizes the error) with respect to the matches. However, when matches are noisy or — worse — when some of them are outliers (such as in the region around the tumor in Fig. 6), the recovered displacement is disturbed and does not follow the displacement of the tissue. Some of the mesh tetrahedra can even flip, modeling

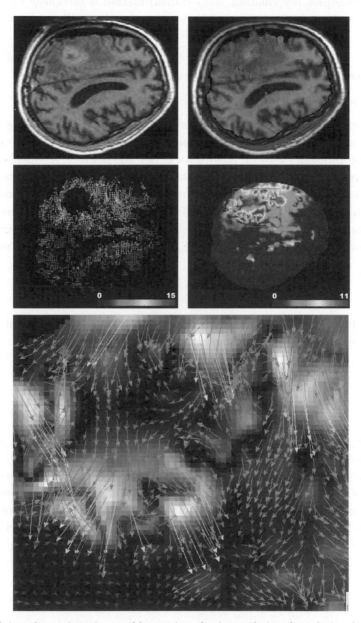

Fig. 6. Solving the registration problem using the interpolation formulation leads to poor matches. Top left: intraoperative MR image intersecting the tumor. Top right: result of the registration of the preoperative on the intraoperative image using the interpolation formulation (Eq. 14). Middle left: estimated displacement using the block-matching algorithm (same slice). Middle right: norm of the recovered displacement field using the interpolation formulation. Bottom: zoom on the registration displacement field around the tumor region (red box) indicates disturbed displacements.

a non-diffeomorphic deformation. This transformation is obviously not physically acceptable, and emphasizes the need for selecting mechanically realistic matches.

### 2.4. Robust gradual transformation estimate

#### 2.4.1. Formulation

We have seen in Sec. 2.3. that the approximation formulation performs well in the presence of noise but suffers from a systematic error. Alternatively, solving the exact interpolation problem based on noisy data is not adequate.

We developed an algorithm which takes advantage of both formulations to iteratively estimate the deformation from the approximation to the interpolation based formulation while rejecting outliers. The gradual convergence to the interpolation solution is achieved through the use of an external force $F$ added to the approximation formulation of Eq. 8, which balances the internal mesh stress:

$$[K + H^T S H]U = H^T S D + F. \tag{15}$$

This force $F_i$ is computed at each iteration $i$ to balance the mesh internal force $KU_i$. This leads to the iterative scheme:

$$F_i \Leftarrow KU_i, \tag{16}$$
$$U_{i+1} \Leftarrow [K + H^T S H]^{-1}[H^T S D + F_i]. \tag{17}$$

The transformation is then estimated in a coarse to fine approach, from large deformations to small details up to the interpolation.

This new formulation combines the advantages of robustness to noise at the beginning of the algorithm and accuracy when reaching convergence. Because some of the measured displacements are outliers, we propose to introduce a robust block-rejection step based on a least-trimmed squares algorithm.[45] This algorithm rejects a fraction of the total blocks based on an error function $\xi_k$ measuring for block $k$ the error between the current mesh displacement and the matching target:

$$\xi_k = \|S_k[(HU)_k - D_k]\|, \tag{18}$$

where $D_k$, $(HU)_k$, and $[(HU)_k - D_k]$, respectively define the measured displacement, the current mesh-induced displacement, and the current displacement error for block $k$. $\xi_k$ is thus simply the displacement error weighted according to the direction of the intensity gradient in block $k$. However, our experiments showed that the block-matching error is rather multiplicative than additive (i.e. the larger the displacement of the tissue, the larger the measured displacement error is). Therefore, we modified

$\xi$ to take into account the current estimate of the displacement:

$$\xi_k = \frac{\|S_k[(HU)_k - D_k]\|}{\lambda\|(HU)_k\| + 1}, \tag{19}$$

where $\lambda$ is a parameter of the algorithm tailored to the error distribution on matches. Note that a log-error function could also have been used. With such a cost function, the rejection criterion is more flexible with points that account for larger displacements. Matrices $S$ and $H$ now have to be recomputed at each iteration involving an outlier rejection step.

The number of rejection steps based on this error function, and the fraction of blocks rejected per iteration are defined by the user. The algorithm then iterates the numerical scheme defined by Eqs. 16 and 17 until convergence. Figure 7

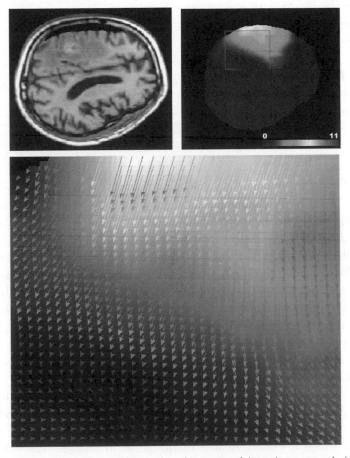

Fig. 7. Solving the registration problem using the proposed iterative approach (Algorithm 1.). Top left: result of the registration of the preoperative on the intraoperative image using the iterative formulation (same slice as Fig. 6). Top right: norm of the recovered displacement field. Bottom: zoom on the registration displacement field around the tumor region (red box) indicates realistic displacements.

gives an example of the registered image and the associated displacement field at convergence. The final registration scheme is given in Algorithm 1..

---

**Algorithm 1.** Registration scheme

1: Get the number of rejection steps $n_R$ from user
2: Get the fraction of total blocks rejected $f_R$ from user
3: **for** $i = 0$ to $n_R$ **do**
4:     $F_i \Leftarrow KU_i$
5:     $U_{i+1} \Leftarrow [K + H^T SH]^{-1} [H^T SD + F_i]$
6:     **for all** Blocks $k$ **do**
7:         Compute error function $\xi_k$
8:     **end for**
9:     Reject $\frac{f_R}{n_R}$ blocks with highest error function $\xi$
10:    Recompute $S$, $H$, $D$
11: **end for**
12: **repeat**
13:    $F_i \Leftarrow KU_i$
14:    $U_{i+1} \Leftarrow [K + H^T SH]^{-1} [H^T SD + F_i]$
15: **until** Convergence

---

### 2.4.2. Parameter setting

We used $7 \times 7 \times 7$ blocks, searching in an $11 \times 11 \times 25$ window (we used a larger window in the direction of larger displacement: following gravity as observed in Roberts et al.[46]) with an integral translation step of $1 \times 1 \times 1$.

Although the least-trimmed squares algorithm is a robust estimator up to 50% of outliers,[45] we experienced that a cumulated rejection rate representing 25% of the total initial selected blocks is sufficient to reject every significant outlier. Figure 8 shows the evolution in the ouliers rejection scheme. A variation of $\pm5\%$ does not have a significant influence on the registration. Below 20%, a quantitative examination of the matches reveals that some outliers could remain. Over 30%, relevant information is discarded in some regions; the displacement then follows the mechanical model in these regions.

$\lambda$ defines the breakup point between an additive and a multiplicative error model: with displacements less (respectively more) than $\frac{1}{\lambda}$ mm, the model is additive (respectively multiplicative). This value thus has to be adapted to the accuracy of the matches, which is closely related to the noise in images. The value of $\lambda$ has been estimated empirically: $\frac{1}{2}$ gave best results, but we encountered significant changes (average difference on the displacement of $2 \times 10^{-2}$ mm, standard deviation of $4 \times 10^{-2}$ mm and maximum displacement difference of $1.1$ mm on the dataset) for variations of $\lambda$ up to $\pm\frac{1}{10}$.

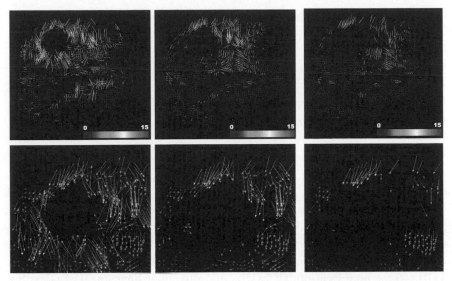

Fig. 8. Visualization of the block-rejection step on the same patient as Fig. 6 (2.5% of blocks rejected per iteration). Left: initial matches. Middle: after five iterations (12.5% rejection). Right: final selected matches after 10 iterations of block rejection (25% of the total blocks are rejected). The region around the tumor seems to have a larger rejection rate than the rest of the brain (especially below the tumor). A closer look at this region (bottom row) reveals that lots of matches around the tumor point toward a wrong direction.

The last parameter is the matching stiffness $\alpha$. Even if it does not influence the convergence, its value might indeed disturb the rejection steps if the convergence rate is too slow. The largest displacements could indeed be considered as outliers if the matching energy does not balance fast enough the mechanical one. Therefore, we choose a matching stiffness $\alpha = \frac{\text{trace}(K)}{n}$, reflecting the average vertex stiffness (note that this value does not depend on the number of vertices used to mesh the volume) so that at least half of the displacement is already recovered after the first iteration. Experiments showed that the results are almost unchanged (max. difference <0.1 mm) when $\alpha$ is scaled (multiplied of divided) by a factor of 5.

### 2.4.3. *Implementation issues and time constraint*

The mechanical system was solved using the conjugate gradient (see Saad *et al.* for details[47]) method with the GMM++ sparse linear system solver.[c] The rejected block fraction for one iteration was set to 2.5% and the number of rejection steps to 10. The following computation times have been recorded on the first

---

[c]http://www.gmm.insa-tlse.fr/getfem/gmm_intro.

patient of our database, using a Pentium IV 3 Ghz machine running the sequential algorithm:

- block-matching computation $\longmapsto$ 162 s.
- Building matrices $S, H, K$ and vector $D \longmapsto 1.8$ s.
- Computing external force vector (Eq. 16) $\longmapsto 7 \times 10^{-2}$ s/iteration.
- Solve system (Eq. 17) $\longmapsto 9 \times 10^{-2}$ s/iteration.
- Blocks rejection $\longmapsto 12 \times 10^{-2}$ s/iteration.
- Update $H, S, D \longmapsto 25 \times 10^{-2}$ s/iteration.

Most of the computation time is spent in the block-matching algorithm. We developed a parallel version of it using PVM[d] able to run on an heterogeneous cluster of PCs, and taking advantage of the sparse computing resource available in a clinical environment. This version reduced the block-matching computation time to 25 s on a heterogeneous group of 15 PCs, composed of three dual Pentium IV 3 GHz, three dual Pentium IV 2 GHz, and nine dual Pentium III 1 GHz. Similar hardware is widely available in hospitals and additionally very inexpensive compared to high-performance computers. The full 3D registration process (including the image update time) could thus be achieved in less than 35 s, after 15 iterations of the algorithm. We think that this time is compatible with the constraint imposed by the procedure.

## 3. Experiments

We evaluated our algorithm on six pairs of pre- and intraoperative MR T1 weighted images. For every patient, the intraoperative registered image is always the last full MR image acquired during the procedure (acquired 1–4 h after the opening of the dura). The skin, skull, and dura are opened, and significant brain resection was performed at this time. The six experiments have been run using the same set of parameters. Figure 9 presents the six preoperative image registrations compared with the intraoperative images on the slice showing the largest displacement (which does not necessarily show the resection cavity).[e] Preoperative, intraoperative, and warped images are shown on corresponding slices after rigid registration.

The registration algorithm shows qualitatively good results: the displacement field is smooth and reflects the tissue behavior, and the algorithm can still recover large deformations (up to 14 mm for patient 5). The algorithm does not require manual intervention, making it fully automatic following the intraoperative MR scan.

---

[d]http://www.csm.ornl.gov/pvm/.
[e]More result images can be seen on the website:
   http://splweb.bwh.harvard.edu:8000/pages/ppl/oclatz/registration/results.html.

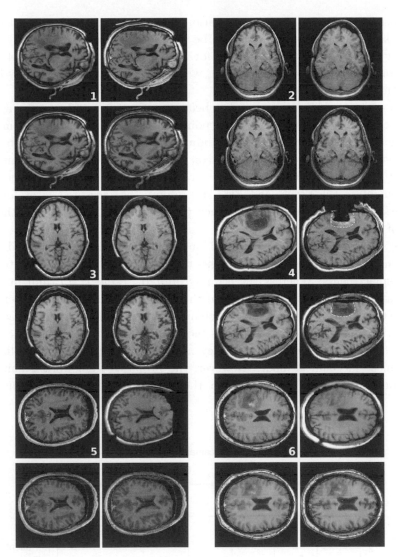

Fig. 9.    Result of the nonrigid registration of the preoperative image on the intraoperative image. For each patient: (top left) preoperative image; (top right) intraoperative image; (bottom left) result of the registration: deformation of the preoperative image on the intraoperative image; (bottom right) gradient of the intraoperative image superimposed on the result image. The enhanced region on the patient 4 image indicates that the resection is incomplete. The white dotted line shows where the outline of the tumor is predicted to be after deformation (top right). It shows a reasonable matching with the tumor margin in the deformed image (bottom right).

We can observe that the quality of the brain segmentation has a direct influence on the deformed image, for example patient 3 of Fig. 9 had a brain mask eroded on the frontal lobe which misses in the registered image. The deformation field, however, should not suffer from the mask inaccuracy, since the brain segmentation is not directly used to guide the registration. The assumption of local translation in the block-matching algorithm seems to be well adapted to the motion of the brain parenchyma. It shows some limitations for ventricles expansion (patients 4 and 6 of Fig. 9) or collapse (patient 5 of Fig. 9), where the error is approximately between 2 and 3 mm.

The accuracy of the algorithm has been quantitatively evaluated by a medical expert selecting corresponding feature points in the registration result image and the target intraoperative image. This landmark-based error (not limited to in-plane error) estimation has been performed on every image for nine different points. Figure 10 presents the measured error for the 54 landmarks as a function of the displacement of the tissue, and Fig. 11 presents the measured error for the 54 landmarks as a function of the distance to the tumor. Table 1 gives the global values of the registration error.

The error distribution presented in Fig. 10 looks uncorrelated to the displacement of the tissue. This highlights the potential of this algorithm to recover large displacements. Whereas the error is limited (Table 1: 0.75 mm in average, 2.5 mm at maximum), Fig. 11 shows that the error somewhat increases when getting closer to the tumor. Because a substantial number of matches are rejected as outliers around the tumor, the displacement is more influenced by the mechanical model in this region. The decrease of accuracy may be a consequence of the limitation of the linear mechanical model. However, the proposed framework is suitable for more complex *a priori* knowledge on the behavior of the brain tissue or the tumor.

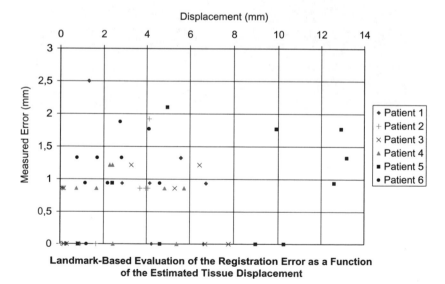

**Landmark-Based Evaluation of the Registration Error as a Function of the Estimated Tissue Displacement**

Fig. 10.    Measure of the registration error for 54 landmarks as a function of the initial error (i.e. as a function of the real displacement of tissue, estimated with the landmarks).

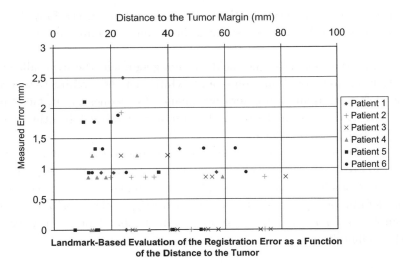

Fig. 11.   Measure of the registration error for 54 landmarks as a function of the distance to the tumor margin.

Table 1.   Quantitative assessment of the registration accuracy using manual selection of corresponding feature points. (A) Maximum displacement (mm). (B) Mean displacement ± standard deviation (mm). (C) Mean error ± standard deviation (mm). (D) Maximum error (mm). (E) Mean relative error (%).

|   | All patients | Patient 1 | Patient 2 | Patient 3 | Patient 4 | Patient 5 | Patient 6 |
|---|---|---|---|---|---|---|---|
| A | 13.18 | 6.73 | 4.10 | 7.77 | 5.74 | 13.18 | 4.60 |
| B | 3.77±3.3 | 3.63±2.4 | 2.41±1.9 | 2.89±3.0 | 2.71±1.9 | 8.06±4.5 | 2.36±1.3 |
| C | 0.75±0.6 | 0.73±0.8 | 0.69±0.6 | 0.45±0.5 | 0.58±0.5 | 0.88±0.8 | 1.16±0.5 |
| D | 2.50 | 2.50 | 1.92 | 1.21 | 1.21 | 2.10 | 1.88 |
| E | 19 | 20 | 28 | 15 | 21 | 10 | 49 |

## 4. Conclusion

We present a new registration algorithm for nonrigid registration of intraoperative MR images. The algorithm has been motivated by the concept of moving from the approximation to the interpolation formulation while rejecting outliers. It could easily be adapted to other interpolation methods, e.g. parametric functions (splines, radial basis functions, etc.) that minimize an error criterion with respect to the data (typically the sum of the squared errors).

The results obtained with the six patients demonstrate the applicability of our algorithm to clinical cases. This method seems to be well suited to capture the mechanical brain deformation based on a sparse and noisy displacement field, limiting the error in critical regions of the brain (such as in the tumor segmentation). The remaining error may be due to the limitation of the linear elastic model.

Regarding the computation time, this algorithm successfully meets the constraints required by a neurosurgical procedure, making it reliable for a clinical use.

This algorithm extends the field of image-guided therapy, allowing the visualization of functional anatomy and white matter architecture projected onto the deformed brain intraoperative image. Consequently, it facilitates the identification of the margin between the tumor and critical healthy structures, making the resection more efficient.

In the future, we will explore the possibility to extend the framework developed in this chapter to other organs such as the kidney or the liver. We also wish to adapt multiscale methods to our problem, as proposed in Hellier et al.,[48] to compute near real-time deformations. In addition, we will investigate the possibility to include more complex a priori mechanical knowledge in regions where the linear elastic model shows limitations.

## References

1. D. Kacher, S. Maier, H. Mamata, Y. M. A. Nabavi and F. Jolesz, Motion robust imaging for continuous intraoperative MRI, *J. Magn. Reson. Imaging* **1**(13) (2001) 158–161.

2. F. Jolesz, Image-guided procedures and the operating room of the future, *Radiology* **204**(3) (1997) 601–612.

3. E. Grimson, R. Kikinis, F. Jolesz and P. Black, Image-guided surgery, *Sci. Am.* **280**(6) (1999) 62–69.

4. L. Platenik, M. Miga, D. Roberts, K. Lunn, F. Kennedy, A. Hartov and K. Paulsen, In vivo quantification of retraction deformation modeling for updated image-guidance during neurosurgery, *IEEE Trans. Biomed. Eng.* **49**(8) (2002) 823–835.

5. C. Nimsky, O. Ganslandt, S. Cerny, P. Hastreiter, G. Greiner and R. Fahlbusch, Quantification of, visualization of and compensation for brain shift using intraoperative magnetic resonance imaging, *Neurosurgery* **47**(5) (2000) 1070–1079.

6. T. Hartkens, D. Hill, A. Castellano-Smith, D. Hawkes, C. M. Jr, A. Martin, W. Hall, H. Liu and C. Truwit, Measurement and analysis of brain deformation during neurosurgery, *IEEE Trans. Med. Imaging* **22**(1) (2003) 82–92.

7. D. Hill, C. Maurer, R. Maciunas, J. Barwise, J. Fitzpatrick and M. Wang, Measurement of intraoperative brain surface deformation under a craniotomy, *Neurosurgery* **43**(3) (1998) 514–526.

8. M. Knauth, C. Wirtz, V. Tronnier, N. Aras, S. Kunze and K. Sartor, Intraoperative MR imaging increases the extent of tumor resection in patients with high-grade gliomas, *Am. J. Neuroradiol.* **20**(9) (1999) 1642–1646.

9. F. Jolesz, Future perspectives for intraoperative MRI, *Neurosurg. Clin. North Am.* **16**(1) (2005) 201–213.

10. T. Poggio, V. Torre and C. Koch, Computational vision and regularization theory, *Nature* **317** (1985) 314–319.

11. K. Miller, *Biomechanics of Brain for Computer Integrated Surgery* (Warsaw University of Technology Publishing House, 2002). ISBN 83-7207-347-3.

12. M. Miga, K. Paulsen, J. Lemry, F. Kennedy, S. Eisner, A. Hartov and D. Roberts, Model-updated image guidance: Initial clinical experience with gravity-induced brain deformation, *IEEE Trans. Med. Imaging* **18**(10) (1999) 866–874.

13. M. Miga, D. Roberts, F. Kennedy, L. Platenik, A. Hartov, K. Lunn and K. Paulsen, Modeling of retraction and resection for intraoperative updating of images, *Neurosurgery* **49**(1) (2001) 75–84.
14. A. Castellano-Smith, T. Hartkens, J. Schnabel, D. Hose, H. Liu, W. Hall, C. Truwit, D. Hawkes and D. Hill, Constructing patient specific models for correcting intraoperative brain deformation, in *Medical Image Computing and Computer-Assisted Intervention (MICCAI'01)*, Vol. 2208, LNCS, (Springer, 2001), pp. 1091–1098.
15. C. Davatzikos, D. Shen, A. Mohamed and S. Kyriacou, A framework for predictive modeling of anatomical deformations, *IEEE Trans. Med. Imaging* **20**(8) (2001) 836–843.
16. K. Lunn, K. Paulsen, D. Roberts, F. Kennedy, A. Hartov and L. Platenik, Nonrigid brain registration: Synthesizing full volume deformation fields from model basis solutions constrained by partial volume intraoperative data, *Comput. Vision Image Understanding* **89**(2) (2003) 299–317.
17. P. Hastreiter, C. Rezk-Salama, G. Soza, M. Bauer, G. Greiner, R. Fahlbusch, O. Ganslandt and C. Nimsky, Strategies for brain shift evaluation, *Med. Image Anal.* **8**(4) (2004) 447–464.
18. T. Rohlfing and C. Maurer, Nonrigid image registration in shared-memory multiprocessor environments with application to brains, breasts and bees, *IEEE Trans. Inform. Tech. Biomed.* **7**(1) (2003) 16–25.
19. D. Rueckert, L. Sonoda, C. Hayes, D. Hill, M. Leach and D. Hawkes, Nonrigid registration using free-form deformations: Application to breast MR images, *IEEE Trans. Med. Imaging* **18**(8) (1999) 712–721.
20. M. Audette, Anatomical Surface Identifcation, Range-Sensing and Registration for Characterizing Intrasurgical Brain Deformations, PhD thesis, McGill University (2003).
21. M. Miga, T. Sinha, D. Cash, R. Galloway and R. Weil, Cortical surface registration for image-guided neurosurgery using laser-range scanning, *IEEE Trans. Med. Imaging* **22**(8) (2003) 973–985.
22. O. Skrinjar, A. Nabavi and J. Duncan, Model-driven brain shift compensation, *Med. Image Anal.* **6**(4) (2002) 361–374.
23. H. Sun, D. Roberts, A. Hartov, K. Rick and K. Paulsen, Using cortical vessels for patient registration during image-guided neurosurgery: A phantom study, in *Medical Imaging 2003: Visualization, Image-Guided Procedures and Display*, eds. J. Galloway and L. Robert, Vol. 5029, Proceedings of the SPIE (May 2003), pp. 183–191.
24. M. Ferrant, A. Nabavi, B. Macq, P. Black, F. Jolesz, R. Kikinis and S. Warfield, Serial registration of intraoperative MR images of the brain, *Med. Image Anal.* **6**(4) (2002) 337–360.
25. J. Rexilius, S. Warfield, C. Guttmann, X. Wei, R. Benson, L. Wolfson, M. Shenton, H. Handels and R. Kikinis, A novel nonrigid registration algorithm and applications, in *Medical Image Computing and Computer-Assisted Intervention (MICCAI'01)*, Vol. 2208, LNCS, (Springer, 2001) pp. 923–931.
26. J. Ruiz-Alzola, C.-F. Westin, S. K. Warfield, C. Alberola, S. E. Maier and R. Kikinis, Nonrigid registration of 3d tensor medical data, *Med. Image Anal.* **6**(2) (2002) 143–161.
27. F. Yeung, S. Levinson, D. Fu and K. Parker, Feature-adaptive motion tracking of ultrasound image sequences using a deformable mesh, *IEEE Trans. Med. Imaging* **17**(6) (1998) 945–956.
28. N. Hata, R. Dohi, S. Warfield, W. Wells, R. Kikinis and F. A. Jolesz, Multimodality deformable registration of pre- and intraoperative images for MRI-guided brain surgery, in *International Conference on Medical Image Computing and*

*Computer-Assisted Intervention*, Vol. 1496, Lecture Notes in Computer Science (1998), pp. 1067–1074, ISBN 3-540-65136-5.

29. W. Wells, P. Viola, H. Atsumiand, S. Nakajima and R. Kikinis, Multi-modal volume registration by maximization of mutual information, *Med. Image Anal.* **1**(1) (1996) 35–52.

30. K. Rohr, H. Stiehl, R. Sprengel, T. Buzug, J. Weese and M. Kuhn, Landmark-based elastic registration using approximating thin-plate splines, *IEEE Trans. Med. Imaging* **20**(6) (2001) 526–534.

31. D. Shen and C. Davatzikos, Hammer: Hierarchical attribute matching mechanism for elastic registration, *IEEE Trans. Med. Imaging* **21**(11) (2002) 1421–1439. ISSN 0278-0062.

32. J.-F. Mangin, V. Frouin, I. Bloch, J. Régis and J. López-Krahe, From 3D magnetic resonance images to structural representations of the cortex topography using topology preserving deformations, *J. Math. Imaging Vision* **5**(4) (1995) 297–318. ISSN 0924-9907.

33. S. Ourselin, X. Pennec, R. Stefanescu, G. Malandain and N. Ayache, Robust registration of multi-modal medical images: Toward real-time clinical applications. Research report 4333, INRIA (2001). URL http://www.inria.fr/rrrt/rr-4333.html.

34. S. Ourselin, R. Stefanescu and X. Pennec, Robust registration of multi-modal images: Toward real-time clinical applications, in *Medical Image Computing and Computer-Assisted Intervention (MICCAI'02)*, eds. T. Dohi and R. Kikinis, Vol. 2489, LNCS, (Springer, 2002), pp. 140–147.

35. S. Ourselin, Recalage d'images médicales par appariement de régions - Application à la construction d'atlas histologiques 3D. Thèse de sciences, Université de Nice Sophia-Antipolis (January 2002). URL http://www.inria.fr/rrrt/tu-0744.html.

36. W. Lorensen and H. Cline, Marching cubes: A high resolution 3D surface construction algorithm, in *SIGGRAPH 87 Conference Proceedings*, Vol. 21, *Computer Graphics*, (July, 1987), pp. 163–170.

37. P. J. Frey, Yams a fully automatic adaptive isotropic surface remeshing procedure, Technical Report RT-0252 INRIA (November 2001).

38. P. J. Frey and P. L. George, *Mesh Generation* (Hermes Science Publications, 2000).

39. Y.-C. Fung, *Biomechanics: Mechanical Properties of Living Tissues* (Springer-Verlag, 1993). ISBN 0387979476.

40. O. Clatz, P. Bondiau, H. Delingette, M. Sermesant, S. Warfield, G. Malandain and N. Ayache, Brain tumor growth simulation, Research report 5187, INRIA (2004). URL http://www-sop.inria.fr/rapports/sophia/RR-5187.html.

41. M. Bierling, Displacement estimation by hierarchical blockmatching, in *Proc. SPIE Conf. Visual Commun. Image Proc. '88*, Vol. 1001 (1988), pp. 942–951.

42. J. Boreczky and L. Rowe, Comparison of video shot boundary detection techniques, in *Storage and Retrieval for Image and Video Databases (SPIE)* (1996), pp. 170–179.

43. A. Roche, G. Malandain and N. Ayache, Unifying maximum likelihood approaches in medical image registration, *Int. J. Imaging Syst. Technol.: Special Issue on 3D Imaging* **11**(1) (2000) 71–80.

44. H. Delingette and N. Ayache, Soft tissue modeling for surgery simulation, in *Computational Models for the Human Body*, ed. N. Ayache, Handbook of Numerical Analysis, ed. Ph. Ciarlet (Elsevier, 2004), pp. 453–550.

45. P. Rousseeuw, Least median-of-squares regression, *J. Am. Stat. Assoc.* **79** (1984) 871–880.

46. D. Roberts, A. Hartov, F. Kennedy, M. Miga and K. Paulsen, Intraoperative brain shift and deformation: A quantitative analysis of cortical displacement in 28 cases, *Neurosurgery* **43**(4) (1998) 749–760. ISSN 1077-3142.
47. Y. Saad, *Iterative Methods for Sparse Linear Systems* (PWS Publishing, Boston, MA, 1996).
48. P. Hellier, C. Barillot, E. Mémin and P. Pérez, Hierarchical estimation of a dense deformation field for 3D robust registration, *IEEE Trans. Med. Imaging* **20**(5) (2001) 388–402.

## CHAPTER 5

# OPTICAL IMAGING IN CEREBRAL HEMODYNAMICS AND PATHOPHYSIOLOGY: TECHNIQUES AND APPLICATIONS

QINGMING LUO, SHANGBIN CHEN, PENGCHENG LI, and SHAOQUN ZENG

*The Key Laboratory of Biomedical Photonics of Ministry of Education — Wuhan National Laboratory for Optoelectronics, Huazhong University of Science and Technology*
*Wuhan 430074, China*
*qluo@mail.hust.edu.cn*

This chapter outlines the basic principles and instrumentation of two functional neuroimaging techniques: optical intrinsic signal imaging and laser speckle imaging. The major application fields and advantages of them are reviewed. The application cases in our lab are especially, addressed: functional activation by sciatic nerve stimulation, cortical spreading depression, and focal cerebral ischemia. The two techniques are easy to implement but it is challenging to study the cerebral hemodynamics and pathophysiology with high spatial and temporal resolution.

## 1. Introduction

The great Greek philosopher Socrates quoted: "Know Yourself." Advancing the understanding of the brain and nervous system is critically important. Great success has been obtained with neuroimaging techniques in the fields of neuroscience research and clinical diagnosis.[1-3] Modern neuroimaging techniques use signals originating from microcirculation to map brain function.[4] More than a century ago (1890), Roy and Sherrington postulated that "the brain possesses an intrinsic mechanism by which its vascular supply can be varied locally in correspondence with local variations of functional activity".[5] This concept is a basis for modern functional brain imaging technologies including functional magnetic resonance imaging (fMRI), positron emission tomography (PET), optical intrinsic signal imaging (OISI), laser speckle imaging (LSI), and near infrared optical tomography.[6-8] In this chapter, we will focus on OISI and LSI.

There is no organ in the body as dependent as the brain on a continuous supply of blood.[9] If cerebral blood flow (CBF) is interrupted, brain function ceases within seconds and irreversible damage to its cellular constituents ensues within minutes. Lack of fuel reserves and high energy demands are responsible for the brain's dependence on blood flow. So, monitoring the cerebral hemodynamics is crucial during normal and pathophysiologic conditions.

As we know, optical measurements are classified as either extrinsic (using exogenous contrast agents) or intrinsic (without exogenous contrast agents).[1,10] Both OISI and LSI have no need to use exogenous contrast agents. Generally, the optical reflectance imaging of brain surface is recorded with a charge-coupled device (CCD) camera that provides high resolution imaging based on changes of cerebral blood volume (CBV), oxygenation, and cerebral blood flow (CBF)[11–18] (see Fig. 1). The technique of OISI is developed by Grinvald and co-workers,[2,4,11,14,19,20] which uses noncoherent light to illuminate the brain surface and mainly acquire the information of CBV and oxygenation. A more comprehensive description of the OISI technique can be found in Refs. 2 and 21. On the other hand, LSI suggested as a method for blood flow imaging almost 20 years ago by Fercher and Briers,[22] needs coherent light source and uses the same OISI system (i.e. coherent-OISI). Since LSI is sensitive to the speed of flow (including CBF), it is also named as laser speckle flowmetry (LSF).[23–26]

Both OISI and LSI have been used very successfully to study the interrelationship of neural, metabolic, and hemodynamic processes in normal and diseased brain (not only in animals but also in human beings).[23,27–31] By different sensory stimulation, cortical functional architecture and sensory information processing have been mapped.[4,11,13,14,25,32–35] Even for neurovascular disease, including migraine, epilepsy, and focal cerebral ischemia, great progresses have been obtained.[31,36–39]

OISI and LSI offer several advantages over conventional electrophysiological and anatomical techniques. The optical imaging methods are noninvasive and do not require dyes, a clear benefit for clinical applications.[19] Although, both autopsy and biopsy are being used in the neuroscience field (for example, in determination

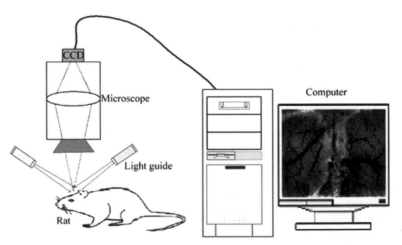

Fig. 1.   The schematic system of OISI and LSI. A charge-coupled device (CCD) camera collects the reflected light from the area of interest through microscope and digitized the light intensity into image.

of the functional column of vision), optical biopsy based on OISI and LSI would be more attractive.[19,40] They can map a relatively large region *in vivo* with tens of milliseconds temporal resolution and microns spatial resolution.[3,11,20,23,29,39,41–45] Although PET and fMRI have the capability to collect three-dimensional spatial information at multiple timepoints in one subject, the spatial resolution of these techniques is on the order of millimeters. Additionally, OISI and LSF are implemented with simple instruments, so the costs are low. Thus, OISI and LSF are two minimally invasive procedures for monitoring short- and long-term changes in cerebral activity.[11]

## 2. Theory

### 2.1. *Spectroscopic imaging*

#### 2.1.1. *Absorption spectrum of oxyhemoglobin and deoxyhemoglobin*

First of all, we will discuss some principles on OISI. Generally, the OISI technique recorded the reflected light intensity from the cortex with a few exceptions of tansmission.[16,17] When photons enter the brain tissue, two main types of interactions may occur[1]: (1) absorption which may lead to radiationless loss of energy to the medium, or induce either fluorescence (or delayed fluorescence) or phosphorescence; and (2) scattering at unchanged frequency when occurring in stationary tissue or accompanied by a Doppler shift due to scattering by moving particles in the tissue (for example, red blood cells). Importantly, the changes in optical properties of brain tissue are associated with brain activity. At least three characteristic physiological parameters affect the degree to which incident light is reflected by the active cortex.[46] These are: (a) changes in the blood volume; (b) chromophore redox, including the oxy/deoxy-hemoglobin ratio (oxymetry); intracellular cytochrome oxidase and electron carriers and; (c) light scattering. All these components have different absorbance spectra, so it is possible to emphasize different physiological phenomena by filtering the incident or reflected light at various wavelengths. For brain imaging, the dominant tissue absorber for visible wavelengths is hemoglobin with its oxygenated and deoxygenated components.[47] The absorption spectra of oxyhemoglobin (HbO) and deoxyhemoglobin (HbR) in the wavelength range 250–1000 nm are given in Fig. 2. In fact, the original data of the above absorption spectra of oxyhemoglobin and deoxyhemoglobin can be found in the website: http://omlc.ogi.edu/spectra/hemoglobin/summary.html.[48]

At some isobestic points of hemoglobin (approximately 550 nm, 570 nm), deoxygenated hemoglobin and oxygenated hemoglobin have the same absorbance and therefore changes in total hemoglobin concentration or cerebral blood volume (CBV) are emphasized.[11,13,41] In the low 600-nm range, oxyhemoglobin absorbance is negligible compared with that of deoxyhemoglobin absorbance. By imaging

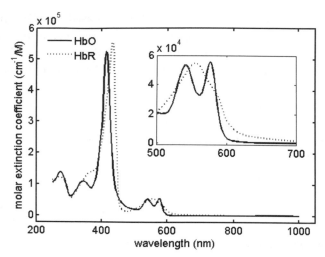

Fig. 2.   Extinction spectra of HbO and HbR in the wavelength range 250–1000 nm. In the inset, the spectra in the range 500–700 nm are enlarged.

at 600–630 nm, one emphasizes changes in deoxyhemoglobin concentration or hemoglobin oximetry.[11,41] Light scattering occurs over the entire visible spectrum and near infrared. At 700–850 nm wavelengths, the light scattering component dominates the intrinsic signal, while hemoglobin absorption is low.[11,41] Usually, cellular swelling would reduce light scattering.[1] However, under "normal" conditions of somatosensory stimulation, the hemoglobin and blood volume contribution appears to be much larger than light scattering.[35] Thus, OISI can be used to map different physiological processes depending on the specific wavelength chosen for illumination. Band-pass interference filters are used to limit the wavelength of the illuminating light. In the review paper,[46] the most frequently used filters are listed: (1) green filter, 546 nm (30 nm wide) — best for obtaining the blood vessel/surface picture; (2) orange filter, 605 nm (5–15 nm wide) — at this wavelength the oxymetry component dominates the signal; (3) red filter, 630 nm (30 nm wide) — at this wavelength the intrinsic signal is dominated by changes in blood volume and the oxygenation saturation level of hemoglobin; (4) near infrared filters, 700–850 nm (30 nm wide)—at these wavelengths, the light scattering component dominates the intrinsic signal, while the contribution of hemoglobin signals is much reduced.

### 2.1.2. *Physical model for the spectroscopic data analysis*

Commonly, the effect of light scattering changes is ignored in a spectroscopic imaging under 700 nm wavelength. The reflectance changes were dominated by the contribution of only two chromophores: oxyhemoglobin and deoxyhemoglobin. In a simplified form, changes in attenuation ($OD = \log 10(R_0/R)$, where $R$ is the reflected light intensity) and changes in concentrations ($\Delta C$) are related by a modified Lambert–Beer law:[13,34,47]

$$OD(\lambda, t) = -\log_{10}\left[R(\lambda, t)/R_0(\lambda)\right]$$
$$= [\varepsilon_{\mathrm{HbO}}(\lambda)\Delta C_{\mathrm{HbO}}(t) + \varepsilon_{\mathrm{HbR}}(\lambda)\Delta C_{\mathrm{HbR}}(t)]L(\lambda), \tag{1}$$

where $R$ is the reflected light intensity, $R_0$ is the incident intensity, $C$ is the concentration of the absorbing molecules (in mM), $\varepsilon$ is the molar extinction coefficient (in $\mathrm{molar}^{-1}\mathrm{mm}^{-1}$) at the selected wavelength, and $L$ is the differential pathlength factor (in mm), accounting for the fact that each wavelength travels slightly different pathlengths through the tissue due to the wavelength dependence of scattering and absorption in the tissue, and was estimated through Monte Carlo simulations of light propagation in tissue.[47] So, if two wavelengths are used, Eq. (1) can determine the two vascular parameters $\Delta C_{\mathrm{HbO}}$ and $\Delta C_{\mathrm{HbR}}$ quantitatively. If multi-wavelengths are used, $\Delta C_{\mathrm{HbO}}$ and $\Delta C_{\mathrm{HbR}}$ can be solved from Eq. (1) using a least-squares approach.[34]

## 2.2. *Laser speckle flowmetry*

### 2.2.1. *Introduction of laser speckle phenomenon*

LSI is also named as laser speckle flowmetry (LSF),[39,49] since it is sensitive to the speed of bioflow, including blood flow[29,39,42−44] and lymph flow.[50] LSF shares almost the same system with OISI (see Fig. 1). The major difference lies in the illuminating light source (laser light).

In the early 1960s the inventors and first users of the laser had a surprise: when laser light fell on a diffusing (nonspecular) surface, they saw a high-contrast grainy pattern, i.e. speckle.[51] The fact that speckle patterns only came into prominence with the invention of the laser suggests that the cause of the phenomenon might be the high degree of coherence of the laser.[49] Further investigation shows that this is indeed the case. Laser speckle was an interference pattern produced by the light reflected or scattered from different parts of the illuminated rough (i.e. nonspecular) surface. When the area illuminated by laser light was imaged onto a CCD camera, there produced a granular or speckle pattern[39,49] (see Fig. 3.) If the scattered particles were moving, a time-varying speckle pattern was generated at each pixel in the image. The intensity variations of this pattern contained information of the scattered particles.[49]

### 2.2.2. *Laser speckle contrast analysis for full field blood flow mapping*

Since the spatial and temporal intensity variation of time-varying speckle pattern contains information on the scattered particles, statistics of speckle patterns has been developed to quantify the speed of scatters.[52] Briers has done some pioneering works in this field.[22,49,53] Through analyzing the spatial blurring of the speckle image obtained by CCD, the two-dimensional velocity distribution with a high

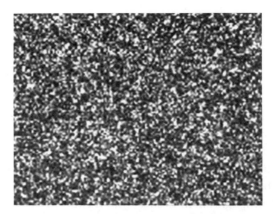

Fig. 3.   A typical speckle pattern. It is acquired by imaging the surface of a porcelain plate with the laser illumination.

spatial and temporal resolution has been shown.[29,32,39,42–44,54,55] This blurring is represented as a local speckle contrast, which is defined as the ratio of the standard deviation to the mean intensity:

$$C = \frac{\sigma_s}{\langle I \rangle}, \tag{2}$$

where $C$, $\sigma_s$, and $\langle I \rangle$ stand for speckle contrast, the standard deviation of light intensity, and the mean value of light intensity, respectively. The speckle contrast lies between the values of 0 and 1. The higher the velocity, the smaller the contrast is; the lower the velocity, the larger the contrast is. A speckle contrast of 1 demonstrates no blurring of speckle, namely, no motion, whereas a speckle contrast of 0 indicates rapidly moving scatterers. The link between the speckle contrast and the correlation time can be manifested by the following equation[39]:

$$C = \frac{\sigma_s}{\langle I \rangle} = \left[ \frac{\tau_c}{2T} \left\{ 1 - \exp\left( \frac{-2T}{\tau_c} \right) \right\} \right]^{\frac{1}{2}}, \tag{3}$$

where $\tau_c = 1/(ak_0v)$, is inversely proportional to the velocity, $v$ is the mean velocity, $k_0$ is the light wavenumber, and $a$ is a factor that depends on the Lorentzian width and scattering properties of the tissue. The value of $\tau_c$ can be computed from the corresponding value of $C$ to get the relative velocity. The above method is also called as laser speckle spatial contrast analysis (LASSCA). Dunn *et al.* have implemented laser speckle imaging for monitoring cerebral blood flow.[29,34,39] Cheng *et al.* have extended this technique to study regional blood flow in the rat mesentery.[42,43]

Further, our lab has provided a modified laser speckle imaging method with laser speckle temporal contrast analysis (LASTCA).[44] The speckle temporal contrast image was constructed by calculating the speckle temporal contrast of each image pixel in the time sequence. The value of speckle temporal contrast $C_t(x, y)$ at pixel

$(x, y)$ is calculated as[56]:

$$C_t(x,y) = \frac{\sigma_{x,y}}{\langle I_{x,y} \rangle} = \sqrt{\left[\sum_{n=1}^{N}(I_{x,y}(n) - \langle I_{x,y} \rangle)^2\right] \bigg/ (N-1)}/\langle I_{x,y} \rangle. \qquad (4)$$

Some advantages of LASTCA have been shown, including imaging obscured subsurface inhomogeneity[57] and even imaging CBF through the intact rat skull[56] (Fig. 4).

## 3. Instrumentation

### 3.1. *Multi-wavelength reflectance imaging*

OISI has provided numerous insights into the functional organization[20] and pathophysiology[38] of the cortex by mapping the changes in cortical reflectance arising from the hemodynamic changes. The majority of these studies have previously been performed at single wavelength band. For multi-wavelengths reflectance imaging, the spectroscopic information would be provided (i.e. multi vascular parameters).[27,29,34] Acquisition of this spectroscopic information has been achieved by sacrificing spatial information,[4] which has precluded full field imaging of HbO, HbR, and total hemoglobin (HbT). While a few studies have utilized intrinsic optical imaging at more than one wavelength, the spectral information was acquired in separate trials[41,45] and was not combined with a physical model of light propagation through a tissue to quantify the spatiotemporal changes in hemoglobin concentrations and oxygenation. Recently, Dunn *et al.* have developed a spectroscopic imaging method that enables full field imaging of reflectance changes at multiple wavelengths by rapid switching of the illumination wavelength using a continuously rotating filter wheel.[29] This technique allows quantitative imaging of the concentration changes in HbO, HbR, and HbT with the same spatial and temporal resolution as traditional intrinsic optical imaging. They have used this instrument to study the relationship between the hemodynamic changes and electrical activity during whisker stimulation in rats by combining the imaging technique with simultaneous electrophysiology recordings.[27] As a supplement, we also developed an electrical switch to drive different wavelength LED to implement the multi-wavelength OISI.[58] In fact, the instrumentation of multi-wavelength reflectance imaging has no substantial difference with the conventional OISI at the single wavelength band. The key is the synchronization of illumination of special wavelength light and acquisition of image frame. In other words, it is important for multi-wavelength OISI to control the switch of illuminating wavelength and the timing to acquire the fames. Dunn *et al.* used the timing signal of filter wheel to trigger the CCD camera.[29] We used a common timing signal produced by an electrical controller to trigger the CCD camera and flash the light at different wavelength.[58]

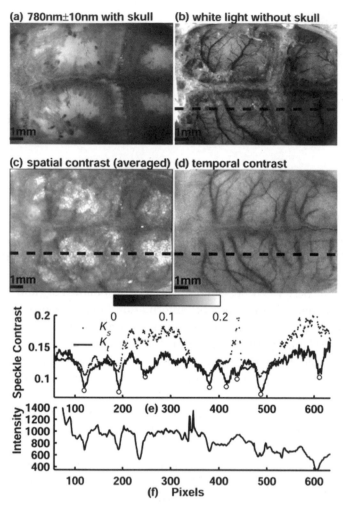

Fig. 4.   Imaging cerebral blood flow through the intact rat skull with temporal laser speckle imaging. (a) Incoherent light reflection image recorded from an intact rat skull. (b) White light reflection image recorded from the exposed cortex of the same rat. (c) Averaged speckle spatial contrast image constructed from 40 speckle images recorded from the intact rat skull. (d) Speckle temporal contrast image constructed from the same data set producing (c). (e) Profiles of the speckle spatial and temporal contrast values along the horizontal dash line in (c) and (d). (f) Profile of the optical intensity along the indicated horizontal dash line in (b). The grayscale bar indicates the value of speckle contrast in (c) and (d) which share the same scale (from Ref. 56).

The typical system of OISI mainly consists of: (1) light source, (2) microscope (macroscope), (3) CCD camera, (4) frame grabber, and (5) computer. In Fig. 1, the schematic setup of OISI has been shown. Of course, the system should work in a dark room or in a dark box in order to avoid the aberrant light effect. Preferably, the OISI system should be placed on a vibration isolator table. For practical cases, we still need use stereotactic frame to fix the experimental animal. Here, we would like to explain the components of the OISI system.

**Light source:** Optimal illumination of the area of interest is crucial for the quality of the maps.[46] Even illumination is best achieved by using at least two fiber-optic light guides directed at the region of interest with an oblique angle of about 30°,[59] whereas a high quality regulated DC power supply is essential for guaranteeing a stable light intensity. Commonly, the halogen lamp[2] and mercury xenon arc lamp[29] are used as the light source. Band-pass interference filters are used to limit the wavelength of the illuminating light. An alternative to the use of light guides (in combination with band-pass filters) is the illumination by a ring of light-emitting diodes (LEDs) of specific wavelengths.[60]

**Microscope:** Although conventional microscope has been used for OISI, the macroscope with its large numerical aperture for a low magnification and the large working distance offers the following considerable advantages[2]: 1. It is easier to use microelectrodes for intracellular or extracellular recordings which record the direct neural activities.[12,27,28,61] 2. The signal-to-noise ratio is better because of the macroscope's high numerical aperture. Under some conditions the total gain in light intensity may be more than 100-fold relative to a standard objective for low magnification. In many of the *in vivo* applications, the sub-micron spatial resolution of objectives and condensers far exceeds the requirements for optical imaging of neuronal activity and the macroscope with low magnification is more than adequate. For barrel columns, the clusters of neurons, approximately $200\,\mu$m in diameter, on the contralateral somatosensory cortex are related with each whisker in a one-to-one fashion.[29]

**CCD camera:** Different types of cameras, such as photodiode arrays[19] and video-cameras[62] have been used for functional brain imaging. Nowadays, most OISI systems contain CCD camera. Photons reflected from the cortex strike the CCD faceplate liberating electrons that accumulate in $SiO_2$ "wells," at a rate proportional to incident photon intensity. Slow-scan digital CCD cameras have been widely used for intrinsic signal imaging. They provide good signal-to-noise ratios at a high spatial resolution, and their main disadvantage, the low image acquisition or frame rate ($<10\,$Hz), is not critical for imaging of the rather slow intrinsic signals. In contrast, video-cameras with CCD-type sensors are much faster ($25\,$Hz) and have an even better signal-to-noise ratio at the light levels typical of an optical imaging (OI) experiment. In the past, they were hampered by eight-bit frame grabbers, which could not digitize intensity changes of $<1/256$ (with the typical signal amplitude in OI being only about $1/1000$). However, this problem can be overcome by differential subtraction of a stored (analog) reference image, resulting in an effective 10- to 12-bit digitization. This image enhancement is no longer necessary, as precision video cameras with 12-bit digitization have been developed, allowing optical imaging up to $40\,$Hz.[13]

**Frame grabber:** The optical reflectance changes are digitized by CCD camera. And the image frames are acquired by frame grabber and stored temporarily in the random-access memory (RAM) of computer. Aided by some certain software, the image frames can be exported to hard disk for off-line analysis.

**Computer:** Computer is used as a controller of OISI. The imaging mode parameters are set in some imaging software. The computer should enable the CPU power to control the stimulation, image acquisition, and the adequate space memory to store the images.

Here, we give a paradigm of OISI system in our work.[13] In each trial, the images of backscattered and reflected light were collected and stored in the RAM of computer over a period of 9 s at 40 Hz using a 12-bit 640×480 pixels video-camera (PixelFly VGA, Germany) attached to a microscope (Olympus SZ6045TRCTV, Japan). After the acquisition of all the 360 frames images was completed, the images were transferred from RAM to the hard disk. Frames were recorded 1 s before the stimulation onset. The stimulations were generated with a stimulator (STG1004, Germany) and the stimulator was triggered by the CCD busy output signal of CCD camera. The rat hindlimb somatosensory cortex was illuminated with light at 570 nm through a dual light guide (Olympus LG-DI, Japan) (for optical imaging setup see Fig. 1). The two-dimensional optical spatial resolution and time resolution applied in the present optical imaging studies were 5 $\mu$m/pixel (over a 3.2 mm × 2.4 mm field) and 25 ms, respectively. In fact, the cost of our whole system of OISI is less than \$20,000.

### 3.2. *Laser speckle imaging*

The system of LSI shares almost the same system with OISI. Most importantly, a laser is used in LSI instead of the noncoherent light used for OISI. The instrument developed for the laser speckle measurements is introduced in Ref. 39. In our work,[44] a He–Ne laser ($\lambda = 632.8$ nm, 3 mW) was coupled into a fiber bundle with 8 mm diameter, which was adjusted to illuminate the area of interest evenly. The illuminated areas are imaged through a zoom stereo microscope (SZ6045TRCTV, Olympus, Japan) onto a CCD camera (Pixelfly, PCO Computer Optics, Germany) with 640 × 480 pixels. Raw images are acquired at 40 frames per second, which is controlled by the computer. And the exposure time of CCD is 20 ms. This system offers a high spatial resolution (25 ms), temporal resolution (13 $\mu$m), and the discrimination of 9% change of velocity. Of course, a laser diode (LD) with different wavelength and intensity power is also a suitable choice. For example, in Ref. 39, a LD (Sharp LTO25MD; $\lambda = 780$ nm, 30 mW; Thorlabs, Newton, NJ, USA) is used. Because the original laser beam is concentrated, it should be expanded before using to illuminate the area of interest.

### 3.3. *Combination of multi-wavelength reflectance imaging and laser speckle imaging*

The common ground of the instrumentation of multi-wavelength OISI and LSI provides the possibility to combine them in a complete system. This work has been

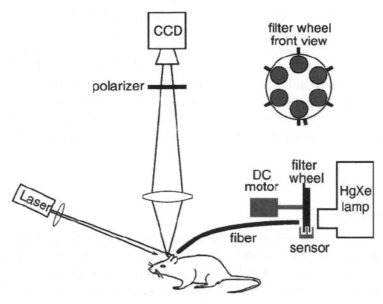

Fig. 5. Schematic of instrument used for multi-wavelength OISI and LSI. A DC motor is operated continuously to drive the filter wheel for the different wavelengths. A radial extension is attached to the filter wheel at each filter position, providing a trigger signal for the camera at each filter position. For interleaved spectral and speckle imaging, one of the filter positions is blocked, and the trigger signal for that filter position is used to switch the diode laser on for LSI (from Ref. 29).

accomplished by Dunn *et al.*[29] The instrument is depicted in Fig. 5. An expanded diode laser ($\lambda = 785$ nm) illuminates the cortex at an angle of approximately $30°$, and the resulting speckle pattern is imaged onto a cooled 12-bit CCD camera. For multiwavelength imaging a mercury xenon arc lamp is directed through a six-position filter wheel and is coupled into a 12-mm fiber bundle that illuminates the cortex. The filters were 10-nm bandpass filters centered at wavelengths of 560, 570, 580, 590, 600, and 610 nm. The filter wheel is mounted on a DC motor and is operated continuously at approximately 3 revolutions per second, resulting in a frame rate of about 18 Hz. A radial extension is attached to the filter wheel at each filter position, and, as the filter wheel rotates, each extension passes through an optical sensor, providing a trigger signal for the camera at each filter position. In addition, a second extension attached to the filter wheel at one of the filter positions serves as a reference for the other filter positions. The output of the sensors, as well as a signal from the CCD indicating when an image is acquired, is recorded by a separate computer. These timing signals are necessary to account for the fact that the camera occasionally misses a trigger signal from the filter wheel, with the result that the order of acquired images can vary slightly. Software was written to analyze the timing signals to determine the filter position and time of acquisition for each image. For interleaved spectral and speckle imaging, one of the filter positions is blocked, and the trigger signal for that filter position is used to switch the diode laser on for approximately 5 ms. Therefore, five spectral images and one speckle image are acquired during interleaved operation. Since images at each filter position are not acquired simultaneously, the time series for each set of images was interpolated onto a common time base. This system is capable of simultaneously imaging both CBF and HbT concentration and oxygenation changes in the brain through a thinned skull preparation. Blood flow is imaged by use of laser speckle contrast imaging, and a six-wavelength filter wheel is used to acquire spectral images for the calculation of HbO and Hb images.

## 4. Applications

OISI was firstly developed to investigate and understand the detailed functional architecture of cat and monkey visual cortex.[11,19,20] In a recent review,[46] some major applications of OISI were outlined: (i) studying the functional architecture of motor, somatosensory, auditory cortices, and the olfactory bulb, (ii) assessing cortical maps in awake animals, and (iii) investigating functional cortical development and plasticity under normal and pathological conditions and following environmental manipulations. Lately, the technique has also been used to visualize the spread of focal epileptic seizures and the reorganization of functional cortical maps in the surrounding of a focal ischemic injury, and it has been adapted to image the human cortex intraoperatively.[1,3,30,46]

LSF has been used extensively to study CBF in normal and diseased brain in rat and mouse. It can acquire the full field CBF in real time, and a representative result is shown in Dunn et al.'s work.[39] The applications also include functional activation by forepaw[25,34] and whisker[23,29] stimulation and temperature variation,[44] pathophysiological model of migraine (cortical spreading depression, CSD)[24,29,31,39,63] and focal cerebral ischemia.[23,39]

Combination of multi-wavelength OISI with LSF has distinct advantages to study the changes of the changes in HbO, HbR, HbT, CBF, and the cerebral metabolic rate of oxygen (CMRO$_2$).[27,29,34] For example, during forepaw and whisker stimulation, the spatial extents of the response of each hemodynamic parameter and CMRO$_2$ were found to be comparable at the time of peak response, and at early times following stimulation onset, the spatial extent of the change in HbR was smaller than that of HbO, HbT, CBF, and CMRO$_2$.[34] With our implemented system, multi-parameter vascular changes during CSD were described.[58] Certainly, multi-parameter full field imaging of the functional response provides a more complete picture of the hemodynamic response to functional activation including the spatial and temporal estimation of CMRO$_2$ changes.[34]

Although many great progresses have been obtained by OISI and LSF, they are still potential and power tool to study hemodynamics and pathyophsiology of brain. In the following, we introduce some of the work in our lab.

## 4.1. *Spatiotemporal quantification of cerebral hemodynamic and metabolism change during functional activation*

As we all know, the combination of multi-wavelength OISI with LSF has the capability to quantify cerebral hemodynamic and metabolism changes.[27,29,34] In the following two examples we only address the CBV[13] and CBF[54] changes during functional activation.

## Case 1: Spatiotemporal characteristics of cerebral blood volume changes in rat somatosensory cortex evoked by sciatic nerve stimulation using optical imaging[45]

The spatiotemporal characteristics of changes in cerebral blood volume associated with neuronal activity were investigated in the hindlimb somatosensory cortex of $\alpha$-chloralose/urethane anesthetized rats ($n = 10$) with optical imaging at 570 nm through a thinned skull. Activation of cortex was carried out by electrical stimulation of the contralateral sciatic nerve with 5 Hz, 0.3 V pulses (0.5 ms) for a duration of 2 s.

The stimulation evoked a monophasic optical reflectance decrease at the cortical parenchyma and arteries sites rapidly after the onset of stimulation, whereas no similar response was observed at the vein compartments. Spatial patterns and time courses of stimulus-induced optical reflectance changes are given in Figs. 6 and 7, respectively. The optical signal changes reached 10% of the peak response $0.70 \pm 0.32$ s after stimulation onset and no significant time lag in this 10% start latency time was observed between the response at the cortical parenchyma and arteries compartments. The evoked optical reflectance decrease reached the peak ($0.25\% \pm 0.047\%$) $2.66 \pm 0.61$ s after the stimulus onset at the parenchyma site, $0.40 \pm 0.20$ s earlier ($P < 0.05$) than that at the arteries site ($0.50\% \pm 0.068\%$, $3.06 \pm 0.70$ s). The temporal characteristics of the cortical parenchyma and arteries compartments are listed in Table 1. Variable location within the cortical parenchyma and arteries compartment themselves did not affect the temporal characteristics of the evoked signal significantly. These results suggest that the sciatic nerve stimulation evokes a local blood volume increase at both capillaries (cortical parenchyma) and arterioles rapidly after the stimulus onset but the evoked blood volume increase in capillaries could not be entirely accounted for by the dilation of arterioles.

## Case 2: Temporal clustering analysis of cerebral blood flow activation maps measured by laser speckle contrast imaging[54]

Temporal and spatial orchestration of neurovascular coupling in brain neuronal activity is the crucial comprehending mechanism of functional cerebral metabolism and pathophysiology. Laser speckle contrast imaging (LSCI) through a thinned skull over the somatosensory cortex was utilized to map the spatiotemporal characteristics of local cerebral blood flow (CBF) in anesthetized rats during sciatic nerve stimulation (Fig. 8). The time course of signals from all spatial loci among

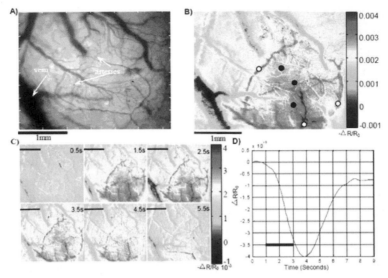

Fig. 6. Spatial pattern of stimulus-induced optical reflectance changes ($\Delta R/R_0$) at 570 nm.
(A) Raw image of exposed somatosensory cortex through a thinned skull at illumination of 570 nm.
Parietal branches of the superior cerebral vein and arteries are clearly distinguishable. (B) Spatial
pattern of stimulation evoked vascular response. The image is obtained by averaging the activation
maps from 2.5 to 3 s after the onset of stimulation. The activation map is a visualization of optical
reflectance difference between an individual frame after stimulus onset and the mean intensity
of frames prior to the stimulation onset. The color bar indicates the amplitude of signal change
$\Delta R/R_0$, where $R$ = optical reflectance collected during an individual image and $\Delta R = R_i - R_0$
denotes the reflectance difference between $i$th frame and the baseline level. (C) Time course of
activation maps in one experimental animal. Among the top images, the left, middle, and right
images correspond respectively to the mean activation maps during: 0.5 s (averaged from 0 to
0.5 s), 1.5 s (averaged from 1 to 1.5 s), 2.5 s (averaged from 2 to 2.5 s); the left, middle, and right
images shown at the bottom correspond respectively to the mean activation maps during: 3.5 s
(averaged from 3 to 3.5 s), 4.5 s (averaged from 4 to 4.5 s) and 5.5 s (averaged from 5 to 5.5 s);
the horizontal bars indicate 1 mm. (D) Mean temporal response of optical reflectance changes over
the whole activated region across animals ($n = 10$). The horizontal bar indicates the duration of
stimulation (Refs. 13 and 45).

the massive dataset is hard to analyze, especially for the thousands of images, each
of which is composed of millions of pixels. We introduced a temporal clustering
analysis[54,64–68] (TCA) method, which was proved as an efficient method to analyze
functional magnetic resonance imaging (fMRI) data in the temporal domain. The
timing and location of CBF activation showed that contralateral hindlimb sensory
cortical microflow was activated to increase promptly in less than 1 s after the
onset of 2 s electrical stimulation and was evolved in different discrete regions
(Fig. 9). This pattern is slightly elaborated similar to the results obtained from laser
Doppler flowmetry (LDF) and fMRI. We presented this combination to investigate
interacting brain regions, which might lead to a better understanding of the nature
of brain parcellation and effective connectivity.

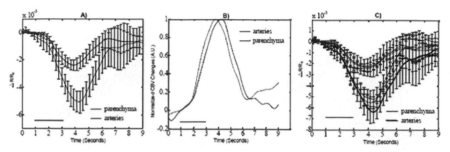

Fig. 7. Time course of stimulus-evoked optical reflectance changes at 570 nm in different microvascular compartments across animals ($n = 10$): cortical parenchyma and arteries. The horizontal bars indicate the duration of stimulation. (A) Mean temporal dynamics over the marked regions in Fig. 6(b) (white dots are for arteries compartment, whereas black dots are for cortical parenchyma compartment). Both the parenchyma and arteries plots are the average result of the time courses of their three 0.01 mm² "sampling" regions. (B) Normalized changes of blood volume over the marked "sampling" regions in Fig. 6(b). The blood volume changes were normalized to the peak amplitude of the signal changes. (C) Time courses of changes of optical reflectance in the six selected regions. Each plot results from averaging the intensity changes of all the pixels within the region of interest across 10 experimental animals (Refs. 13 and 45).

Table 1. Temporal characteristics of optical reflectance changes in somatosensory cortex evoked by sciatic nerve stimulation.

|  | Peak amplitude (%) | Start latency (s) | Peak latency (s) | Termination time (s) |
|---|---|---|---|---|
| Cortical parenchyma | 0.25% ± 0.047% | 0.70 ± 0.32 | 2.66 ± 0.61 | 5.90 ± 1.20 |
| Arteries | 0.50% ± 0.068% |  | 3.06 ± 0.70 | 6.70 ± 1.30 |

## 4.2. Cortical spreading depression

Cortical spreading depression (CSD) was discovered more than 60 years ago.[69] Related to migraine and ischemia, it attracts intensive attention and research[31,70–72]. CSD is characterized by a depolarization of a band of glia and neurons in the cortex (gray matter), and is associated with transient increases of cerebral blood flow, neurotransmitters (glutamate), and extracelluar ions (K⁺), as well as dramatic shifts in cortical steady potential (DC) and EEG depression.[73–75] CSD spreads out from the initiation site like a wave at a rate of 3–5 mm/min on the cortical surface.[71]

The relationship between the neuronal functional changes and cerebral blood flow changes remains unclear during CSD.[76] Hemodynamic response to CSD was extensively studied with a wide variety of methodologies including PET,[77] MRI,[78] LDF,[79] autoradiography, and observation of pial vessel diameter.[80] These techniques have either high spatial or high temporal resolution but not both, and they generally show an increase in blood flow and blood volume that lasts for 1–2 min, followed by a reduction in blood flow that lasts for up to 1 hour. However, with respect to

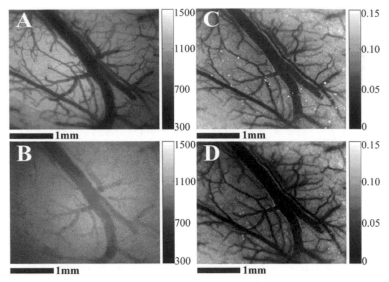

Fig. 8.   LSCI of a representative animal. (A, B) A vascular topography illuminated with green
light (540 ± 20 nm) and a raw speckle image with laser. (A) The vascular pattern is referenced
in case loss of computation occurred. (C, D) Speckle-contrast images under the pre-stimulus and
post-stimulus levels demonstrate response pattern of cerebrocortical microflow, in which arteriolar
and venous blood flow increased clearly due to sciatic nerve stimulation. The gray intensity bar
(C, D) indicates the speckle-contrast values. The darker values correspond to the higher blood
flow (Ref. 54).

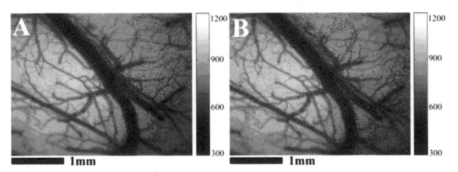

Fig. 9.   Spatial activation map of CBF induced by sciatic nerve stimulation. Two representative
images are selected from the relative blood-flow images with the labeled extremal pixels at double-
peak in temporal domain to display spatial evolution of CBF response across the imaged area.
(A, B) Activated locations of CBF at the first and second peaks. The dotted areas stand for those
changes of CBF that reached extrema at the peak moment (Ref. 54).

early vascular changes, the findings were rather inconsistent.[16,17] During the onset
of CSD, vasoconstriction was found variable and usually brief.[76]

OISI is a neuroimaging technique that allows monitoring of a large region of
the cortex with both high temporal and spatial resolution.[4,11,14] It is particularly
suitable for the investigation of CSD wave propagation.[15,41,61,81]

**Case 3: Simultaneous imaging intrinsic optical signals and cerebral vessel responses during cortical spreading depression in rats[82]**

We investigated the spatiotemporal characteristics of the intrinsic optical signals (IOS) at 570 nm and the cerebral blood vessel responses during CSD simultaneously by optical reflectance imaging *in vivo*. The CSD as induced by pinprick in 10 $\alpha$-chloralose/urethane anesthetized Sprague-Dawley rats. A four-phasic IOS decreased (N1, amplitude: $-2.1\% \pm -1.2\%$, duration: $16.2\,\mathrm{s}\pm 3.8\,\mathrm{s}$), increased (P2, amplitude: $2.9\%\pm 1.6\%$, duration: $13.8\,\mathrm{s}\pm 2.2\,\mathrm{s}$), decreased (N3, amplitude: $-14.2\% \pm -4.5\%$, duration: $40.6\,\mathrm{s}\pm 8.4\,\mathrm{s}$), and then increased (P4, $146.2\,\mathrm{s}\pm 40.3\,\mathrm{s}$). The spatiotemporal evolution of CSD is shown in Fig. 10. Optical reflectance was observed at pial arteries and parenchymal sites, and an initial slight pial arteries dilation $(21.5\%\pm 13.6\%)$ and constriction $(-14.2\%\pm 11.5\%)$ preceding the dramatic dilation $(69.2\% \pm 26.1\%)$ of pial arterioles was recorded. Our experimental results show a high correlation $(r = 0.89 \pm 0.025)$ between the IOS response and the diameter changes of the cerebral blood vessels during CSD in rats. A typical result is shown in Fig. 11.

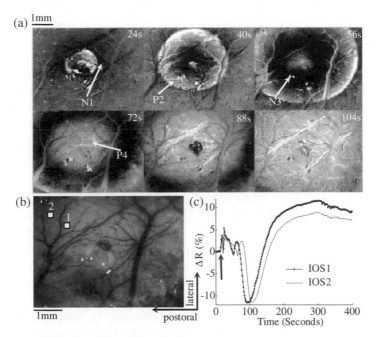

Fig. 10. (a) Spatial pattern of ratio images ($\Delta$ Image) and its progress during the CSD at every 16 s in a rat. The pinprick was induced at the center of the field of view. The four-phasic IOS responses spread from center to periphery. The number labeled at the right top of each graph is the time elapsed after the onset of CSD induction. The arrows of N1, P2, N3, P4 indicate the ring pattern of the four phases of IOS changes. (b) Raw optical reflectance image. (c) The time courses of the optical reflectance changes ($\Delta R$) during CSD in the two parenchymal ROIs marked with white squares in (b). The arrow indicates the time when the CSD was induced (Ref. 82).

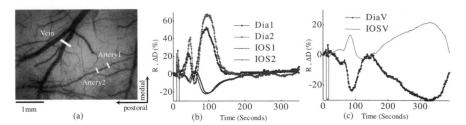

Fig. 11.   Correlation of the temporal pattern of IOS response and the changes of cerebral vessel diameter during CSD in a rat. (a) Raw optical reflectance image. (b) Time course of changes of pial artery diameters ($\Delta D$) in the two chosen section marked in (a) and the corresponding time course of IOS ($\Delta R$) at the arteries site. (c) Time course of changes of vein diameter in the chosen section marked in (a) and the corresponding time course of IOS at the vein site (Ref. 82).

## Case 4: Time-varying spreading depression waves in rat cortex revealed by optical intrinsic signal imaging[61]

The following study aimed to investigate the variation of propagation patterns of successive CSD waves induced by $K^+$ in rat cortex. CSD was elicited by 1 M KCl solution in the frontal cortex of 18 Sprague-Dawley rats under $\alpha$-chloralose/urethane anesthesia. We applied OISI at an isosbestic point of hemoglobin (550 nm) to examine regional CBV changes in the parieto-occipital cortex. In 6 of the 18 rats, OISI was performed in conjunction with the DC potential recording of the cortex. CBV changes appeared as repetitive propagation of wave-like hyperemia at a speed of $3.7 \pm 0.4$ mm/min, which was characterized by a significant negative peak ($-14.3 \pm 3.2\%$) in the reflectance signal (Fig. 12). Among the observed 186 CSDs, the first wave always propagated through the entire imaged cortex in every rat, whereas the following waves that followed were likely to bypass the medial area of the imaged cortex (partially propagated waves, $n = 65$, 35%). A representative result is given in Fig. 13. Correspondingly, DC potential shifts were nonuniform in the medial area, and they seemed closely related to the changes in reflectance.

For partially propagated CSD waves, the mean time interval to the previous CSD wave ($217.0 \pm 24.3$ s) was significantly shorter than that for fully propagated CSD waves ($251.2 \pm 29.0$ s). The results suggest that the propagation patterns of a series of CSD waves are time-varying in different regions of rat cortex, and the variation is related to the interval between CSD waves.

Recently, we also induced a series of CSD waves by pinprick with different intervals as 4 min and 8 min. Qualitatively, we only find the partially propagated CSD waves with 4 min interval's induction of pinprick, but not 8 min. The results imply that the time-varying propagation patterns of a series of CSD waves are not patents of $K^+$. The interval of successive CSD waves affects the spatial pattern of CSD waves. Importantly, the results have shown the inhomogeneous spatiotemporal evolution of CSD. This is an important supplement to the traditional notion, which considers CSD as an "all or none" process.

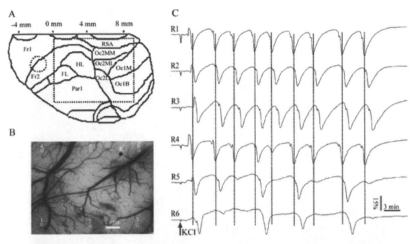

Fig. 12. (A) Schematic dorsal view of the rat brain (Fr1 and Fr2 are frontal cortex area 1 and 2; Par1 is parietal area 1; FL is forelimb area; HL is hind limb area; RSA is regio retrosplenial agranularis; Oc2MM, Oc2ML are occipital cortex area 2 mediomedial part and mediolateral part, respectively; Oc1B and Oc1M are occipital cortex area 1 binocular part and monocular part), the dashed circle (∅ 2 mm) denotes the area of $K^+$ application, and the rectangle corresponds to the imaging area (6.4 × 8.5 mm). (B) A raw optical image and 6 ROIs (5 × 5 pixels, refers to all rats) selected in the parenchyma. The black circle (•) indicates where the electrode was inserted into the cortex (only for six rats). (C) Percent changes of reflectance at 550 nm relative to pre-CSD reflectance, taken from six ROIs (R1–R6). Nine CSDs are observed in these signals; each CSD is characterized with a pronounced negative peak (−14.3 ± 3.2%). The dashed lines indicate the timepoints of the negative peaks in ROI1, and the latency of ROIs 2 and 3 indicates the propagation of CSD waves. Interestingly, the peaks of some CSD waves disappear in ROIs 4, 5 and 6. Calibration: 3 min and 15% (Ref. 61).

### 4.3. *Focal cerebral ischemia*

Focal cerebral ischemia, clinically called stroke, may result in severe or lethal neurological deficits. Ischemia results from a transient or permanent reduction in cerebral blood flow that is restricted to the territory of a major brain artery.[83] Experimental models of stroke have been developed in many species using numerous procedures.[84] Middle cerebral artery occlusion (MCAO) is usually used to model the focal cerebral ischemia in both rodents and primates.[85-88] Due to differences in residual cerebral blood flow (CBF) and metabolism, the ischemic hemisphere consists of ischemic core, ischemic penumbra, and normal tissue.[9,83] The ischemic penumbra is functionally impaired but retains morphological integrity.[83] It is potentially destined for infarction but not irreversibly damaged. The evolution of the ischemic penumbra into infarction is of particular interest.[9,89,90] The primary goal of neuroprotection in focal cerebral ischemia is to salvage the penumbra.[83]

During focal cerebral ischemia, a complex series of pathophysiological events evolve in time and space, including excitotoxicity, cortical spreading depression

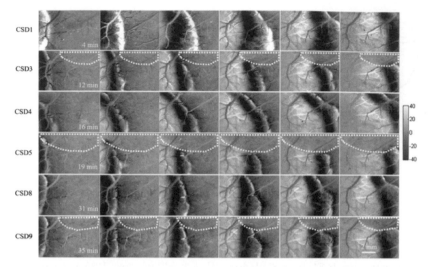

Fig. 13. The spatiotemporal evolution of CSD waves was revealed by subtracting consecutive images. Each row denotes a single CSD wave (the same data with Fig. 12(c), CSD*i* stands for the *i*th CSD wave); the time when the image series was acquired is shown in the leftmost images. The interval between consecutive images is 20 s. Generally, CSD waves showed a bright and sharp arc-shaped wavefront followed first by a dark and broad band and then a dispersive light area. However, some waves (No. 3, 5, and 9) did not spread fully in the observed cortex, bypassing the medial area, primarily RSA, Oc2MM and Oc2ML. Grayscales represent the change in reflectance signal intensity. The scale bar is 2 mm, as given in the last image. (Ref. 61).

(CSD), inflammation, and apoptosis.[83] Among them, CSD is attracting intensive attention for its underlying role in ischemia. It is characterized by a band of neuronal and glial depolarization that propagates like a wave on the cortical surface at a speed of 2–5 mm/min.[75] Peri-infarct depolarization and ischemic depolarization are terms used synonymous to CSD in the ischemic cortex.[72,91] The intermittent CSD waves which spread from the vicinity of the infarcted area have in the past shown to cause a stepwise expansion of the infarct core.[72,92,93] Moreover, therapeutic suppression of CSD minimizes infarct size.[94] Surprisingly, however, pre-conditioning of the normal cortex with CSD enhances the tolerance to focal ischemia.[70]

Although many imaging techniques, including PET,[86,95] MRI,[87,96] laser speckle contrast imaging,[23,39] near infrared spectroscopy[97,98] and autoradiography,[93,99] have been used to study ischemic penumbra, previous studies concentrated on the residual CBF and water flow in the tissue but not on the spontaneous CSD waves. Since CSD has shown to both promote and indicate the evolution of the ischemic lesion, the direct current (DC) potential waves of CSD have been used for acute and long-term monitoring of the penumbral zone.[100] CSD wave propagation was strongly damped in the partial cortex and completely stopped in the infarcted tissue. However, the electrophysiological recording of DC potentials has an inherently low resolution, and thus the origin of CSD waves cannot be exactly determined. On the other hand, OISI is a novel neuroimaging technique that can map a large region of cortex both with high temporal and spatial resolution.[15,17,41,45,81] It is particularly suitable for investigating CSD wave propagation. OISI at 550 nm wavelength is commonly used at least for two reasons: (1) the reflectance is related to the changes in regional cerebral blood volume (CBV) as deoxyhemoglobin and oxyhemoglobin have the same absorbance; (2) the changes in reflectance caused by CSD waves are very prominent at that wavelength.[41] OISI has previously been applied to study the induced CSD by pinprick and $K^+$ in the normal cortex,[15,17,41,45,81] but to our knowledge not to monitor spontaneous developing CSD in the ischemic cortex. So the primary objective of this study is to apply OISI to characterize the series of spontaneous CSD waves following MCAO. In the future, we hope to use these determined characteristics of CSD waves to monitor the evolution of focal cerebral ischemia.

### Case 5: *In vivo* optical reflectance imaging of spreading depression waves in rat brain with and without focal cerebral ischemia[59]

Optical reflectance imaging at $550 \pm 10$-nm wavelength provides high resolution imaging of CSD waves based on the changes in blood perfusion. We present optical images of CSD waves in normal rat brain induced by pinprick (results not shown), and the spontaneous CSD waves that follow MCAO (Fig. 14).

Following MCAO, a series of $n$ spontaneous CSD waves ($n = 10 \pm 4$) developed within 4 h in the animals. For a typical rat, there were 15 CSD episodes. The images of change in reflectance are calculated as $A = (I - I_0)/I_0$, where I is pixel intensity at some timepoint and $I_0$ is the initial intensity just prior to a CSD wave. Time courses of ischemia-induced $A$ signals for six sites in the representative rat are shown in Fig. 15.

Statistically, the signals were primarily characterized by negative peaks ($-12.5\% \pm 2.8\%$) in the medial cortical region near the midline (0.3–2 mm lateral), which were quite similar to peaks observed during induced CSD in the normal cortex. In the lateral cortical region (3.5–6.3 mm lateral), the signal remained flat ($3.1\% \pm 2.5\%$), although the baseline increased. In the intermedial region (2–3.5 mm lateral), the signals showed a transient increase ($12.1 \pm 3.6\%$). The three types of changes implicated the heterogeneity of the ischemic hemisphere, which

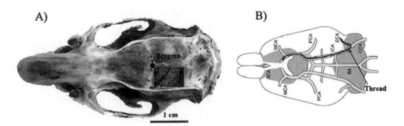

Fig. 14. (A) Top view of the rat skull. The rectangle shows the area of the thinned skull used for optical imaging, located just lateral to the Bregma. (B) A monofilament nylon thread was inserted into the ICA via the ECA to occlude the left medial carotid artery (MCA) (Ref. 59).

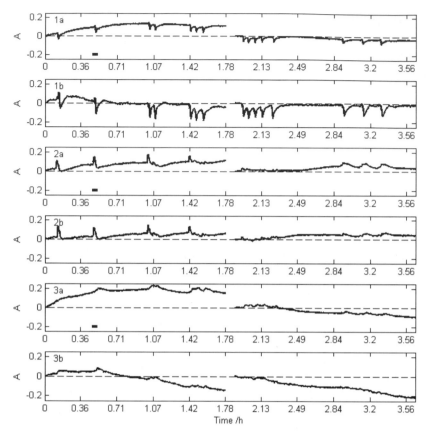

Fig. 15.   Time course of ischemia-induced $A$ signals for six sites (1a, 1b, 2a, 2b, 3a, and 3b in Figs. 16 and 17) to illustrate the reproducibility of the CSD wave signals. Horizontal bar shows the time domain of the data shown in Fig. 18 (Ref. 59).

consisted of normal tissue, ischemic penumbra, and ischemic core. In Fig. 16, the image sequence of ischemia-induced CSD wave was shown as $A$ images. The spatial patterns were consistent with the time courses. In another way, difference in images $B = [I(i) - I(i-1)]/I_0$, where $I(i)$ is the image at time $i$ and $I(i-1)$ is the previous image at time $i - 1$ (a 6.4-s interval), significantly sharpen the boundaries between the leading and trailing edges of the CSD wave (Fig. 17).

Time courses of $A$ and $B$ signals during an ischemia-induced CSD wave corresponding to normal brain, penumbra, and infarct (labeled 1a, 2a, and 3a corresponding to sites in Figs. 16 and 17) are shown in Fig. 18. The penumbra showed a rapid initial rise in the rate-of-change $B$ signal (frames 7–9) that was a signature for the penumbra, corresponding to a rapid constriction of blood volume. The normal brain did not present this initial rise in $B$ signal, but later showed a drop in $B$ signal (frames 16 through 19) due to hyperperfusion. The infarct did not change.

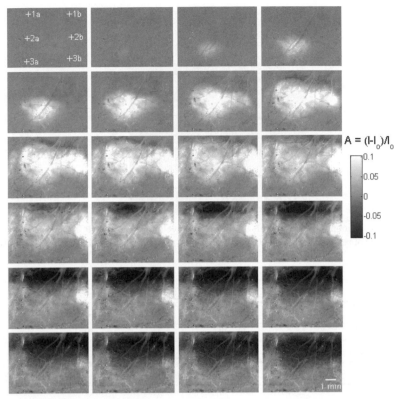

Fig. 16. Image sequence of an ischemia-induced CSD wave in brain after MCAO procedure (A images of relative reflectance), showing one CSD wave. Top region is normal brain (contains sites 1a and 1b), intermediate region is penumbra (2a and 2b), and the lower region is the infarct area (3a and 3b). The CSD wave originates in the penumbra, presenting a white region of increased reflectance due to a drop in cerebral blood volume (CBV). Subsequently, normal brain darkens quickly as reflectance drops below the initial reflectance level due to the hyperperfusion. In contrast, the penumbra returns slowly to normal reflectance with very little hyperperfusion. The infarct area shows no changes (Ref. 59).

Maximum rate-of-change images $C = \max(B)$ display the maximum pixel value of $B$ within the duration of a single CSD wave, and provide an image that visualizes the entire penumbra (Fig. 19). The penumbra appears bright due to a rapid drop in perfusion, while the normal brain and infarct area appear dark. In fact, the results from 2,3,5-triphenyltetrazolium chloride (TTC) staining proved that the brain that suffered spontaneous CSD waves showed infarction in the ipsilateral hemisphere of ischemia (Fig. 21). The pallid area indicated the location of an infarcted region, which was located around the territory of the MCA and accounted for about 70% of the whole left hemisphere area. In the dorsal view of the brain, the infarct area was localized in the lateral region, and the medial area seems physiologically intact.

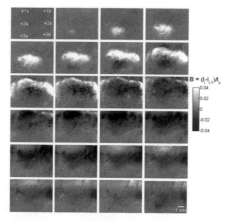

Fig. 17.    Image sequence of an ischemia-induced SD wave in brain after MCAO procedure (*B* images
of rate of change of reflectance). The *B* images highlight the changes seen in Fig. 16. (Ref. 59).

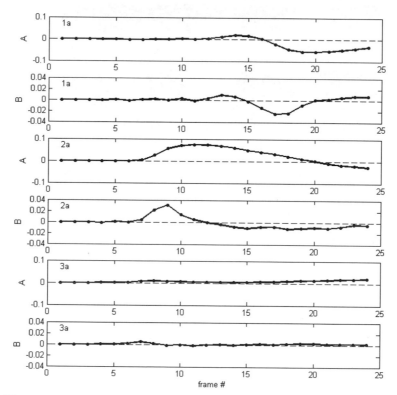

Fig. 18.    Time course of *A* and *B* signals from an ischemia-induced CSD wave corresponding to
normal brain, penumbra, and infarct (labeled 1a, 2a, and 3a corresponding to sites in Figs. 16 and
17). The penumbra shows a rapid initial rise in the rate-of-change *B* signal (frames 7–9) that is
a signature for the penumbra, corresponding to a rapid constriction of blood volume. The normal
brain does not present this initial rise in *B* signal, but later shows a drop in *B* signal (frames 16
through 19) due to hyperperfusion. The infarct does not change (Ref. 59).

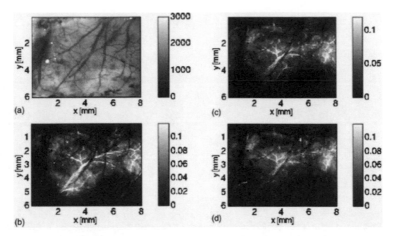

Fig. 19. Maximum rate-of-change images ($C$ images) of the first three CSD waves induced by ischemia. (a) Original image just prior to first CSD wave, shown in units of counts/pixel. (b) First CSD wave, as $C$ image. (c) Second CSD wave. (d) Third CSD wave. Each wave requires about 3 min to propagate over the field of view. These $C$ images show the maximum $B$ signal of each pixel over that time duration. The penumbra (intermediate region of image) shows bright, because each CSD wave elicits a rapid initial rise in reflectance due to a sudden constriction of microvasculature. The normal brain (top region) and infarct (lower region) remain dark. Note that the lower penumbra–infarct boundary is slowly moving upward in (b), (c), and (d), indicating the slow expansion of the infarct and shrinkage of the penumbra. The upper penumbra–normal boundary is stable (Ref. 59).

We were able to prove, for the first time to our knowledge, the useful applicability of OISI based on CSD to distinguish nonischemic cortex, penumbra, and infarct core in the ischemic hemisphere and investigate the evolution of focal cerebral ischemia with high spatial resolution. We believe that OISI can be employed as an efficient tool to assess the efficacy of neuroprotective drugs and treatment methods *in vivo*.

## Case 6: Origin sites of spontaneous cortical spreading depression migrated during focal cerebral ischemia in rats[101]

CSD has been found to occur in the penumbral zone of the brain in rats with focal cerebral ischemia, and has shown to promote expansion of infarction. Electrophysiological recording of CSD has been used for monitoring the penumbral zone,[100] but with an inherently low spatial resolution; consequently, OISI was applied to characterize the spontaneous CSD waves following permanent left side MCAO in rats under $\alpha$-chloralose/urethane anesthesia. Besides the previous report about the regional variation of optical reflectance during spontaneous CSD following MCAO,[36,59] the origin site of CSD was easily determined using OISI with the benefit of high resolution in the present study. Those origin points ($n = 82$) were dynamically located in the ipsilateral hemisphere cortex: sometimes outside of the 6 mm × 8 mm observation area in the parietal cortex ($n = 19$, 23%), and sometimes

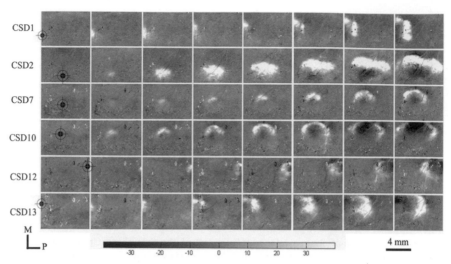

Fig. 20. Origin sites of CSD waves were revealed in the subtracting consecutive images. Each row denotes a single CSD wave (CSD$i$ stands for the $i$th CSD wave). The leftmost image is taken just before CSD appeared in the imaging field (accurate time not shown), and the interval between consecutive images is 6.4 s. Usually, CSD waves began from a small light area (shown in the second image in every row), and then an arc-shaped wavefront spread out from this point peripherally. So the onset spot is defined as the origin site of the CSD wave, which is shown in the first image as the target symbol (⊕). Sometimes the origin of CSD occurred outside of the imaged area. The first landing area of CSD was considered as the origin for easy consideration (examples of CSD1, CSD12, and CSD13). The data shows that the initiation points of those waves were dynamically located in the left hemisphere cortex and the general trend was toward the medial cortex. Notably, the lateral area, which showed few entries of CSD waves, may be infarcted (Fig. 21). Grayscales represent the changes in the intensity of reflectance signal as CCD camera counts. M: medial; P: posterior. The scale bar is 4 mm (Ref. 101).

inside ($n = 63$, 77%). The data showed a general trend toward the medial cortex ($0.40 \pm 0.15$ mm per CSD). Because the lateral cortex of the rat brain proved to be infarcted with 2% TTC staining after 4 h occlusion, the migration of the origin sites implied a growth of the infarcted area. Hence, the determination of the origins of spontaneous CSD using OISI would contribute to the continued study of stroke.

Origin sites of CSD waves were revealed in the subtracting consecutive images in Fig. 20. Usually, CSD waves began from a small light area (shown in the second image in every row), and then an arc-shaped wavefront spread out from this point peripherally. So the onset spot was defined as the origin site of the CSD wave, which was shown in the first image as the target symbol (⊕). In a representative rat (see Fig. 21), all of the 15 origins were drawn as filled circles in a rectangular area on the brain surface corresponding to the imaged area (6 mm × 8 mm) (including the six examples in Fig. 20).

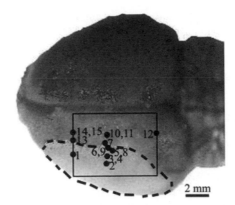

Fig. 21.   Origins of spontaneous CSD migrated during focal cerebral ischemia in a representative rat. All of the 15 origins (including the six examples in Fig. 20.) are drawn as filled circles in a rectangular area on the brain surface corresponding to the imaged area (6 mm × 8 mm). The nearby numbers indicate the order of the 15 waves, and some points of origins overlapped. Although those origin points sometimes were out of the observed area (CSD1, 12, 13, 14, 15) and sometimes were inside (CSD2~11), a general trend toward the medial cortex is shown. Despite the differences resulting from different animals, a reliable phenomenon was the migration of CSD waves' origins. And the general feature was similar: the common trend was toward the medial cortex. These results imply that the growth pattern of the infarction of the lateral area of the rat cortex will be similar. TTC staining proves the infarct of the lateral zone in a rat brain showed few entries of CSD (see Fig. 20). Bar: 2 mm (Ref. 101).

## Acknowledgments

This work was supported by the National Science Fund for Distinguished Young Scholars (Grant No. 60025514), the National Natural Science Foundation of China (Grant Nos. 60478016, 30500115) and the Major Program of Science and Technology Research of Ministry of Education (Grant No. 10420). The authors express their deep gratitude to Weihua Luo, Songlin Ni, and Wenjia Wang for their useful discussion and suggestions.

## References

1. A. Villringer and B. Chance, Non-invasive optical spectroscopy and imaging of human brain function, *Trends Neurosci.* **20**(10) (1997) 435–442.
2. A. Grinvald, *et al.*, *In vivo* optical imaging of cortical architecture and dynamics in *Modern Techniques In Neuroscience Research*, eds. U. Windhorst and H. Johansson (Springer-Verlag, Heidelberg, 1999), pp. 893–969.
3. N. Pouratian, *et al.*, Shedding light on brain mapping: Advances in human optical imaging, *Trends Neurosci.* **26**(5) (2003) 277–282.
4. D. Malonek and A. Grinvald, Interactions between electrical activity and cortical microcirculation revealed by imaging spectroscopy: Implications for functional brain mapping, *Science* **272**(5261) (1996) 551–554.
5. C. S. Roy and C. S. Sherrington, On the regulation of the blood-supply of the brain, *J. Physiol.* **1** (1890) 85–108.

6. A. Villringer and U. Dirnagl, Coupling of brain activity and cerebral blood flow: Basis of functional neuroimaging. *Cerebrovasc. Brain Metab. Rev.* **7**(3) (1995) 240–276.

7. D. Attwell and C. Iadecola, The neural basis of functional brain imaging signals, *Trends Neurosci.* **25**(12) (2002) 621–625.

8. S. G. Kim, Progress in understanding functional imaging signals, *Proc. Natl. Acad. Sci. USA* **100**(7) (2003) 3550–3552.

9. K. A. Hossmann, Viability thresholds and the penumbra of focal ischemia, *Ann. Neurol.* **36**(4) (1994) 557–565.

10. B. Chance, *et al.*, Optical investigations of physiology: A study of intrinsic and extrinsic biomedical contrast, *Philos. Trans. Roy. Soc. Lond. B Biol. Sci.* **352**(1354) (1997) 707–716.

11. R. D. Frostig, *et al.*, Cortical functional architecture and local coupling between neuronal activity and the microcirculation revealed by *in vivo* high-resolution optical imaging of intrinsic signals, *Proc. Natl. Acad. Sci. USA* **87**(16) (1990) 6082–6086.

12. M. Guiou, *et al.*, Cortical spreading depression produces long-term disruption of activity-related changes in cerebral blood volume and neurovascular coupling, *J. Biomed. Opt.* **10**(1) (2005) 11004.

13. P. Li, *et al.*, Spatiotemporal characteristics of cerebral blood volume changes in rat somatosensory cortex evoked by sciatic nerve stimulation and obtained by optical imaging, *J. Biomed. Opt.* **8**(4) (2003) 629–635.

14. D. Malonek, *et al.*, Vascular imprints of neuronal activity: Relationships between the dynamics of cortical blood flow, oxygenation, and volume changes following sensory stimulation, in *Proc. Natl. Acad. Sci. USA* **94**(26) (1997) 14826–14831.

15. A. M. O'Farrell, *et al.*, Characterization of optical intrinsic signals and blood volume during cortical spreading depression, *Neuroreport* **11**(10) (2000) 2121–2125.

16. M. Tomita, *et al.*, Initial oligemia with capillary flow stop followed by hyperemia during K+-induced cortical spreading depression in rats, *J. Cereb. Blood. Flow. Metab.* **25**(6) (2005) 742–747.

17. Y. Tomita, *et al.*, Repetitive concentric wave-ring spread of oligemia/hyperemia in the sensorimotor cortex accompanying K(+)-induced spreading depression in rats and cats, *Neurosci. Lett.* **322**(3) (2002) 157–160.

18. I. Vanzetta, R. Hildesheim and A. Grinvald, Compartment-resolved imaging of activity-dependent dynamics of cortical blood volume and oximetry, *J. Neurosci.* **25**(9) (2005) 2233–2244.

19. A. Grinvald, *et al.*, Functional architecture of cortex revealed by optical imaging of intrinsic signals, *Nature* **324**(6095) (1986) 361–364.

20. D. Y. Ts'o, *et al.*, Functional organization of primate visual cortex revealed by high resolution optical imaging, *Science* **249**(4967) (1990) 417–420.

21. A. Kharlamov, *et al.*, Heterogeneous response of cerebral blood flow to hypotension demonstrated by laser speckle imaging flowmetry in rats, *Neurosci. Lett.* **368**(2) (2004) 151–156.

22. A. Fercher and J. Briers, Flow visualization by means of single exposure speckle photography, *Opt. Commum.* **37** (1981) 326–329.

23. C. Ayata, *et al.*, Laser speckle flowmetry for the study of cerebrovascular physiology in normal and ischemic mouse cortex, *J. Cereb. Blood. Flow. Metab.* **24**(7) (2004) 744–755.

24. C. Ayata, *et al.*, Pronounced hypoperfusion during spreading depression in mouse cortex, *J. Cereb. Blood Flow Metab.* **24**(10) (2004) 1172–1182.

25. T. Durduran, *et al.*, Spatiotemporal quantification of cerebral blood flow during functional activation in rat somatosensory cortex using laser-speckle flowmetry, *J. Cereb. Blood. Flow. Metab.* **24**(5) (2004) 518–525.

26. A. J. Strong, *et al.*, Evaluation of laser speckle flowmetry for imaging cortical perfusion in experimental stroke studies: quantitation of perfusion and detection of peri-infarct depolarisations. *J. Cereb. Blood Flow Metab.* **26**(5) (2006) 645–653.

27. A. Devor, *et al.*, Coupling of the cortical hemodynamic response to cortical and thalamic neuronal activity, *Proc. Natl. Acad. Sci. USA* **102**(10) (2005) 3822–3827.

28. A. Devor, *et al.*, Coupling of total hemoglobin concentration, oxygenation, and neural activity in rat somatosensory cortex, *Neuron* **39**(2) (2003) 353–359.

29. A. K. Dunn, *et al.*, Simultaneous imaging of total cerebral hemoglobin concentration, oxygenation, and blood flow during functional activation, *Opt. Lett.* **28**(1) (2003) 28–30.

30. K. Sato, *et al.*, Intraoperative intrinsic optical imaging of neuronal activity from subdivisions of the human primary somatosensory cortex, *Cereb. Cortex.* **12**(3) (2002) 269–280.

31. H. Bolay, *et al.*, Intrinsic brain activity triggers trigeminal meningeal afferents in a migraine model, *Nat. Med.* **8**(2) (2002) 136–142.

32. J. Cang, *et al.*, Optical imaging of the intrinsic signal as a measure of cortical plasticity in the mouse, *Vis. Neurosci.* **22**(5) (2005) 685–691.

33. J. G. Dubroff, *et al.*, Use-dependent plasticity in barrel cortex: intrinsic signal imaging reveals functional expansion of spared whisker representation into adjacent deprived columns, *Somatosens. Mot. Res.* (2005) **22**(1–2) 25–35.

34. A. K. Dunn, *et al.*, Spatial extent of oxygen metabolism and hemodynamic changes during functional activation of the rat somatosensory cortex, *Neuroimage* **27**(2) (2005) 279–290.

35. M. Nemoto, *et al.*, Analysis of optical signals evoked by peripheral nerve stimulation in rat somatosensory cortex: Dynamic changes in hemoglobin concentration and oxygenation, *J. Cereb. Blood Flow. Metab.* **19**(3) (1999) 246–259.

36. Z. Feng, *et al.*, Dynamic evolution of focal cerebral ischemia in rats observed by optical imaging, *Prog. Biochem. Biophysics* **32**(9) (2005) 871–875.

37. C. Iadecola, From CSD to headache: A long and winding road, *Nat. Med.* **8**(2) (2002) 110–112.

38. T. H. Schwartz and T. Bonhoeffer, *In vivo* optical mapping of epileptic foci and surround inhibition in ferret cerebral cortex, *Nat. Med.* **7**(9) (2001) 1063–1067.

39. A. K. Dunn, *et al.*, Dynamic imaging of cerebral blood flow using laser speckle, *J. Cereb. Blood Flow. Metab.* **21**(3) (2001) 195–201.

40. E. Shtoyerman, *et al.*, Long-term optical imaging and spectroscopy reveal mechanisms underlying the intrinsic signal and stability of cortical maps in V1 of behaving monkeys, *J. Neurosci.* **20**(21) (2000) 8111–8121.

41. A. M. Ba, *et al.*, Multiwavelength optical intrinsic signal imaging of cortical spreading depression, *J. Neurophysiol.* **88**(5) (2002) 2726–2735.

42. H. Cheng, *et al.*, Laser speckle imaging of blood flow in microcirculation, *Phys. Med. Biol.* **49**(7) (2004) 1347–1357.

43. H. Cheng, *et al.*, Efficient characterization of regional mesenteric blood flow by use of laser speckle imaging, *Appl. Opt.* **42**(28) (2003) 5759–5764.

44. H. Cheng, *et al.*, Modified laser speckle imaging method with improved spatial resolution, *J. Biomed. Opt.* **8**(3) (2003) 559–564.

45. P. C. Li, *et al.*, *In vivo* optical imaging of intrinsic signal during cortical spreading depression in rats, *Prog. Biochem. Biophys.* **30**(4) (2003) 605–611.

46. A. Zepeda, C. Arias and F. Sengpiel, Optical imaging of intrinsic signals: recent developments in the methodology and its applications, *J. Neurosci. Methods.* **136**(1) (2004) 1–21.

47. M. Kohl, *et al.*, Physical model for the spectroscopic analysis of cortical intrinsic optical signals, *Phys. Med. Biol.* **45**(12) (2000) 3749–3764.

48. S. A. Prahl, Optical absorption of hemoglobin, http://omlc.ogi.edu/spectra/hemoglobin/summary.html. (1999).

49. J. Briers, Time-varying laser speckle for measuring motion and flow, in *Proc. SPIE* (2001) 4242.

50. S. S. Ulyanov, *et al.*, The applications of speckle interferometry for the monitoring of blood and lymph flow in microvessels, *Lasers. Med. Sci.* **12** (1997) 31–41.

51. J. D. Rigden and E. I. Gordon, The granularity of scattered optical maser light, in *Proc. IRE.* **50** (1962) 2367–2368.

52. J. W. Goodman, "Statistical properties of laser speckle patterns", in *Laser Speckle and Related Topics*, ed. J. C. Dainty, 2nd edn. (Springer-Verlag, Berlin, 1984).

53. J. D. Briers, Laser Doppler, Speckle and related techniques for blood perfusion mapping and imaging, *Physiol. Meas.* **22**(4) (2001) R35–R66.

54. Q. Liu, Z. Wang and Q. Luo, Temporal clustering analysis of cerebral blood flow activation maps measured by laser speckle contrast imaging, *J. Biomed. Opt.* **10**(2) (2005) 024019.

55. J. S. Paul, *et al.*, Imaging the development of an ischemic core following photochemically induced cortical infarction in rats using Laser Speckle Contrast Analysis (LASCA), *Neuroimage* **29**(1) (2006) 38–45.

56. P. Li, *et al.*, Imaging cerebral blood flow through the intact rat skull with temporal laser speckle imaging, *Opt. Lett.* **31**(12) (2006) 1824–1826.

57. R. Nothdurft and G. Yao, Imaging obscured subsurface inhomogeneity using laser speckle, *Optics. Express.* **13**(25) (2005) 10034–10039.

58. S. Ni, *et al.*, Hemodynamic responses to functional activation accessed by optical imaging, in *Proc. SPIE*, **6026** (2006) 602607.

59. S. Chen, *et al.*, *In vivo* optical reflectance imaging of spreading depression waves in rat brain with and without focal cerebral ischemia, *J. Biomed. Opt.* **11**(3) (2006) 13.

60. J. E. Mayhew, *et al.*, Cerebral vasomotion: A 0.1-Hz oscillation in reflected light imaging of neural activity, *Neuroimage* **4**(3, P1) (1996) 183–193.

61. S. Chen, *et al.*, Time-varying spreading depression waves in rat cortex revealed by optical intrinsic signal imaging, *Neurosci. Lett.* **396**(2) (2006) 132–136.

62. G. G. Blasdel and G. Salama, Voltage-sensitive dyes reveal a modular organization in monkey striate cortex. *Nature* **321**(6070) (1986) 579–585.

63. S. Chen, *et al.*, *In vivo* optical imaging of cortical spreading depression in rat, in *Proc. SPIE* **5254** (2004) 262.

64. Y. Liu, *et al.*, The temporal response of the brain after eating revealed by functional MRI, *Nature* **405**(6790) (2000) 1058–1062.

65. S. H. Yee and J. H. Gao, Improved detection of time windows of brain responses in fMRI using modified temporal clustering analysis, *Magn. Reson. Imaging* **20**(1) (2002) 17–26.

66. J. H. Gao and S. H. Yee, Iterative temporal clustering analysis for the detection of multiple response peaks in fMRI, *Magn. Reson. Imaging* **21**(1) (2003) 51–53.

67. V. L. Morgan, *et al.*, Resting functional MRI with temporal clustering analysis for localization of epileptic activity without EEG, *Neuroimage* **21**(1) (2004) 473–481.

68. S. Chen, *et al.*, Combine temporal clustering analysis with least square estimation to determine the dynamic pattern of cortical spreading depression, in *Proc. SPIE* (2006) **6085** 60850D.

69. A. A. P. Leão, Spreading depression of activity in the cerebral cortex, *J. Neurophysiol.* **7** (1944) 359–390.

70. T. Otori, J. H. Greenberg and F. A. Welsh, Cortical spreading depression causes a long-lasting decrease in cerebral blood flow and induces tolerance to permanent focal ischemia in rat brain, *J. Cereb. Blood Flow Metab.* **23**(1) (2003) 43–50.
71. M. Lauritzen, Cortical spreading depression in migraine, *Cephalalgia* **21**(7) (2001) 757–760.
72. K. A. Hossmann, Peri-infarct depolarizations, *Cerebrovasc. Brain Metab. Rev.* **8**(3) (1996) 195–208.
73. G. G. Somjen, Aristides Leao's discovery of cortical spreading depression, *J. Neurophysiol.* **94**(1) (2005) 2–4.
74. H. Martins-Ferreira, M. Nedergaard and C. Nicholson, Perspectives on spreading depression, *Brain Res. Rev.* **32**(1) (2000) 215–234.
75. G. G. Somjen, Mechanisms of spreading depression and hypoxic spreading depression-like depolarization, *Physiol. Rev.* **81**(3) (2001) 1065–1096.
76. M. Lauritzen, Pathophysiology of the migraine aura, The spreading depression theory, *Brain* **117** (Pt 1) (1994) 199–210.
77. Y. Kuge, *et al.*, Effects of single and repetitive spreading depression on cerebral blood flow and glucose metabolism in cats: A PET study, *J. Neurol. Sci.* **176**(2) (2000) 114–123.
78. M. F. James, *et al.*, Cortical spreading depression in the gyrencephalic feline brain studied by magnetic resonance imaging, *J. Physiol.* **519** (Pt 2) (1999) 415–425.
79. A. N. Nielsen, M. Fabricius and M. Lauritzen, Scanning laser-Doppler flowmetry of rat cerebral circulation during cortical spreading depression, *J. Vasc. Res.* **37**(6) (2000) 513–522.
80. A. A. P. Leão, Pial circulation and spreading depression of activity in the cerebral cortex, *J. Neurophysiol.* **7** (1944) 391–396.
81. R. S. Yoon, *et al.*, Characterization of cortical spreading depression by imaging of intrinsic optical signals, *Neuroreport* **7**(15–17) (1996) 2671–2674.
82. P. Li, *et al.*, Simultaneous imaging of intrinsic optical signals and cerebral vessel responses during cortical spreading depression in rats, in *Proc. SPIE* **5254** (2004) 145.
83. U. Dirnagl, C. Iadecola and M. A. Moskowitz, Pathobiology of ischaemic stroke: An integrated view, *Trends Neurosci.* **22**(9) (1999) 391–397.
84. G. Z. Feuerstein and X. Wang, Animal models of stroke, *Mol. Med. Today.* **6**(3) (2000) 133–135.
85. A. J. Strong, *et al.*, Factors influencing the frequency of fluorescence transients as markers of peri-infarct depolarizations in focal cerebral ischemia, *Stroke* **31**(1) (2000) 214–222.
86. P. Frykholm, *et al.*, A metabolic threshold of irreversible ischemia demonstrated by PET in a middle cerebral artery occlusion-reperfusion primate model, *Acta Neurol. Scand.* **102**(1) (2000) 18–26.
87. K. Takano, *et al.*, The role of spreading depression in focal ischemia evaluated by diffusion mapping, *Ann. Neurol.* **39**(3) (1996) 308–318.
88. E. Z. Longa, *et al.*, Reversible middle cerebral artery occlusion without craniectomy in rats, *Stroke* **20**(1) (1989) 84–91.
89. O. W. Witte, *et al.*, Functional differentiation of multiple perilesional zones after focal cerebral ischemia, *J. Cereb. Blood. Flow Metab.* **20**(8) (2000) 1149–1165.
90. W. D. Heiss, Experimental evidence of ischemic thresholds and functional recovery, *Stroke* **23**(11) (1992) 1668–1672.
91. H. Nallet, E. T. MacKenzie and S. Roussel, The nature of penumbral depolarizations following focal cerebral ischemia in the rat, *Brain Res.* **842**(1) (1999) 148–158.

92. G. Mies, T. Iijima and K. A. Hossmann, Correlation between peri-infarct DC shifts and ischaemic neuronal damage in rat, *Neuroreport* **4**(6) (1993) 709–711.
93. M. Nedergaard and J. Astrup, Infarct rim: Effect of hyperglycemia on direct current potential and [14C]2-deoxyglucose phosphorylation, *J. Cereb. Blood Flow Metab.* **6**(5) (1986) 607–615.
94. R. Gill, *et al.*, The effect of MK-801 on cortical spreading depression in the penumbral zone following focal ischaemia in the rat, *J. Cereb. Blood Flow Metab.* **12**(3) (1992) 371–379.
95. S. Pappata, *et al.*, PET study of changes in local brain hemodynamics and oxygen metabolism after unilateral middle cerebral artery occlusion in baboons, *J. Cereb. Blood Flow Metab.* **13**(3) (1993) 416–424.
96. Q. Shen, *et al.*, Pixel-by-pixel spatiotemporal progression of focal ischemia derived using quantitative perfusion and diffusion imaging, *J. Cereb. Blood Flow Metab.* **23**(12) (2003) 1479–1488.
97. J. P. Culver, *et al.*, Diffuse optical measurement of hemoglobin and cerebral blood flow in rat brain during hypercapnia, hypoxia and cardiac arrest, *Adv. Exp. Med. Biol.* **510** (2003) 293–297.
98. T. Wolf, *et al.*, Noninvasive near infrared spectroscopy monitoring of regional cerebral blood oxygenation changes during peri-infarct depolarizations in focal cerebral ischemia in the rat, *J. Cereb. Blood Flow Metab.* **17**(9) (1997) 950–954.
99. M. D. Ginsberg, *et al.*, The acute ischemic penumbra: Topography, life span, and therapeutic response, *Acta Neurochir Suppl.* **73** (1999) 45–50.
100. V. I. Koroleva and J. Bures, The use of spreading depression waves for acute and long-term monitoring of the penumbra zone of focal ischemic damage in rats, in *Proc. Natl. Acad. Sci. USA* **93**(8) (1996) 3710–3714.
101. S. Chen, *et al.*, Origin sites of spontaneous cortical spreading depression migrated during focal cerebral ischemia in rats, *Neurosci. Lett.* **403** (2006) 266–270.

# CHAPTER 6

# THE AUDITORY BRAINSTEM IMPLANT

HIROKAZU TAKAHASHI

*Research Center for Advanced Science and Technology*
*The University of Tokyo*
*4-6-1 Komaba, Megruro-ku, Tokyo 153-8904, Japan*
*takahashi@i.u-tokyo.ac.jp*

MASAYUKI NAKAO

*Department of Engineering Synthesis, Graduate School of Engineering*
*The University of Tokyo*
*7-3-1 Hongo, Bunkyo-ku, Tokyo 113-8656, Japan*
*nakao@hnl.t.u-tokyo.ac.jp*

KIMITAKA KAGA

*National Institute of Sensory Organs*
*2-5-1 Higashigaoka, Menguru-ku*
*Tokyo 152-0021, Japan*
*kimikaga-tky@umin.ac.jp*

Auditory brainstem implants (ABI) that electrically stimulate the surface of cochlear nucleus have been clinically used for the rehabilitation of deaf patients typically with bilateral vestibular schwannomas. This chapter reviews the history and presents status of ABIs, as well as our recent animal studies that show the promising capability of the neural prosthesis. At present, the change of pitch perception with an active electrode location is not as clear in ABIs as in cochlear implants, a factor which might play a role in poorer speech performance in ABIs. On the other hand, our experimental results demonstrated that microstimulation of both the dorsal and the ventral cochlear nucleus (DCN and VCN) could reproduce a similar cortical place code of intensity and frequency to the acoustically produced code. We also found that the cortical dynamic range was wider for the DCN than VCN stimulation and for the low-frequency pathway than for the high-frequency pathway. These results shed light on future studies on the primary problem about how to produce clear pitch percepts, and they have great implications for improved ABI performance.

## 1. Clinical Study

Cochlear implants and auditory brainstem implants (ABIs) have been clinically used as auditory neural prostheses in order to restore a sense of hearing.[1] The cochlear implant electrically stimulates auditory nerves, whereas ABI stimulates a secondary processing center in the auditory neural system, i.e. the cochlear nucleus. ABI is an option for patients who have no intact auditory nerves and thereby cannot benefit from the cochlear implant.

More than 650 ABIs (approximately 600 by Cochlear Corp., the leading company for ABI development) have been implanted at present (2006) since the first implantation in 1979. According to clinical reports, ABI is able to elicit some hearing senses, but shows poorer performance of an understanding of speech as compared to the cochlear implant. Extensive studies are still required to improve the performance from both clinical and physiological aspects. In this section, we will overview ABI from a clinical aspect.

## 1.1. *History and system description*

Figure 1 illustrates a normal auditory system from an ear to the auditory cortex, and the ABI system that bypasses the auditory pathway. In a normal auditory system, a sound wave is amplified and transmitted through an outer and middle ear to a cochlea, a snail-shaped transducer, where sensory hair cells in lymph convert the vibration into electrical impulses, which are then transmitted to the cochlear nucleus in the medulla through the auditory nerves. Because the cochlea has a low resonance frequency at the apical turn and high resonance frequency at the basal turn, hair cells and their postsynaptic afferent fibers, i.e. auditory nerves, at the cochlear base discharge preferentially to high-frequency sound, whereas those at the cochlear apex respond to low-frequency sound.[2-4] Thus, the cochlea maps frequency contents of sound along an epithelial array of receptors, producing a place code of frequency, referred to as a tonotopic map or tonotopic organization. This tonotopic analysis is used in the higher-order auditory brainstem pathway from the cochlear nucleus through the superior olivary nuclei in the medulla, inferior colliculus in the midbrain, and the medial geniculate nucleus in the thalamus to the auditory cortex.

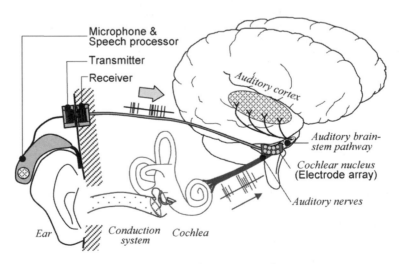

Fig. 1.   Auditory brainstem implant.

Deficits in the auditory system can cause many different hearing losses. Depending on the causes, different auditory prostheses have been developed so far. A hearing aid acoustically amplifies sounds, and can remedy a conductive hearing loss due to defects in either the outer or the middle ear.[5,6] Middle ear prosthesis has been designed as another option for a conductive hearing loss that directly vibrates the oval window of the cochlea.[7,8] For profound deafness due to loss of the sensory hair cells, the cochlear implant directly activates the auditory nerve by an electrode array inserted in the cochlea.[1,9–11] The cochlear implant is one of the most successful neural prostheses. A significant proportion of the recipients can converse on the phone, and most children with the device can learn in mainstream classrooms. The cochlear implant, however, does not bring any benefit to some profoundly deaf individuals without intact auditory nerves. For these individuals, ABI targets the upstream cochlear nucleus with an implanted electrode array analogous to the cochlear implant.[12–26] A tonotopic map found in the cochlear nucleus like in the cochlea is a rationale of ABI feasibility.[27–32]

The pioneer of ABI is the House Ear Institute in the United States, and Cochlear Corp. in Australia has led the development. The ABI system is basically similar to the cochlear implant system, which is composed of an implantable electrode array, a transcutaneous coil transmitter/receiver system, and an external speech processor and microphone (Fig. 1). The current ABI electrode array available from Cochlear Corp. since 1998 has 21 platinum disk electrodes each with a diameter of 0.7 mm in an 8.5-mm by 3-mm silicone elastomer substrate. Fibrous tissue, called Dacron, encapsulated the array in order to enhance the stabilization on the brainstem (Fig. 2(a)). In addition to these surface electrode arrays, implantation of a penetrating microelectrode array, which may better access the tonotopic organization in the cochlear nucleus, has been approved for the clinical trial by Food and Drug Administration (FDA) in the United States since 2002 (Fig. 2(b)). Other ABIs are produced by MED-EL Corp. in Austria[33] and MXM Medical Technologies in France.[34]

Figure 3 shows the history of the ABI electrode array.[14] In 1979, a pair of ball electrodes was implanted for the first time into the substance of the cochlear nucleus.[12] Although the stimulation with the electrode could produce useful auditory sensations, migration of the electrode resulted in lower extremity sensory

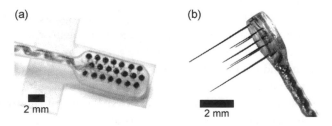

Fig. 2.   ABI electrode array. Courtesy of Nihon Cochlear Co. Ltd.

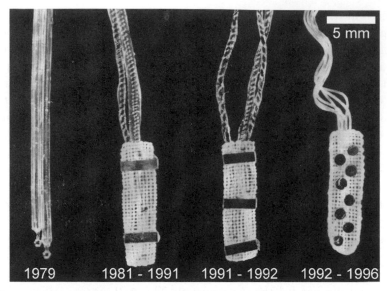

Fig. 3. History of the ABI electrode array. Reprinted from Ref. 14 with permission from American Academy of Otolaryngology — Head and Neck Surgery Foundation, Inc.

side effects. In 1981, a pair of surface plate electrode replaced the ball electrodes,[13] and a three-plate electrode array was developed in 1991. These designs allowed inserting the electrode array into the lateral recess of the fourth ventricle. The Dacron mesh carrier was also introduced in this model. In 1992, a current form of ABI with eight disk electrodes was developed and used in more than 100 cases until 1999. Through these clinical trials, FDA approved ABI in 2000.

## 1.2. *Implantation*

The candidates for ABI are mostly diagnosed as having bilateral vestibular schwannomas, the Schwann cell tumors which bilaterally invade on the vestibular branch of the eighth cranial nerves (the auditory nerves). Their damage of bilateral auditory nerves results in complete hearing loss. Among 50,000 patients worldwide afflicted with this condition, the most common type of neuromas is of neurofibromatosis type 2 (NF2), a genetic disease occurring approximately in one out of 40,000 births (Fig. 4).[35–37] Recently, research has expanded the indications for ABI implantation to subjects with other cochlear or cochlear nerve malfunctions who cannot benefit from the cochlear implant (e.g. cochlear nerve aplasia, avulsion, cochlear ossification, and cochlear fracture).[23,24]

Prior to the implantation, tumors are usually removed through an opening in the mastoid bone behind the ear down to the lateral recess of the fourth ventricle, which is close to the cochlear nucleus. This translabyrinthine surgical approach can provide the best access and visualization of the target region.[38,39] When the tumors

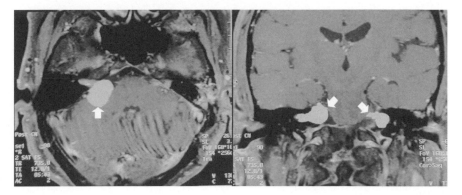

Fig. 4.   MRI image of NF2. Arrows indicate tumors.

are too large to keep the brainstem in a normal position, the implantation of ABI is performed on another day. The cochlear nucleus is unfortunately invisible to the surgeon, and therefore must be explored in relation to some anatomical landmarks (Fig. 5(a)). Once the electrode array is placed around the cochlear nucleus, evoked potentials by electrical stimulation through the tentatively implanted electrodes (electrically evoked auditory brainstem responses; e-ABR) are monitored to examine

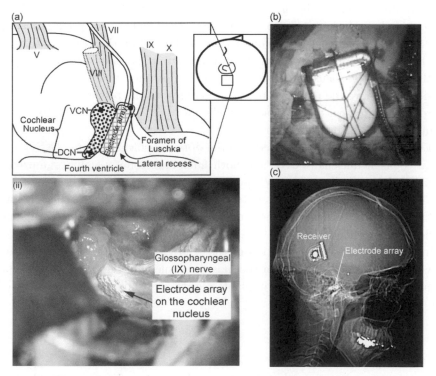

Fig. 5.   Implantation of ABI. (a) Electrode array. (i) Illustration of anatomical landmarks. (ii) View of implantation. (b) Internal receiver. (c) X-ray image of a skull of the ABI recipient.

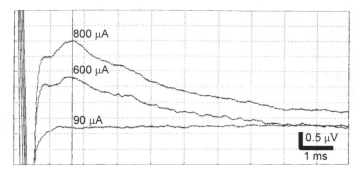

Fig. 6. Intraoperative e-ABR. Responses develop with increasing current of brainstem stimulation.

whether the array is correctly placed on the cochlear nucleus (Fig. 6).[14,40-42] The presence of e-ABR is a sign that the stimulation activates the auditory system, whereas the stimulation-induced myogenic activities in the ipsilateral masseter or pharyngeal muscles indicate that the electrodes are incorrectly placed on other cranial nerves. Incorrect positioning leads to postsurgical side effects. Thus, the placement of ABI electrodes is finally determined so that e-ABR is maximized and other myogenic activities are minimized.

In animal studies, the non-toxic fluorescent axonal tracers, Fast Blue or Fluorogold, have been tested to intraoperatively identify the proximal auditory nerves and cochlear nucleus.[43] Four to seven days after the tracers are injected into the cochlea, appropriate ultraviolet illumination can label the auditory nerve and the cochlear nucleus as colored fluorescence on the living brain. This kind of technique will have the potential to aid surgeons with the proper positioning of the electrode array in near future especially when a brain is anatomically distorted due to tumor growth or preceding surgery.

The cochlear nucleus is divided into the dorsal cochlear nucleus (DCN) and the ventral cochlear nucleus (VCN), and both nuclei are tonotopically organized.[27-32] Existing ABIs usually stimulate the posterior part of VCN, because VCN is considered the mainstream of auditory pathways. More ventral placement, i.e. directly over VCN, tends to produce non-auditory stimulation of other cranial nerves and flocculus of the cerebellum.

In addition to the implantation of the ABI electrode array, a transcutaneous receiver is implanted and fixed in the mastoid bone (Fig. 5(b)). This procedure is the same as that in the cochlear implant. Figure 5(c) shows an X-ray image of the skull after the surgery.

### 1.3. Rehabilitation

Six or eight weeks after the surgery, audiologists adjust electrical currents for each electrode through the speech processor so that the stimuli produce adequate auditory percepts. This procedure is called "mapping" of ABI electrodes.

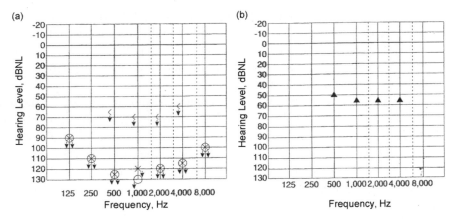

Fig. 7.   Audiograms of the ABI recipient. (a) Presurgery audiogram showing that complete loss of hearing bilaterally. (b) Postsurgery audiogram demonstrating improvement of hearing threshold.

The mapping is repeated every three months in our institute. Figure 7 shows an example of pre and postsurgery audiograms. The results indicate that ABI produced some kind of auditory percepts when each electrode was pulsed. However, an understanding of speech by ABI hearing was impossible. This performance level is similar to that of a single channel cochlear implant that was attempted three decades ago.

According to other recent reports, ABI electrodes in an adequate position can elicit auditory percepts in most cases. The threshold charge per pulse to evoke the percepts is 30–50 nC on average, which is similar or slightly higher than the cochlear implant.[16]

ABI recipients describe that the quality of the sound percept produced by ABI can be likened to a bass guitar, a horn, a bell, a honking car, and so on.[16,20] In terms of pitch perception, in approximately half of recipients, a percept pitch tends to increase in a lateral-to-medial direction across the electrode array.[18,20] In a significant number of the remaining recipients, however, a percept pitch was random or flattened across electrodes.

ABI hearing generally improves abilities of detection and discrimination of environmental sounds. In addition, in terms of communication ability, ABI can significantly improve speech recognition under a lip-reading condition. On sentence recognition tests, the discrimination scores increase by 25%–50% for lip-reading with ABI hearing as compared to lip-reading only. Thus, auditory perception by ABI can be useful cues for lip-reading.[14–22] However, ABI hearing without lip-reading cannot generally bring speech recognition ability. Exceptionally, a small number of ABI recipients can achieve free speech understanding, and use a telephone as recipients of cochlear implant do.[18] These reports suggest the potential of ABI and encourage the continuing efforts to improve the average performance.

There is a significant correlation between modulation detection thresholds and speech understanding, suggesting that the cochlear nucleus has a separate pathway specialized for modulated sounds. In addition, non-NF2 ABI recipients show significantly higher performance of modulation detection and speech understanding than NF2 ABI recipients.[24] There is a possibility that, in NF2 patients, the tumor and surgery selectively damage the pathway responsible for modulated sounds, resulting in poor speech recognition with ABI.

Positron emission tomography (PET) imaging demonstrates that functional speech processing of ABI recipients elicits activation in the auditory cortex and other cortical regions classically associated with speech processing.[44−47] The degrees of success in speech processing of ABI are reflected in the resultant PET images. In contrast, subjects who could not achieve functional speech processing had activation in the frontal cortex, suggesting that other cognitive strategies are used to assist speech processing.

In general, electrical stimulation from ABI does not result in any serious complication. However, there are two major postoperative problems. First, ABI recipients must take long lasting auditory rehabilitation and lip-reading training because the auditory perception is incomplete. Generally, lip-reading enhancement improves within the first six months, which is required for relearning and adaptation of the central auditory system to the altered form of auditory information by ABI.[19] Second, there are considerable non-auditory side effects of ABI, which are described as mild tingling or twinge sensations in the head and body, because the electrodes have to be placed near non-auditory cranial nerves (see Fig. 5(a)). Approximately 60% of these side effects are in the head ipsilateral to the implantation.[16,17] Electrodes are deactivated when the stimulation elicits non-auditory side effects or when the stimulation fails to elicit auditory perception. The number of activated electrodes is 40%–70% of the total on average, and recently increasing up to 60%–80% owing to the surgical improvements.[21,22] Once the ABI electrode array is implanted and fixed, there are almost no observable shifts in the electrode position over a decade or longer.[13,14]

Although the efficacy of ABIs is only limited to lip-reading enhancement today, 83% of the recipients have agreed that they benefit from the use of ABIs, and 85% have agreed that their decision to avail of ABI was the right one, according to a recent survey ($n = 88$).[18,20] The survey indicates that ABI improves the quality of life of the recipients. At the same time, it also indicates their high hopes of obtaining any auditory information however poor the quality is, and encourages the continuing development of better ABIs.

## 2. Animal Study

### 2.1. *Overview*

A successful development of a neural prosthesis will depend on well-balanced efforts on clinical studies, animal studies, and device designs. In particular, animal studies have provided a number of useful design parameters that improve the safety and performance of ABI for the chronic use. These studies mainly included the identification of the safe stimulation level on the basis of histological observations of stimulation-induced tissue injury,[48–58] and the design of the penetrating array.[59–64] In addition, of great value in developing a neural prosthesis involving the central nervous system is the development of animal models that can directly demonstrate the possibility and capability and provide clues to the better strategies of microstimulation on the basis of physiological data. Such animal models can encourage the continuing development of the prosthesis in spite of poor results of pilot clinical trials.

### 2.1.1. *Safety viewpoint*

Prolonged electrical stimulation of even moderate intensity could damage nervous tissue histologically. Several evidences imply that these damages are caused by neuronal hyperactivity due to repeated passage of the stimulus current through neural tissues, rather than by electrochemical reactions at the electrode–tissue interface.[49] First, prolonged stimulation for a few weeks by faradic electrodes produces neural damages, while capacitor electrode stimulation does not. Second, short-term stimulation for 4–7 hours selectively damages neurons resulting in stellate shrunken hyperchromic forms or intracellular edema, while Glia cells appear normal. The selective damage of neurons can be the consequence of metabolic events associated with hyperactivity. Prolonged stimulation for 50 hours also induces considerable gliosis with an increased number of astrocytes,[50] and calcification in neurons.[51] High-intensity stimulation can affect all type of cells and produce an infarct.

A number of animal studies attempted to identify the safe level of electrical stimulation in the brain. First, charge-balanced biphasic pulses proved better than monophasic pulses to avoid neural damages.[52,53] Second, both the charge and the charge density per phase of the stimulus waveform have been considered as important parameters to identify the threshold of neural damage.[48,49,54,55] The charge per phase is defined as the integral of the stimulus current over one phase of one cycle. The charge density is defined as the charge per phase divided by the electrode surface area. The boundary between safe and unsafe charge injections is empirically described as

$$\log(D) = k - \log(Q),$$

where $D$ is the charge density in $\mu C/cm^2/phase$, $Q$ is the charge in $g\mu C/phase$, and $k$ is a constant.[56] Neural damages are observed at $k = 2$ or larger, while $k = 1.5$ is considered safe (Fig. 8). These results can serve as a useful guideline for designing the electrode dimension and stimulation protocol.

Even below the safe stimulation level, the electrical excitability of neurons becomes suppressed without histologically detectable tissue injury when the stimulation rate is high, i.e. on the order of 250 Hz, and when the localization

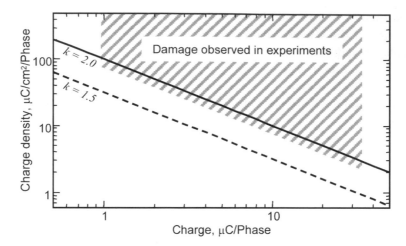

Fig. 8.   Charge and charge density that induce neural damage.

of stimulus current is so high that neurons close to microelectrodes are excited repeatedly.[57,58] A few hours of high-rate microstimulation in the cochlear nucleus causes prolonged stimulation-induced depression of neuronal excitability (SIDNE), and short-acting neuronal refractivity (SANR) in evoked potentials in the upstream nucleus, the inferior colliculus. SIDNE persists for many hours or even days after the end of the high-rate stimulation, while SANR is apparent only during the stimulation. Although the consequences of both SIDNE and SANR are still unclear, these effects may cause degradation of the ABI performance at the safe level. A stimulation protocol should be designed so as to minimize the sum of the SIDN and SANR specifically for the penetrating microelectrode array, which produces localized high-density currents as compared with the conventional surface electrode stimulation and repeated excitations of a particular neuronal population.

### 2.1.2. Functional viewpoint

As mentioned previously, the quality of the sound percept reported by ABI recipients can be likened to a bass guitar, a horn, or a bell, suggesting that ABI stimuli unselectively and broadly activate auditory neurons corresponding to a wide frequency range. In addition, stimulation via different electrodes of the array evokes different auditory sensations, but continues to produce ambiguous pitch perception.

The limitations of the surface electrode array may be the cause of poor performance of ABI. Intuitively, a surface array may have a poor access to the three-dimensional place code of frequency information, i.e. the tonotopic organization, in the cochlear nucleus. Moreover, surface stimulation requires a high-amplitude current to activate neural populations and, due to the spread of the electrical current, may not be able to target a distinct population of neurons. Thus, previous works have pointed out that a penetrating array is more efficient than a surface array in terms of accessing the tonotopic organization, and achieving a lower threshold, wider dynamic range, and higher selectivity of activation.[59–64] However, the penetration itself may trade off a risk of irreversible tissue injury.[64] Moreover, the stimulation produces localized high-density currents as compared with the conventional surface electrode stimulation, resulting in SINDE and SANR.[57,58] The optimization of these design parameters is still a challenging work to improve the ABI performance.

In addition, we are in desperate need of electrophysiological studies that demonstrate the neurological consequences of cochlear nuclear stimulation and optimize the microstimulation. First, we need to confirm whether the micro-stimulation can precisely target the appropriate place code of both intensity and frequency, i.e. the ampli-tonotopic organization, and trigger the corresponding intrinsic neuronal responses after the targeted information has been relayed at least once. Indeed, some earlier works have recorded tonotopically localized activation in the inferior colliculus following electric stimulation of the cochlear nucleus, suggesting a successful creation of pitch perception.[59,60,65] However, this may simply reflect the fact that the cochlear nucleus partly has direct projections to the inferior colliculus,[66,67] and there is a possibility that other pathways are crucial to relay the tonotopic information accurately to the upstream nuclei. In addition, the encoding of intensity perception in combination with pitch perception is poorly understood to date. Thus, further studies are necessary to support the claim that sound information of frequency and intensity can accurately reach the higher-level auditory nuclei, e.g. the auditory cortex.

Furthermore, we need to establish a model of where and how to microstimulate the cochlear nucleus such that intended frequency and intensity information are most efficiently encoded. For example, although VCN is considered as the mainstream in the auditory system and targeted in ABI, there is little direct evidence showing that the microstimulation of VCN is more efficient than that of DCN in evoking accurate and distinguishable nerve activation representing frequency and intensity. The stimulation strategy of ABI, which is currently adopted from that of cochlear implant and thereby designed for auditory nerve stimulation, may not be optimized for the cochlear nuclear stimulation. In the following sections, we review our recent works that attempted to answer these questions.[68–71]

## 2.2. Animal model of ABI

Obviously, extensive works are still required to develop the next-generation ABI, which may produce clearer pitch perception and improve the performance on speech recognition. Toward this end, we designed a rat model of ABI to obtain much needed physiological data, which can compare cortical activities elicited by tone bursts and those by microstimuli presented to the cochlear nucleus (Fig. 9). In the model, we first need to objectively interpret the auditory perception that animals experience.

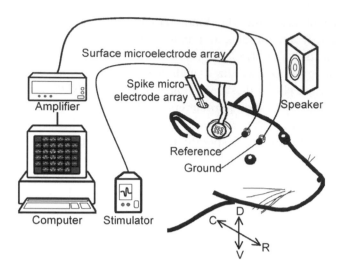

Fig. 9. An animal model of ABI. Reprinted from Ref. 68. © 2005 IEEE.

As a solution to this problem, we have developed a surface microelectrode array to acquire the evoked-potential patterns over the auditory cortex and unravel the cortical representation of intensity and frequency. Second, for the microstimulation to the cochlear nucleus, we have also developed a penetrating microelectrode array.

In the following experiments, we first characterize the auditory cortical representation of intensity and frequency by dense AEP mapping. Second, we show the direct evidence of the feasibility of ABI; the microstimulation can trigger the intrinsic neuronal processing of frequency and intensity information, and this information can reach the auditory cortex. Third, in order to derive further implication for the development of future ABI, we expand the stimulating target from VCN to DCN, and compare the cortical activities evoked by the microstimulation of DCN and those of VCN.

### 2.2.1. Auditory cortex of rat

In the ABI animal model, we first need to know the detailed auditory cortical representation of frequency and intensity information. The place code of frequency made in the cochlea is inherited in the higher systems, and the auditory cortex also represents sound information tonotopically. The auditory cortex, however, has several tonotopically organized auditory fields, and the entire cortical representation is not satisfactorily identified to date. In addition, how the auditory cortex handles other modalites of sound such as intensity remains unknown.

Cytoarchitectonic, connectional, and physiological studies have so far delineated multiple auditory fields in mammalian cortices, suggesting the parallel and hierarchical processing of auditory information.[72] These studies, for example, have first showed that the rat auditory cortex can be subdivided into the core and belt areas[73] (see Fig. 17). The core cortex, located in area $41^{74,75}$ or TE1,[76] features a large number of granular cells in layer IV, dense myelinated fibers, and direct projections mainly from the ventral division of the medial geniculate body (MGv).[77–79] In contrast, the belt cortex, usually labeled in areas 20 and 36, or TE2 and TE3, has less granular cells, less myelination, and main projections from the dorsal division of the medial geniculate body (MGd). The direct stimulation of MGv and MGd also evoked confined responses in area 41, and areas 20 and 36, respectively, suggesting that the multiple fields are originated from parallel auditory pathways with separate thalamocortical inputs.[80,81] These evidences for multiple fields suggest that each field plays a different role in the encoding of sound information.

In fact, many unit studies have elucidated that both the core and belt areas contain multiple fields, each of which has a different tonotopic organization. Earlier works on rats have first demonstrated a clear tonotopic organization within the primary auditory field (AI), and some tonotopic discontinuity around AI suggesting multiple fields.[82,83] Other studies have then noted an additional tonotopic organization within the anterior[84,85] and the posterior fields.[86] These studies have also found interfield differences in a tuning property and responsive latency at a single neuron level. Furthermore, some unit studies have noted interfield differences in the sensitivity to particular temporal changes and aspects of sound intensity, suggesting that each field serves as a different temporal filter that extracts a particular dynamic temporal change.[87,88] These evidences at a single neuron level suggest that interfield differences are important for the integration of auditory information.

At a field level, however, the existence of the interfield difference in a place code of intensity, i.e. amplitopic organization, has been controversial for years,[88–92] since such an organization was found in a particular part of the bat auditory cortex.[93] Previous works characterized auditory neurons as having non-monotonic properties of discharge rates with respect to sound pressure level (SPL) of test tones and explored the orderly distribution of the so-called best SPLs that induced the highest discharge rate. Since high-intensity tones generally activate monotonic neurons rather than non-monotonic neurons, the best SPL is often hard to be found at a high SPL. Rather, a few studies using techniques other than unit recording, e.g. extrinsic optical recording[94] and auditory evoked potential (AEP) recording,[95,96] implied that the spatial coordinate of intensity may exist in a different form from the best SPL.

## 2.2.2. *Auditory evoked potentials*

In order to further address the encoding of sound in the multiple fields in the auditory cortex, we attempt to rough out the cortical representation by densely mapping AEP. Tone bursts produced AEP patterns reflecting spatiotemporally synchronized activities over the auditory cortex. Typically, a high-intensity tone

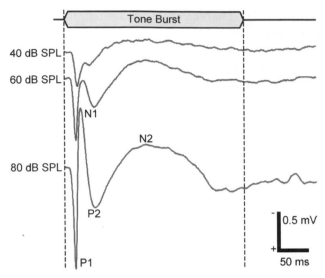

Fig. 10.    Auditory evoked potential and definition of the wave (P1, N1, P2, N2). Reprinted from Ref. 69 with permission from Elsevier.

produces AEP constituting typical peaks of P1, N1, P2, and N2, which are labeled according to their polarity and latency, but low- or moderate-intensity tones sometimes resulted in irregular AEP waveforms with a small N1 (Fig. 10).

Extensive studies have unraveled that the AEP complex has a biophysical origin in the auditory cortex. First, lesion of the auditory cortex severely affected the AEP.[97] Second, laminar analyses also found major contributors in the depth of the auditory cortex.[97–99] Furthermore, the origin of P1/N1 is probably the direct thalamocortical input. First, the cortical mapping of P1/N1 showed confined foci of activation in the auditory cortex, and some of them demonstrated the tonotopic organization.[68–70,81,99–102] Second, the direct stimulation of the medial geniculate body (MGB) evoked P1/N1 confined within the auditory cortex.[80,81]

The potential reflects immediate effects of thalamocortical input as well as intracortical processing, and is usually dominated by excitatory inputs. In addition, AEP recording is a population measurement of summed activities of neurons with different properties. Recording of spike potentials, on the other hand, characterizes the property of the sortable auditory neuron that reflects intracortical processing; specifically, inhibitory inputs mediate an initiation of spike potential and thereby significantly modify the tuning property of the neuron. AEP therefore can measure only the monotonic growth of responses with increasing SPL as an intensity index, but cannot measure precise intensity tuning, e.g. best SPL. Furthermore, volume conduction effects of the low-frequency local field potential (LFP) decay with a space constant in the order of $500\,\mu$m, while the space constant of spike potentials are in the order of $50\,\mu$m.[103–105] Due to these aspects, AEP-based characterization becomes obscure, and in fact the frequency tuning curve bandwidth of LFP is three to four times wider as compared to those of unit recording.[105,106] Having them in mind, we designed the grid of AEP recording points at 400 μm, and expect the overall characteristics at a field level, which may bridge the previous detailed characterizations at a single neuron level.

### 2.2.3. *Surface microelectrode array*

Stable electromechanical contact of the electrodes to the cortex is one of the most important requirements to reliably measure the cortical evoked potential. The arbitrary curvature of the cortical surface makes it difficult to apply uniform contact. To counter this problem, some previous works using a grid array of conventional microelectrodes filed the arrays into concave shapes to match the convex cortical surface.[99,100] A microelectrode array on a flexible substrate is a better option for the recording because the substrate like material naturally matches the curved surface (Fig. 11).[70] The flexible polyimide ribbon can also follow small movements from breathing or other spontaneous movements, and the recording points can always be in contact with their targets. The array had a conductive gold layer, which was sandwiched by the polyimide substrate and another polyimide insulating layer except for the recording points.

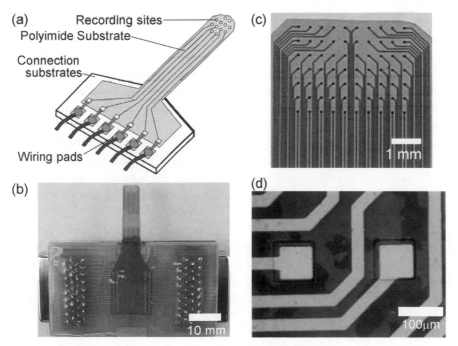

Fig. 11.   Surface microelectrode array. (a) Conceptual scheme. (b) Whole view. (c) Magnification of the recording area. (d) Magnification of the recording sites.

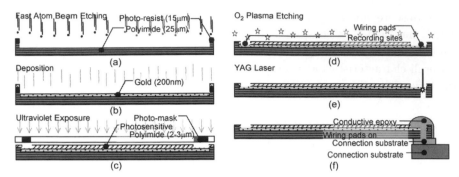

Fig. 12.　Process flow of surface microelectrode array. (a) Groove etching with the fast atom beam. (b) Depositing a conductive layer. (c) Producing an insulating layer pattern. (d) Removing a residual insulating layer over recording points and wiring pads. (e) Opening through-holes for wiring. (f) Wiring pads to connection substrates.

Figure 12 shows the process flow of producing our surface microelectrode array. A 25-$\mu$m thick polyimide film (Toray Du Pont, Kapton 100H) is spin coated with a 15-$\mu$m thick positive photoresist (Tokyo Ohka Kogyo Co. Ltd., AZ4903) and then exposed to ultraviolet light through a photomask. After the developing process, fast atom beams dry-etch the laminate to dig a 1-$\mu$m-deep pattern on the polyimide film (a). A conducting gold layer of thinckness 0.2 $\mu$m is then deposited over the surface after a small quantity of chromium deposition to promote gold–polyimide bond (b). Then the photoresist layer is removed, and sub-micron thick photosensitive polyimide (Toray, Photoneece) is spin coated over the surface as an insulating layer. The laminate is then locally exposed to ultraviolet light (c) to spot remove the last insulating layer over an 80-$\mu$m-square where the recording points are and over a 400-$\mu$m-square where the wiring pads are. Finally, residual photosensitive polyimide over the recording points is completely removed by $O_2$ plasma etching (d). We then connect the polyimide substrate and the connection substrates which are separately designed print-circuit boards. Using YAG laser a 100-$\mu$m-square through-hole in each wiring pad of the polyimide substrate is made (e). After cutting the substrate into a proper size, wiring pads on the substrate are connected to corresponding ones on the connection substrates by filling the holes with conductive epoxy (f).

The surface microelectrode array with polyimide bases had been reported over the past 30 years.[107–112] Our array features a damocene structure of embedding the wiring that significantly improves the process yield and the wiring durability. The array we designed had 70 recording points in a 3.5 by 3-mm area that covered the entire auditory cortex including the primary AI, anterior auditory field (AAF), and ventral auditory field (VAF) (see Fig. 17).[68,69,83–85,96,101,102] Each recording site was 80 by 80 $\mu$m. Figure 13 shows the measured impedance, whose magnitude and phase at 1 kHz was 330 k$\Omega$ and $-66°$ on average with a standard deviation (SD) of 65-k$\Omega$ and 2°, respectively.

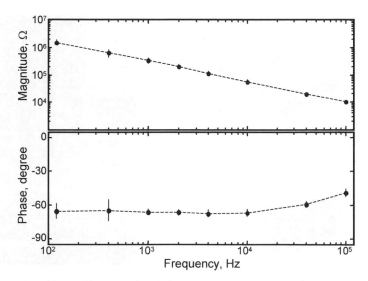

Fig. 13. Impedance spectroscopy of the surface microelectrode in the physiologic saline solution. Means and standard deviations are given ($n = 45$). The multifrequency LCR meter (Yokogawa Hewlett Packard, 4274A) measured the impedance of each recording point at 50 mV. In the measurement, a 3 cm² gold-deposited glass plate served as a counter electrode, and an Ag/AgCl electrode of diameter 1 cm as a reference. Reprinted from Ref. 70. © 2003 IEEE.

### 2.2.4. *Spike microelectrode array*

For microstimulation in the cochlear nucleus, we developed a spike microelectrode array (Fig. 14).[71] The array has tungsten microelectrodes at 400-$\mu$m intervals, and the diameter of the electrode tip was 30 $\mu$m. We designed the fabrication process to minimize routine tasks by separating an initial preparation of a master mold from a routine preparation of substrate replication, array assembly, and tip processing.

Figure 15 shows the process flow of producing our spike microelectrode array. Sandblast processing first produced a glass mold with a pattern of a series of protruding lines at the designed interval of 400 $\mu$m (a). Copying the groove pattern onto polystyrene mass-produced a replica substrate (b). Tungsten probes of diameter 100 $\mu$m (Narishige Co. Ltd. E-3A) were then aligned and fixed on the substrate, and the tips of the probes were finely processed in the block (c). In the tip processing, electrodischarge at 200 V first adjusted the probe tips vertically, and subsequently, electropolish modified their tapers and diameter (d). Tips of tungsten rods were sharpened from 100 $\mu$m in diameter to approximately 80 $\mu$m through 30-s electropolishing at 2 V, and less than 1 $\mu$m through 7-min electropolishing (Fig. 16(a)). The tip of the probes were dipped into polyester resin paint (Cashew Co. Ltd. Cashew Strone Paint), and coated with the insulation paint of a few $\mu$m thickness to form an insulation layer (e). In order to remove the insulation at the tips, we again applied electrodischarge with a direct voltage of 70 V. Finally, the

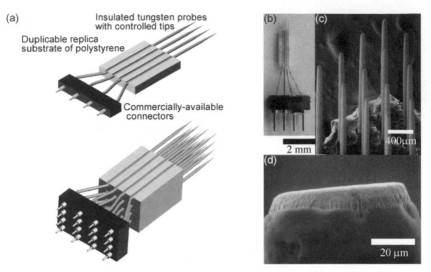

Fig. 14. Spike microelectrode array. (a) Conceptual scheme. (b) Whole view. (c) Magnification of the recording point. Reprinted from Ref. 71. © 2005 IEEE.

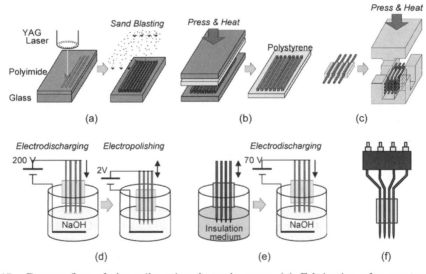

Fig. 15. Process flow of the spike microelectrode array. (a) Fabrication of a master mold. (b) Fabrication of a replica substrate. (c) Assembly of an array. (d) Tip processing. (e) Insulation. (f) Wiring. Reprinted from Ref. 71. © 2005 IEEE.

tails of the processed probes were directly inserted and soldered to commercially available sockets used for integrated circuits (f).

Figure 16(b) shows the measured impedance of probes with diameter $30\,\mu$m. The magnitude and phase at $1\,$kHz was $233\,$k$\Omega$ and $-60°$ on average with a SD of $60\,$k$\Omega$ and $11°$, respectively.

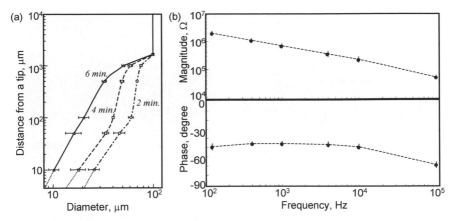

Fig. 16. Characterization of spike microelectrode array. (a) Tip shapes of probes electropolished at 2 V when reciprocating for 1.5 mm at a speed of 60 mm/s. Polishing time ranging from 2 to 6 min served as a parameter. Means and standard deviations are given ($n = 12$). (b) Impedance spectroscopy of the spike microelectrode of diameter 30 μm in the physiologic saline solution ($n = 9$). Reprinted from Ref. 68. © 2005 IEEE.

### 2.2.5. Animal preparation

Wistar rats weighing 200–350 g were used to characterize cortical activation evoked by tone bursts and obtain their ampli-tonotopic organization. Each rat was anesthetized by an intramuscular injection of ketamine (60 mg/kg) and xylazine (5 mg/kg), and fixed to a stereotaxic holder. Supplementary doses (ketamine, 24 mg/kg; xylazine, 2 mg/kg) were administered every hour, or when the heart rate, breathing rate, and/or response to a pinch of the foot showed signs of a light anesthetic level. The agents we used had little effects on the AEP within 100 ms poststimulus latency in the auditory cortex.[113] The ipsilateral eardrum was cut and waxed to ensure unilateral stimulation. The temporal skull and dura mater were partly removed to expose the auditory cortex. The contralateral cerebellum and paraflocculus were partly aspirated to expose DCN. The reference and ground electrodes are implanted at the vertex and 7 mm rostral of the vertex, respectively. These electrodes were 0.5-mm-thick pins used for integrated circuit sockets. They were placed such that they made electrical contacts with the dura mater and fixed to the skull with dental cement.

Figure 17 shows the location of the surface microelectrode array on the auditory cortex, and the putative locations of AI, AAF, and VAF. The vein patterns approximated the location of the auditory cortex, posterior to an ascending branch of the inferior cerebral vein in the caudal part of the temporal cortex.[68,69,83–85] The electrode array was positioned such that it covered AI, AAF, and VAF, and also that the long side of the rectangular recording area was parallel to the flat-skull plane, i.e. the horizontal plane that includes the bregma-lamba axis of the skull.

Following the cortical mapping of the ampli-tonotopic organization, we stimulated the cochlear nucleus and obtained the electrically evoked potentials

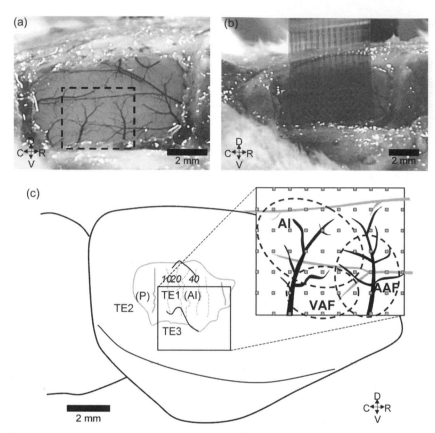

Fig. 17. Auditory cortex of rat and cortical recording using the surface microelectrode array. The right cortex was investigated: C, caudal; D, dorsal; R, rostral; V, ventral. (a) Exposed temporal cortex and the investigated area. (b) The surface microelectrode array mounted on the exposed cortex. (c) Investigated area with respect to the whole cortex. The figure also illustrates cytoarchitectonically defined areas, TE1, TE2, and TE3, with partial boundaries (solid line),[76] and physiologically defined auditory areas, the primary auditory field (AI) and the posterior field (P) from a recent unit study.[86] Isofrequency contours in AI, investigated in the study, are also depicted with digits indicating the characteristic frequency. An inset illustrates recording points and putative auditory fields in an area investigated in the present study. Reprinted from Ref. 69 with permission from Elsevier.

(EEP) over the auditory cortex. The penetrating microelectrode array was first placed in the anteroposterior axis on the lateral part of the DCN surface, and was advanced by a 100-$\mu$m step with a micromanipulator. DCN and VCN have the medial-to-lateral and dorsomedial-to-ventrolateral tonotopic axes from high to low frequencies for both (Fig. 18).[29–32]

### 2.2.6. Recording and test stimuli

Cortical evoked potentials with 0–400 ms poststimulus latency were simultaneously amplified with a gain of 1000 and filtered at a bandpass of 5–1500 Hz, −12 dB/octave

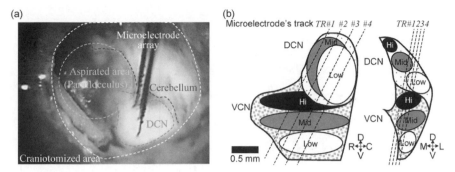

Fig. 18.   Microstimulation of the cochlear nucleus. (a) Spike microelectrode array penetrated into the cochlear nucleus. (b) The cochlear nucleus of rat and the tracks of spike microelectrode array (TR#1–TR#4). The left cochlear nucleus was stimulated. The tonotopic organizations of DCN and VCN are also illustrated. Left, sagittal view; right, section parallel to array tracks. L, lateral; M, medial. Reprinted from Ref. 68. © 2005 IEEE.

(NEC, Biotop 6R12-4), and digitized at a sampling rate of 200 $\mu$s (NEC, DL2300AP) at 64 recording points out of 70. All the data presented were the average of 30 trials or more. During the recording, rats were placed in an anechoic chamber.

For acoustic stimulation, a speaker (Matsushita Electric Industrial Co. Ltd. 10TH800) placed at 20 cm from an ear, contralateral to the exposed cortex, delivered the test stimuli at a rate of 0.7–1 Hz. The stimuli delivered were monitored by a 1/4 inch microphone (Brüel and Kjaer, 4939) placed at the opening of the ear and presented in dB SPL (sound pressure level in dB re 20 $\mu$Pa). Tone bursts with a frequency range of 5–40 kHz, intensity range of 40–80 dB SPL, rise and fall time of 5 ms, and duration of 300 ms were used as test stimuli. Clicks at 80 dB SPL were used as reference stimuli.

For electric stimulation, an electronic stimulator (Nihon Koden, SEN-7203) and isolator (Nihon Koden, SS-202J) generated the test stimuli in the cochlear nucleus at a rate of 0.7–1 Hz. The stimuli were monopolar, negative-first-biphasic, charge-balanced, and constant-current pulses with duration of 100 $\mu$s and amplitude ranging from 1 to 100 $\mu$A.

### 2.3. *Physiological proof of ABI feasibility*

Both tone bursts and microstimulation in the cochlear nucleus elicited spatiotemporally synchronized activities over the auditory cortex. The spatial patterns of activation altered depending on the frequency and intensity of test tones, and the location of microstimulation and applied current, respectively. The typical AEP and EEP waveforms were comparable (Fig. 19), except that EEP had a 0.5–3.0 ms earlier latency than AEP because the direct stimulation of the cochlear nucleus bypassed a middle ear conduction system, cochlear transduction, auditory neural conduction, and relay in the cochlear nucleus.

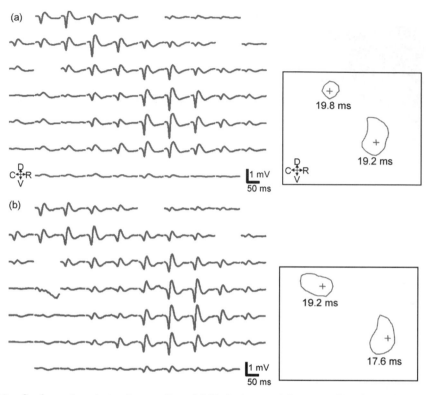

Fig. 19. Surface microelectrode recording. (a) Evoked potentials mapped in the auditory cortex. Each waveform is approximately aligned in the spatial coordinates of recording sites in the auditory cortex. (i) Auditory evoked potentials (AEP). The test tone had a frequency of 20 kHz and intensity of 60 dB SPL. (ii) Electrically evoked potentials (EEP). Microstimulation of 20 $\mu$A was given at a depth of 800 $\mu$m from the surface of the cochlear nucleus. (b) Location of P1 local maxima and foci of activation. Each inset shows the sensing area of 3.5 by 3 mm. Reprinted from Ref. 68. © 2005 IEEE.

In the following experiments, we particularly focus on the earliest P1 waves to characterize the auditory cortex for the following reasons. First, neurons in the rat auditory cortex most synchronously discharge at the stimulus onset within 50 ms poststimulus latency, and these responses have most characterized the functional organizations, so the early P1/N1 components can be of our interest (e.g. Refs. 83–86). Second, the P1 component most consistently appeared even at low intensity (Fig. 10). Third, the characterization of evoked potentials at a long latency becomes obscure because the potentials reflect the successive activations of several distinct but spatially overlapping neuronal populations.[98–102] This difficulty may be lessened as long as we focus on the earliest phase of the responses because of less sequential overlapping. Fourth, previous works demonstrated that both P1 and N1 waves have almost the same areal distribution[99,100] and they are simultaneously evoked by MGB stimulation, suggesting that these components may arise from the same or completely overlapping population of cells.[80,81]

We first explored the recording points exhibiting local maxima of P1, and measured the P1 peak latencies. We then obtained potential distribution patterns at the P1 peak latency with fourfold bicubic interpolation and estimated the location of local maxima in the interpolated grid. In order to visualize the foci of activation intuitively, response areas were clipped at 80% of their peak amplitude, and these iso-contours were called the activated foci in this work (Fig. 19, right insets).

These data sets were used in the following analyses. We first investigate the ampli-tonotopic representation of the auditory cortex on the basis of the AEP patterns. We then characterize how the microstimuli of the cochlear nucleus generate the evoked potentials in the auditory cortex.

### 2.3.1. *Tone-evoked potentials in the auditory cortex*

Figure 20 depicts tonotopicity-based representations from three different animals at 40, 60 and 80, dB SPL, respectively (rat #2–#4). In these representations, AI could

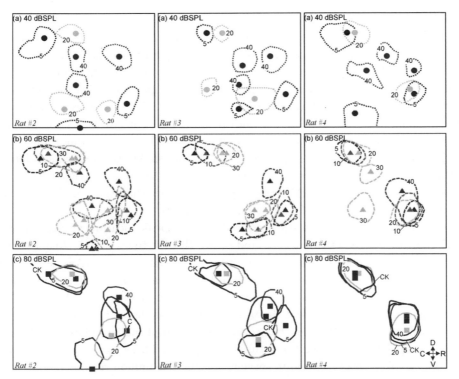

Fig. 20.   Tonotopicity-based representation from three different rats (#2–#4). Test intensity was set at 40 dB SPL (a), 60 dB SPL (b), and 80 dB SPL (c). Digits on the focus contours indicate the test frequency in kHz, and "CK" means the foci produced by a click. Marker types at the P1 peak locations and line types of the activated focus contour indicate the test intensity: circle and dotted line, 40 dB SPL; triangle and broken line, 60 dB SPL; and square and solid line, 80 dB SPL. Reprinted from Ref. 69 with permission from Elsevier.

Table 1. Number of auditory fields identified and investigated in the present work.

| Test tone | | Number of identified fields | | |
| --- | --- | --- | --- | --- |
| Frequency | Intensity | AI | AAF | VAF |
| | 40 dBSPL | 9 | 9 | 9 |
| 5 kHz | 60 dBSPL | 9 | 9 | 7 |
| | 80 dBSPL | 9 | 9 | 4 |
| 10 kHz | 60 dBSPL | 9 | 9 | 5 |
| | 40 dBSPL | 9 | 9 | 7 |
| 20 kHz | 60 dBSPL | 9 | 9 | 5 |
| | 80 dBSPL | 9 | 9 | 2 |
| 30 kHz | 60 dBSPL | 9 | 8 | 5 |
| | 40 dBSPL | 9 | 6 | 6 |
| 40 kHz | 60 dBSPL | 1 | 9 | 3 |
| | 80 dBSPL | 0 | 9 | 0 |

Nine rats were used in total. Reprinted from Ref. 69 with permission from Elsevier.

be identified on the basis of an anterior-to-posterior tonotopic gradient from a high to low frequency, which appeared most distinctly at a low intensity of 40 dB SPL. Another two clusters of foci of activation, which also formed continuous tonotopic gradients, were observed in the anterior and ventral portions with respect to AI, and these were defined as AAF and VAF, respectively. Table 1 shows a summary of P1 local maxima we found from nine auditory cortices. The late P2–N2 amplitudes, on the other hand, had a widespread topography and hence poor tonotopicity.

Figure 21(a) shows the P1 amplitude and latency in AI. No significant difference in the amplitude and latency was noted across test frequencies (two-sided $t$-test, $p < 0.1$). The responses in AAF were larger and earlier than those in AI, while the responses in VAF were smaller and later (Fig. 21(b)).

Clicks at 80 dB SPL always produced the P1 peak location at the center of AAF, halfway between the foci activated by 80-dB SPL tones with 5, 20 and 40 kHz (Fig. 20(c)). The click-evoked P1 amplitude at 80 dB SPL in AAF had a mean of 4.11 mV with a SD of 1.36 mV, and the latency had a mean of 16.0 ms with a SD of 1.9 ms. The amplitude was approximately twice larger than those of 80-dB SPL tone-evoked peak P1s, and the peak location was distinct. In addition, it was comparable to 60-dB SPL-click-evoked peak P1 in amplitude and latency (data not shown), and thus considered as a saturated response. These facts allowed an 80-dB SPL-click-evoked peak location to serve as a reliable common reference point when pooling data across animals.

By superimposing the location of 80 dB-SPL-click-evoked P1 maxima, Fig. 22(a) plots all the P1 peak locations found under all conditions and from all animals investigated. Figure 22(b) shows the general ampli-tonotopic representation by plotting the mean and SD of the P1 locations. Figure 22(c) shows

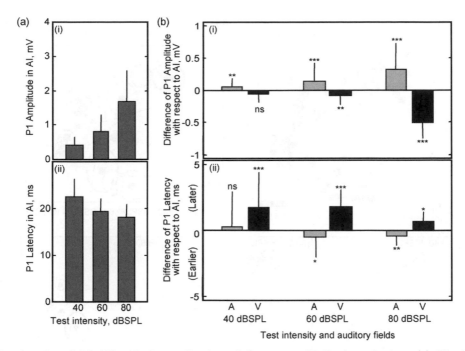

Fig. 21. Interfield difference in amplitude and latency at P1 local maximums. (a) The P1 amplitude (i) and latency (ii) in AI as a function of intensity. Mean and SD are given. (b) Difference in amplitude (i) and latency (ii) in AAF and VAF with respect to AI. Asterisks indicate statistical significance of two-sided t-tests here and hereafter: *$p < 0.1$; **$p < 0.05$; and ***$p < 0.01$. Reprinted from Ref. 69 with permission from Elsevier.

tonotopicity-based representations at indicated intensities, and Fig. 22(d) shows amplitopicity-based representations at each frequency.

Tonotopic organizations were observed in AAF and VAF as well as in AI at a low intensity of 40 dB SPL (Fig. 22(c)(i)). AI represented a zonal tonotopic organization with a high frequency rostrally, and a low frequency caudally, and AAF and VAF represented curvilinear tonotopic organizations with a high frequency dorsocaudally, and a low frequency ventrorostrally, respectively. The P1 peak locations of low-intensity 40-dB SPL tones are called the characteristic frequency (CF) location hereafter according to the test frequency. VAF sometimes missed a complete tonotopic organization because all the responses were not sufficiently large to be identified (Fig. 21(b)). In addition, responses in VAF were often overwhelmed by those in AAF and AI at a moderate or high intensity, and did not exhibit their local maxima and spotlike foci. This trend held across animals and often led to the most typical P1 spatial pattern reflecting AAF and AI activities; high-frequency tones activated the center of the auditory cortex, and low-frequency tones activated both sides, thus forming a mirror image.

The increase of test intensity also altered the foci patterns in each of auditory fields (Fig. 22(d) and Table 2). In AI, higher-intensity tones induced spread

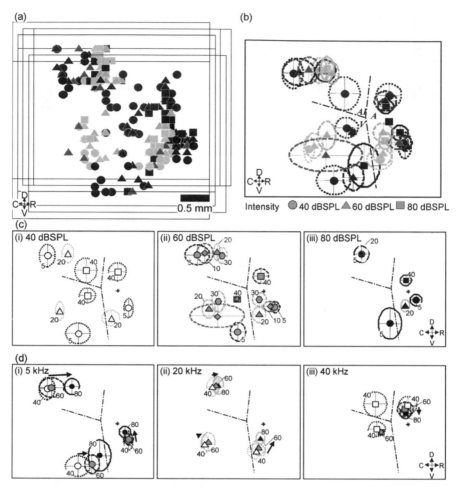

Fig. 22.   Ampli-tonotopic representation from pooled data. (a) P1 local maxima found in nine
rats with respect to an 80-dB-SPL-click-evoked P1 peak location (black square). Thin squares
indicate sensing areas of individual cortices. (b) Mean and standard deviation (SD) of the P1
local maximum across animals. Markers indicate the mean location, and major and minor axes
of elliptic contours correspond to SD in anteroposterior and dorsoventral directions, respectively.
Chain lines depict the putative boundary of auditory fields. (c) Tonotopicity-based representation.
(d) Amplitopicity-based representation. Arrows depict the significant intensity-dependent shifts of
the peak location (at least $p < 0.1$; Table 2). The length and the direction of the arrows indicate
the average distance and angle of the shift, respectively. Reprinted from Ref. 69 with permission
from Elsevier.

activation toward mid- or high-frequency areas, which were usually observed as
a movement of the low-frequency P1 foci toward a rostral portion, and in turn led
to a poor tonotopic representation. This intensity-induced shift of foci was clearly
observed for low-frequency tones, as compared to mid- or high-frequency tones.
Accordingly, the foci activated by 80-dB SPL 5-kHz and 20-kHz tones completely
overlapped (Fig. 22(c)(iii)). Thus, an axis of the intensity-dependent shift in AI

Table 2.  Intensity-dependent shifts of P1 Peak locations.

| Test frequency | Shift of P1 peak | AI | | | AAF | | | VAF | | |
|---|---|---|---|---|---|---|---|---|---|---|
| | | Mean | SD | P | Mean | SD | P | Mean | SD | P |
| 5 kHz | $\Delta x$, $\mu$m | 535 | 193 | ***3.3E-05 | −78 | 92 | **0.0353 | 275 | 228 | **0.0189 |
| | $\Delta y$, $\mu$m | 48 | 109 | 0.225 | 202 | 248 | **0.0401 | 46 | 84 | 0.2 |
| | $\Delta d$, $\mu$m | 549 | 186 | — | 288 | 172 | — | 285 | 236 | — |
| | $\Delta\theta$, ° | 3 | 16.1 | — | 101 | 11.7 | — | 6.6 | 11 | — |
| 20 kHz | $\Delta x$, $\mu$m | 126 | 124 | **0.016 | 88 | 180 | 0.1837 | 105 | 96 | *0.0705 |
| | $\Delta y$, $\mu$m | 36 | 76 | 0.195 | 298 | 191 | ***0.00162 | 64 | 59 | *0.0705 |
| | $\Delta d$, $\mu$m | 159 | 109 | — | 347 | 205 | — | 130 | 103 | — |
| | $\Delta\theta$, ° | 9.1 | 18.5 | — | 59.6 | 37.1 | — | 30.9 | 24.6 | — |
| 40 kHz | $\Delta x$, $\mu$m | NA | NA | NA | −29 | 120 | 0.276 | 175 | 152 | 0.184 |
| | $\Delta y$, $\mu$m | NA | NA | NA | −161 | 148 | **0.0446 | 0 | 0 | 1 |
| | $\Delta d$, $\mu$m | NA | NA | — | 193 | 153 | — | 175 | 152 | — |
| | $\Delta\theta$, ° | NA | NA | — | −90.4 | 41.8 | — | 0 | 0 | — |

In AI and AAF, shifts of the peak locations at 80 dB SPL with respect to those at 40 dB SPL are quantified. In VAF, shifts of the peak locations at 60 dB SPL with respect to those at 40 dB SPL are quantified, because of a small number of samples of 80 dB SPL tones (Table 1). $\Delta x$, shift in a posterior-to-anterior direction; $\Delta y$, shift in a ventral-to-dorsal direction; g$\Delta d$, distance of the alteration; g$\Delta\theta$, angle of the alteration; $P$, significance level under the hypothesis that the distance of shifts, $\Delta x$ or $\Delta y$, is not equal to zero (two-sided $t$-test). Reprinted from Ref. 69 with permission from Elsevier.

was hard to separate from a tonotopic axis. In AAF and VAF, however, intensity-dependent shifts do not parallel the tonotopic axis. In AAF, high-intensity tones generally moved the P1 foci toward the center of the field, keeping the tonotopicity. In VAF, the P1 foci tended to appear rostrally as the test intensity increased, although this alteration was not clear at high intensity because responses in VAF were not sufficiently large as compared to those in AAF and AI.

### 2.3.2. Microstimulation of the cochlear nucleus

Weak microstimulation of the cochlear nucleus could induce the selective activation of the auditory cortex depending on the stimulated location (Figs. 23). The superimposition of the electrically activated foci on the acoustically obtained ampli-tonotopic map suggests that the microstimulation of the cochlear nucleus could selectively activate a cortical region encoding a particular best frequency.

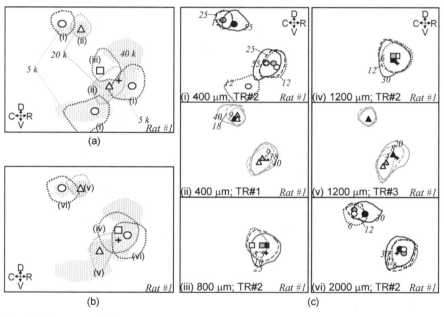

Fig. 23. Auditory cortical activation pattern elicited by microstimulation of the cochlear nucleus. (a) Microstimulation at shallow depths (400–800 μm) in the cochlear nucleus: (i) stimulation at a site in the cochlear nucleus that activated low-frequency regions in the cortex (stimulation at a depth of 400 μm along the penetrating electrode track (TR) #2, which is indicated in Fig. 18); (ii) a mid-frequency regions (at 400 μm along TR#1); and (iii) high-frequency regions (at 800 μm along TR#2). Each inset shows the sensing area of 3.5 by 3 mm. (b) Microstimulation at deep locations (1200–2000 μm): (iv) stimulation at a site that activated low-frequency regions in the cortex (stimulation at depth of 1200 μm along TR#2); (v) mid-frequency regions (at 1200 μm along TR#3); and (vi) high-frequency regions (at 2000 μm along TR#2). Shaded regions in (a) and (b) depict the activated foci of 40-dB-SPL tones with test frequencies of 5, 20, and 40 kHz. In the microstimulation, the current applied was 1 μA above the threshold. (c) Alteration of activated pattern depending on the current applied. Digits on the activated focus contours indicate the current in μA. Reprinted from Ref. 68. © 2005 IEEE.

In addition, an increase in stimulation current shifted the foci in AAF toward the center, and in AI, the foci shifted from low-frequency regions to mid-frequency regions (Fig. 23(c)). This current-dependent alteration of the EEP pattern was comparable to the intensity-dependent AEP pattern alteration, and this trend was commonly observed across animals. Thus, as judged from the activation in AI and AAF, cochlear nuclear microstimulation at an appropriate location and current strength could access the ampli-tonotopic map in the auditory cortex, and possibly evoke selective pitch and intensity sensations, respectively.

Figure 24 shows the maps of the cochlear nuclei of four different rats obtained from the correspondence between the cortical maps of the acoustically evoked and electrically evoked responses. As the stimulating electrode advanced in depth, we often found a tonotopic discontinuity (i.e. a sudden transition from a low- to high-frequency region) at a depth of 500–1000 $\mu$m, which corresponded to the boundary between DCN and VCN. In the shallow location (i.e. DCN), a low-frequency region existed posteriorly, while in the location deeper than the discontinuity (i.e. VCN), a low-frequency region existed in the ventral (deep) portion. This is consistent with the tonotopic organization in the cochlear nucleus, in which DCN has the anteromedial-to-posterolateral tonotopic axis from high to low frequencies and VCN has the dorsomedial-to-ventrolateral axis (Fig. 18(b)).

We stimulated 1860 locations in the cochlear nucleus of 15 rats and obtained auditory cortical responses at 548 locations. The activation of the somatosensory cortex located in the rostrodorsal region with respect to the auditory cortex, or the absence of significant responses to a 30-$\mu$A current pulse, was considered non-auditory responses. Figure 25 lists a breakdown of low-, mid-, and high-frequency regions in the cochlear nucleus at the indicated depth. Since the stimulating electrode was first positioned at a lateral part of the DCN surface, we found more

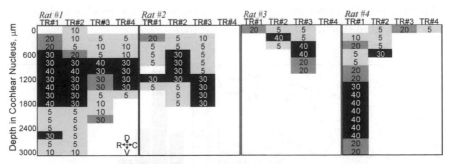

Fig. 24. Cochlear nuclear map on the basis of the correspondence between the cortical maps of acoustically evoked and electrically evoked responses. Digits indicate frequency in kHz (see the method section). The column (TR#1–TR#4) of each map corresponds to the electrode track as indicated in Fig. 18. The inter-electrode spacing is 400 $\mu$m. The stimulated location was also classified as a low-, mid-, or high-frequency region, according to the closest P1 peak location produced by a 5-, 20-, and 40-kHz tone, respectively. The gray levels of shading, i.e. light gray, dark gray and black, correspond to low-, mid-, and high-frequency regions, respectively. Reprinted from Ref. 68. © 2005 IEEE.

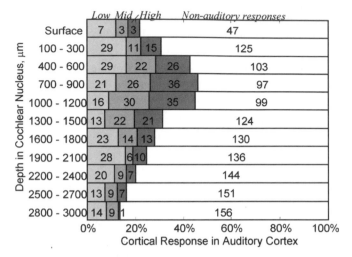

Fig. 25. List of low-, mid-, and high-frequency regions we found in cochlear nuclei of 15 rats. Data presented as described in the legend to Fig. 24. Reprinted from Ref. 68. © 2005 IEEE.

low-frequency regions at a shallow depth, rather than mid- and high-frequency regions. At depths of, 400–600 $\mu$m mid- and high-frequency regions gradually expanded, indicating that the electrode reached VCN. High-frequency regions widely occupied shallow locations in VCN, while low-frequency regions gradually expanded again at deep locations. These results are also consistent with the structure of the cochlear nucleus (Fig. 18(b)).

At 101 locations from nine animals, we examined cortical response amplitudes as a function of stimulation current. To estimate the amplitudes, we determined root mean square (RMS) values within 0–100 ms poststimulus latency and averaged RMS values across the recording sites. An average RMS value was referred to as a cortical activity level hereafter. The cortical activity level was generally an increasing function of current applied (Fig. 26(a)).

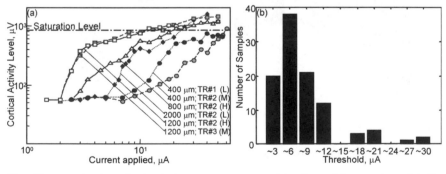

Fig. 26. Characterization of stimulation current presented in the cochlear nucleus. (a) Cortical activity level as a function of current applied. (b) Histogram of threshold current. Reprinted from Ref. 68. © 2005 IEEE.

On the basis of the plots, we measured the threshold current, saturation current, and dynamic current range, and characterized them with respect to the depth and frequency regions. Threshold current was defined as the current above which a cortical activity level was higher than the spontaneous level, and the level could be described as a simple increasing function of stimulation current. Saturation current referred to the current that gave functionally saturated neural activation, i.e. amplitude of response that was as large as percept near maximum comfortable loudness. In the present work, the saturation current was defined as the current that produced 80% of the high-level cortical response, which was evoked by an 80-dB-SPL click. The dynamic current range was defined as the saturation current in decibel with reference to the threshold current (i.e. $20 \log_{10}$ (saturation current/threshold current)).

The threshold currents ranged from 2 to $12 \, \mu A$ (Fig. 26(b)), and 10 locations with threshold currents higher than $12 \, \mu A$ were excluded in the analyses. In addition, at 23 locations, the cortical activity level in response to a $100 \, \mu A$ current pulse did not reach the saturation level (i.e. 80% of 80-dB-SPL-click-evoked cortical activity level), and these locations were also excluded. For the remaining 68 locations, Fig. 27 shows the plots of threshold current, saturation current, and dynamic current range, respectively, as a function of depth in the cochlear nucleus.

We then statistically compared the difference in the threshold current, saturation current, and dynamic current range, between DCN and VCN, and between low- and high-frequency regions, respectively (Fig. 28). The difference between DCN and VCN was determined only in the low-frequency regions, in which DCN and VCN were obviously identified. While no significant difference was observed in a threshold current between DCN and VCN (two-sided $t$-test here and hereafter for statistical analyses, $p < 0.1$), DCN had a significantly higher saturation current ($p < 0.01$) and thus a wider dynamic current range than VCN ($p < 0.01$). In DCN, low-frequency regions had a slightly higher saturation current than high-frequency regions ($p < 0.05$), but no significant difference was observed in the threshold current and dynamic current range. In VCN, low-frequency regions had a slightly higher threshold current ($p < 0.1$) and a wider dynamic current range ($p < 0.05$) than high-frequency regions, while their saturation currents were comparable.

## 3. Discussion

### 3.1. *Cortical mapping of auditory evoked potential*

Figure 29 summarizes the spatial pattern of AEP depending on test frequency and intensity. Each field had a different tonotopic axis and a different manner of intensity-dependent shifts of the activated foci. In AI, the intensity-dependent shifts paralleled the tonotopic axis, while those in AAF and VAF did not parallel. Specifically, the shifts in AAF gravitated toward the central locus of AAF, where

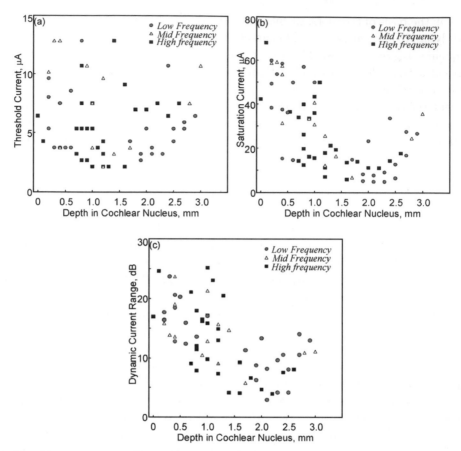

Fig. 27.   Characterization of microstimulation by depths in the cochlear nucleus. (a) Threshold current. (b) Saturation current. (c) Dynamic current range. Reprinted from Ref. 68. © 2005 IEEE.

an 80-dB SPL click produced the largest response, keeping the tonotopicity at a high intensity. The responses in AAF tended to be larger and earlier, while those in VAF were smaller and later, as compared to those in AI.

Unit studies have noted that neurons in the core cortex, including AI and AAF, have a sharper tuning and shorter responsive latency to tones than those in the belt cortex where noise better activates.[83-86] Therefore, in the present result, early and predominant AEPs in AI and AAF as compared to VAF, in combination with the investigated location and size, confirm that both AI and AAF are located in the core cortex while VAF in the belt.

The intensity-dependent change of spatial pattern in AI suggests that AI basically takes over a tuning property of auditory nerves and cochlea. Cortical neurons like auditory nerves constituting a relatively widely tuned excitatory response area with a low-frequency tail at a high intensity can be the cause of a spread of excitation toward high-CF regions as the test intensity increases.

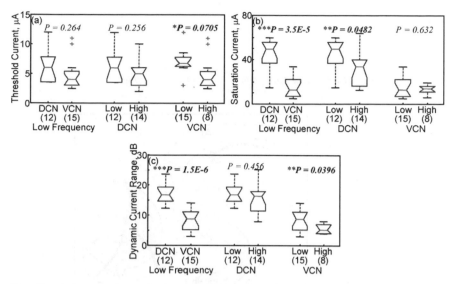

Fig. 28. Boxplot comparison of microstimulation depending on a depth and frequency region. (a) Threshold current. (b) Saturation current. (c) Dynamic current range. The box has lines at the lower quartile, median, and upper quartile values. Lines extending from each end of the box show the extent of the rest of the data. Outliers are data with values beyond the ends of the whiskers. On the basis of data presented in Table 2, We divided the samples into two groups on the basis of depth; the locations between 200 and 1000 $\mu$m presumably corresponding to DCN, and those between 1400 and 3000 $\mu$m corresponding to VCN. The first column compares between DCN and VCN in a low-frequency region. The second column compares between low- and high-frequency regions in DCN, and the third column compares between those in VCN. Digits in parentheses indicate the number of samples. Significance levels of the two-sided $t$-test are also indicated. Reprinted from Ref. 68. © 2005 IEEE.

The tuning property of auditory neurons is basically formed by a non-linearity of basilar membrane motion in the cochlea, by which the sharpness of tuning is reduced at a high intensity and the location of maximal basilar membrane motion moves toward a lower-frequency region.[2,3] In terms of mechanical dynamics, a high-intensity low-frequency tone activates the basal turn, i.e. a high-frequency region, as well as the apical turn, i.e. a low-frequency region, because of higher synchrony of activity for basal regions due to higher traveling wave velocity. In addition, forces generated by the outer hair cells and controlled by their transduction currents, i.e. cochlear amplifier, can be another cause of the non-linearity. These non-linearities are CF-specific, being more prominent at the base of cochlea than at the apex, which was also consistent with the cortical representation we obtained in our study.

In AAF and VAF, the intensity-dependent shifts do not parallel the tonotopic axis, differing from the representation in cochlea and AI. Similar representations were previously found in the guinea pig auditory cortex by extrinsic optical imaging[94] and in the dog cortex by evoked-potential mapping.[95] The direction of shifts in AAF in our study was toward the central locus of the field, where click stimuli, which have a broad spectrum and thereby can activate a wide array of

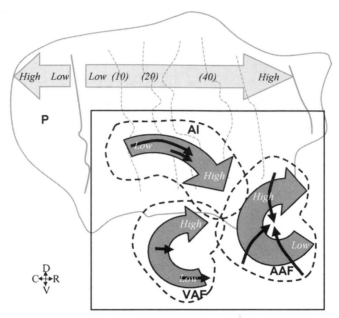

Fig. 29.　Spatial representation of frequency and intensity in AI, AAF and VAF on the basis of the present results. Large arrows indicate tonotopic axes, and small arrows, axes of intensity-dependent spatial change. The illustration is reproduced from Fig. 17c. Reprinted from Ref. 69 with permission from Elsevier.

neurons with different CF, produced the largest response in the AAF central locus. Since high-intensity tones can also activate off-CF neurons, the loci of maximum response could be expected to shift in the middle of AAF. These results therefore reflect how the activation of neurons is summed and spread in those fields as test intensity increases. In the rat AAF at a single neuron level, the proportion of monotonic neurons is higher, and the threshold varies more widely across locations as compared to those in AI,[85] which in turn may mean that the change of response with intensity also varies due to the compressive non-linearity to CF tone. Such properties are required for the intensity-dependent spatial shift that differs from the cochlea, and may cause a spatial coordinate of growth of response amplitude with increasing intensity.

## 3.2. Functional microstimulation in the cochlear nucleus

### 3.2.1. Feasibility of ABI

Our ABI model features the quick surface mapping of the ampli-tonotopic representation in the auditory cortex, which may infer the possible auditory percepts elicited by the microstimulation in the cochlear nucleus. We were able to obtain an AEP-like P1–N1-P2–N2 complex in EEP in the auditory cortex, suggesting that microstimulation evoked a comparable auditory sensation. The AEP mapping demonstrated that the rat auditory cortex was divided into multiple auditory fields, each of which represented a test frequency and intensity differently. The microstimulation of the cochlear nucleus also evoked responses in the multiple fields, and the activation pattern depended on the stimulated region and current strength.

The ampli-tonotopic representation in the auditory cortex could be reproduced by the appropriate microstimulation of both DCN and VCN, suggesting that the stimulation can produce the pitch and intensity sensations. The frequency regions activated in the auditory cortex depended on the frequency region within the tonotopic structure in the cochlear nucleus. Considering that strong currents synchronously activate a broad area of a neuronal population and the activation centers on the stimulated location, the breadth of activation may reflect the intensity of sensation, while the frequency region at the center of activation may correspond to the pitch sensation.

Our study combines previous outcomes from animal to clinical studies and infers further capabilities of ABIs; previous clinical results and imaging studies demonstrate that ABI produces cortical neural activation associated with some auditory percepts,[12–26,44–47] and electrophysiological and connectional studies demonstrating that VCN microstimulation induces the tonotopically localized neural activation in the inferior colliculus.[59,60,65] Expanding from these outcomes, our results first demonstrate that the microstimulation of both VCN and DCN can access the tonotopic organization in the auditory cortex after being relayed at several nuclei in the midbrain and thalamus, thus substantially indicating the ABI capability. Second, the amount of current applied to both VCN and DCN can cover intensity information without losing frequency information.

### 3.2.2. *Implications for developing future ABI*

Microstimulation at the surface of DCN tended to fail to elicit auditory cortical responses as compared to microstimulation at any depth within the cochlear nuclei (Fig. 25). On the other hand, the microstimulation at a shallow depth turned out comparable threshold currents with those at a deep location. These results suggest that the adequate penetration of electrodes, irrespective of the depth, avoids the spread of current fields through conductive cerebrospinal fluid, and enables to distinctly activate neural population close to the electrodes.

The dynamic current range appeared to have dependence on the penetrating depth of the stimulating electrode. However, taking a shallow region at a depth of 200–1000 $\mu$m and a deep region at a depth of 1400–3000 $\mu$m separately, there was no depth dependence in each region, suggesting that these two regions were different nuclei. In addition, the breakdown of low-frequency region in Fig. 25 showed two independent peaks at shallow and deep regions, suggesting two separate nuclei. In terms of the perceptual magnitude, on the other hand, the current applied at VCN in ABI hearing is linearly correlated with the acoustic SPL in normal hearing.[114] On the basis of the AEP amplitude, the discriminable threshold sound level and the maximum comfortable (saturation) sound level of rats can be estimated at 30–40 dB SPL and 80–90 dB SPL, respectively. According to the relation between ABI and normal hearing, we can estimate a saturation current at two to three times the threshold current, and thereby a dynamic current range at 6–9.5 dB, which fits well with VCN microstimulation in our experiments. These results suggest that our microstimulation could successfully access VCN and DCN separately. Nevertheless, since the individual auditory nerve fibers were intact throughout the experiments, there is a possibility that the cortical responses seen when stimulating DCN were relayed through VCN via antidromic activation of the auditory nerves.

The present results suggest that DCN has a wider dynamic current range for microstimulation than VCN. The wide dynamic current range in DCN may lead to a fine adjustment of intensity sensation. Neurons in both DCN and the VCN send ascending projections to the inferior colliculus in the midbrain, while neurons in VCN also provide collateral branches to both the ipsilateral and contralateral superior olivary nuclei in the medulla.[29–32,66,67] Earlier studies mostly focused on VCN as stimulation targets because the auditory pathway from VCN is considered as the mainstream, and in fact the auditory nerves mainly project to VCN. Provided that DCN turns out to be a comparable or better stimulation target than VCN in terms of encoding pitch and intensity information, DCN microstimulation may also have another advantage in terms of reducing non-auditory side effects. Indeed, current surgical improvements have reduced the side effects significantly, but VCN is still close to other cranial nerves, that is, the seventh (facial) and ninth (glossopharyngeal) nerves, and the flocculus of the cerebellum, whose activation induces unnecessary movements and sensations in the head and body.[14,16,17,21,22]

Thus, our results show a possibility that DCN can be a stimulating target, however, cannot lead to a direct evidence of the advantage of DCN. First, recent animal studies suggest that DCN plays an important role on localization of sound sources in space, attention, and multisensory integration, rather than on encoding of the details of sound information.[115–117] In order to carry out these functions effectively, a wide dynamic range and high saturation current may be a prerequisite. Second, in clinical experience, damage to the ventral acoustic stria, the main projection from VCN, results in a profound deficit in speech perception, suggesting that VCN is responsible for conveying speech-related information. In addition, DCN ablation in cats has little effects on the discrimination of test tones.[116,117] Third, the occurrence of stimulation-induced tissue injury depends on both the charge density and the charge per phase of current pulse, and the safe stimulation level limits the advantage of the wide dynamic current range.[48,49,54–56] In particular, the charge density sets a severe limit when using a microelectrode. For example, setting the charge density limit at $100 \, \mu C/cm^2/phase$ and considering a given surface of the stimulating contact at $2 \times 10^{-5} \, cm^2$ (calculated for a minimum active area of $\phi$ $50 \, \mu m$) and a given duration of one phase of current pulse at $50 \, \mu s$, the safe limit of current can be calculated at approximately $40 \, \mu A$, which is lower than the saturation current in VCN. Fourth, as mentioned above, DCN stimulation may induce VCN activation antidromically since the auditory nerve was intact in the experiments.

The dynamic current range of microstimulation also differed when the microstimulation was applied at different points along the tonotopic gradient in the cochlear nucleus, and the range in a low-frequency pathway was relatively wider than in a high-frequency pathway. Such difference was not observed in acoustic tone stimulation,[69,101] so it will be necessary to scale the current amplitude across electrodes. Neuronal recording in the inferior colliculus also provided the same kind of implication in the previous study.[59] Such a scaling is probably needed because the neural activities are adapted to the resonance property of the external ear and the mechanical characteristics of the conduction system from the tympanic membrane through the middle ear to the organ of Corti.

## 4. Summary

In the present chapter, we have reviewed the ABI from both clinical and physiological aspects.

Despite the continuous efforts since the first implantation in 1979, ABI still results in a poor understanding of speech and its benefits are usually limited to a lip-reading enhancement. This ABI performance is likened to a single channel cochlear implant a few decades ago. Nevertheless, most ABI recipients have agreed that they benefit from ABI, indicating that ABI provides useful auditory information and improves their quality of life.

Notable achievements in the earlier animal studies are the identification of safety level for ABI stimulation and other neural prostheses implanted in the brain. The boundary between safe and unsafe injections of the charge-balanced biphasic electrical pulse depends on both the charge and the charge density per phase of the pulse. When using a microelectrode such as the recent penetrating ABI that activates neurons locally and repeatedly, high-rate-SIDNE should be also taken into account the design of the stimulating protocol even under the safety condition.

In order to obtain a physiological proof of ABI capability, we introduced our rat model of ABI, which can compare tone-evoked potentials and EEP by microstimuli presented to the cochlear nucleus.

We first attempted to identify how the auditory cortex represents frequency and intensity information. Our dense mapping of the auditory cortical evoked potential shows that the auditory cortex has multiple independent auditory fields, each with a different ampli-tonotopic organization.

Our animal experiments then demonstrated that microstimulation of both the DCN and the VCN could reproduce similar ampli-tonotopic cortical maps to the tone-evoked maps. These results suggest that the adequate electrical stimulation of DCN and the VCN can activate the intrinsic neuronal processing in the auditory pathway and produce the pitch and intensity sensations, thus substantially indicating a promising ABI capability. The precise access to the tonotopic organization in the cochlear nucleus is the first step for improving the performance.

We also found that the cortical dynamic range was wider for the DCN stimulation than for the VCN stimulation and for the low-frequency pathway than for the high-frequency pathway. These kinds of data can have great implications. Since the current ABI stimulating strategy is adopted from the cochlear implant and thereby designed for auditory nerve stimulation, the data-driven optimization of the ABI strategy will be the next step to boost the ABI performance in the near future.

# References

1. J. P. Rauschecker and R. V. Shannon, Sending sound to the brain, *Science* **295** (2002) 1025–1029.
2. L. Robles and M. A. Ruggero, Mechanics of mammalian cochlea, *Physiol. Rev.* **81** (2001) 1305–1352.
3. M. Ulfendahl, Mechanical responses of the mammalian cochlea; *Prog. Neurobiol.* **53** (1997) 331–380.
4. N. P. Cooper and W. S. Rhode, Basilar membrane mechanics in the hook region of cat and guinea-pig cocheae: Sharp tuning and nonlinearity in the absence of baseline position shifts, *Hear. Res.* **63** (1992) 163–190.
5. B. C. J. Moore, Perceptual consequences of cochlear hearing loss and their implications for the design of hearing, *Ear Hear.* **17** (1996) 133–161.
6. D. J. Vantasell, Hearing-loss, speech and hearing-aids, *J. Speech Hear. Res.* **36** (1993) 228–244.
7. J. L. Dornhoffer, Hearing results with the Dornhoffer ossicular replacement prostheses, *Laryngoscope* **108** (1998) 531–536.
8. J. J. Rosowski and S. N. Merchant, Mechanical and acoustic analysis of middle-ear reconstruction, *Am. J. Otol.* **16** (1995) 486–497.
9. G. E. Loeb, Cochlear prosthetics, *Annu. Rev. Neurosci.* **13** (1990) 357–371.
10. B. S. Wilson, C. C. Finley, D. T. Lawson, R. D. Wolford, D. K. Eddington and W. M. Rabinowitz, Better speech recognition with cochlear implants, *Nature* **352** (1991) 236–238.
11. B. S. Wilson, The future of cochlear implants, *Br. J. Audiol.* **31** (1997) 205–225.
12. B. J. Edgerton, W. F. House and W. Hitselberger, Hearing by cochlear nucleus stimulation in humans, *Ann. Otol. Rhinol. Laryngol.* **91** (suppl.) (1982) 117–124.
13. W. F. House and W. E. Hitselberger, Twenty-year report of the first auditory brain stem nucleus implant, *Ann. Otol. Rhinol. Laryngol.* **110** (2001) 103–105.
14. D. E. Brackmann, W. E. Hitselberger, R. A. Neson, J. Moore, M. D. Waring, F. Portillo, R. V. Shannon and F. F. Telischi, Auditory brainstem implant: I. Issues in surgical implantation, *Otolaryngol. Head Neck Surg.* **108** (1993) 624–633.
15. R. V. Shannon, J. Fayad, J. Moore, W. W. M. Lo, S. Otto, R. A. Neson and M. O'Leary, Auditory brainstem implant: II. Postsurgical issues and performance, *Otolaryngol. Head Neck Surg.* **108** (1993) 634–642.
16. S. R. Otto, R. V. Shannon, D. E. Brackmann, W. E. Hitselberger, S. Stanller and C. Menapace, The multichannel auditory brainstem implant: Performance in twenty patients, *Otolaryngol. Head Neck Surg.* **118** (1998) 291–303.

17. K. Ebinger, S. Otto, J. Arcaroli, S. Staller and P. Arndt, Multichannel auditory brainstem implant: US clinical trial results, *J. Laryngol. Otol.* **114** (2000) 50–53.

18. W. P. Sollmann, R. Laszig and N. Marangos, Surgical experiences in 58 cases using the Nucleus 22 multichannel auditory brainstem implant, *J. Laryngol. Otol.* **114** (2000) 50–53.

19. T. Lenarz, M. Moshrefi, C. Matthies, C. Frohne, A. Lesinski-Schiedat, A. Illg, U. Rost, R. D. Battmer and M. Samii, Auditory brainstem implant: Part I. Auditory performance and its evolution over time, *Otol. Neurotol.* **22** (2001) 823–833.

20. S. R. Otto, D. E. Brackmann, W. E. Hitselberger, R. V. Shannon and J. Kuchta, Multichannel auditory brainstem implant: Update on performance in 61 patients, *J. Neurosurg.* **96** (2002) 1063–1071.

21. B. Nevison, R. Laszig, W. P. Sollmann, T. Lenarz, O. Sterkers, R. Ramsden, B. Fraysse, M. Manrique, H. Rask-Andersen, E. Garcia-Ibanez, V. Colletti, and E. von Wallenberg, Results from a European clinical investigation of the Nucleus (R) multichannel auditory brainstem implant, *Ear Hear.* **23** (2002) 170–183.

22. J. Kuchta, S. R. Otto, R. V. Shannon, W. E. Hitselberger and D. E. Brackmann, The multichannel auditory brainstem implant: How many electrodes make sense? *J. Neurosurg.* **100** (2004) 16–23.

23. V. Colletti, M. Carner, V. Miorelli, M. Guida, L. Colletti and F. Fiorino, Auditory brainstem implant (ABI): New frontiers in adults and children, *Otolaryngol. Head Neck Surg.* **133** (2005) 126–138.

24. V. Colletti and R. V. Shannon, Open set speech perception with auditory brainstem implant? *Laryngoscope* **115** (2005) 1974–1978.

25. K. Kaga, NF2 and auditory brainstem implant, *Curr. Insights Neurol. Sci.* **9** (2000) 10–11.

26. K. Kaga, Auditory cerebral implant. Its feasibility from a view of anatomy and electrophysiology, *Otolaryngol. Head Neck Surg. Jap.* **77** (2005) 194–200.

27. J. K. Moore and K. K. Osen, The cochlear nuclei in man, *Am. J. Anat.* **154** (1979) 393–417.

28. J. K. Moore, The human auditory brain stem, *Hear. Res.* **29** (1987) 1–32.

29. Y. Yajima and Y. Hayashi, Response properties and tonotopical organization in the dorsal cochlear nucleus in rats, *Exp. Brain Res.* **75** (1989) 381–389.

30. J. A. Kaltenbach and J. Lazor, Tonotopic maps obtained from the surface of the dorsal cochlear nucleus of the hamster and rat, *Hear. Res.* **51** (1991) 149–160.

31. J. M. Harrison and R. Irving, Ascending connections of the anterior ventral cochlear nucleus in the rat, *J. Comp. Neurol.* **126** (1966) 51–64.

32. J. M. Harrison and R. Irving, The organization of the posterior ventral cochlear nucleus in the rat, *J. Comp. Neurol.* **126** (1966) 391–402.

33. K. B. Jackson, G. Mark, J. Helms, J. Mueller and R. Behr, An auditory brainstem implant system, *Am. J. Audiol.* **11** (2002) 128–133.

34. C. Vincent, C. Zini, A. Gandolfi, J. M. Triglia, W. Pellet, E. Truy, G. Fischer, M. Maurizi, M. Meglio, J. P. Lejeune and F. M. Vaneecloo, Results of the MXM digisonic auditory brainstem implant clinical trials in Europe, *Otol. Neurotol.* **23** (2002) 56–60.

35. D. G. Evans, S. M. Huson, D. Donnai, W. Neary, V. Blair, D. Teare, V. Newton, T. Strachan, R. Ramsden and R. Harris, A genetic study of type 2 neurofibromatosis in the United Kingdom. I. Prevalence, mutation rate, fitness and confirmation of maternal transmission effect on severity, *J. Med. Genet.* **29** (1992) 841–846.

36. R. L. Marutza and R. Eldridge, Neurofibromatosis 2, *N. Engl. J. Med.* **318** (1988) 684–688.

37. R. J. S. Briggs, D. E. Brackmann, M. E. Baser and W. E. Hitselberger, Comprehensive management of bilateral acoustic neuromas — current perspectives, *Arch. Otolaryngol. Head Neck Surg.* **120** (1994) 1307–1314.

38. D. R. Friedland and P. A. Wackym, Evaluation of surgical approaches to endoscopic auditory brainstem implantation, *Laryngoscope* **109** (1999) 175–180.

39. R. J. S. Briggs, G. Fabinyi and A. H. Kaye, Current management of acoustic neuromas: Review of surgical approaches and outcomes, *J. Clin. Neurosci.* **7** (2000) 521–526.

40. M. D. Waring, Electrically evoked auditory brain-stem response monitoring of auditory brain-stem implant integrity during facial-nerve tumor surgery, *Laryngoscope* **102** (1992) 1293–1295.

41. M. D. Waring, Auditory brain-stem responses evoked by electrical-stimulation of the cochlear nucleus in human-subjects, *Electroencephalogr. Clin. Neurophysiol.* **96** (1995) 338–347.

42. M. D. Waring, Properties of auditory brainstem responses evoked by intra-operative electrical stimulation of the cochlear nucleus in human subjects, *Electroencephalogr. Clin. Neurophysiol.* **100** (1996) 538–548.

43. N. Marangos, R. B. Illing, J. Kruger and R. Laszig, *In vivo* visualization of the cochlear nerve and nuclei with fluorescent axonal tracers, *Hear. Res.* **162** (2001) 48–52.

44. R. T. Miyamoto and D. Wong, Positron emission tomography in cochlear implant and auditory brainstem implant recipients, *J. Comm. Disord.* **34** (2001) 473–478.

45. R. T. Miyamoto, D. Wong, D. B. Pisoni, G. Hutchins, M. Sehgal and R. Fain, Positron emission tomography in cochlear implant and auditory brainstem implant recipients, *Am. J. Otol.* **20** (1999) 596–601.

46. W. W. M. Lo, Imaging of cochlear and auditory brainstem implantation. *Am. J. Neuroradiol.* **19** (1998) 1147–1154.

47. W. Di Nardo, S. Di Girolamo, D. Di Giuda, G. De Rossi, J. Galli and G. Paludetti, SPET monitoring of auditory cortex activation by electric stimulation in a patient with auditory brainstem implant, *Eur. Arch. Oto-Rhino-Laryngol.* **258** (2001) 496–500.

48. W. F. Agnew, D. B. McCreery, T. G. H. Yuen and L. A. Bullara, Effects of prolonged electrical stimulation of the central nervous system, in *Neural Prostheses: Fundamental Studies*, eds. D. B. McCreery and W. F. Agnew (Prentice Hall, Englewood Cliffs, NJ, 1990), pp. 225–252.

49. D. B. McCreery, W. F. Agnew, T. G. H. Yuen and L. A. Bullara, Comparison of neural damage induced by electrical stimulation with faradaic and capacitor electrodes, *Ann. Biomed. Eng.* **16** (1988) 463–481.

50. W. J. Brown, T. L. Babb, H. V. Soper, J. P. Lieb, C. A. Ottino and P. H. Crandall, Tissue reactions to long-term electrical stimulation of the cerebellum in monkeys, *J. Neurosurg.* **47** (1977) 366–379.

51. W. F. Agnew, T. G. H. Yuen, L. A. Bullara, D. Jacques and R. H. Pudenz, Intracellular calcium deposition in brain following electrical stimulation, *Neurol. Res.* **1** (1979) 187–202.

52. S. B. Brummer and J. M. Turner, Electrochemical considerations for safe electrical stimulation of the nervous system with platinum electrodes, *IEEE Trans. Biomed. Eng.* **24** (1977) 59–63.

53. L. S. Robblee and T. L. Rose. Electrochemical guidelines for selection of protocols and electrode materials for neural stimulation, in *Neural Prostheses: Fundamental Studies*, eds. D. B. McCreery and W. F. Agnew (Prentice Hall, Englewood Cliffs, NJ, 1990), pp. 25–66.

54. D. B. McCreery, W. F. Agnew, T. G. H. Yuen and L. A. Bullara, Charge-density and charge per phase as cofactors in neural injury induced by electrical stimulation, *IEEE Trans. Biomed. Eng.* **37** (1990) 996–1001.

55. D. B. McCreery, T. G. H. Yuen, W. F. Agnew and L. A. Bullara, Stimulation parameters affecting tissue injury during microstimulation in the cochlear nucleus of the cat, *Hear. Res.* **77** (1994) 105–115.

56. R. V. Shannon, A model of safe levels for electrical stimulation, *IEEE Trans. Biomed. Eng.* **39** (1992) 424–426.

57. D. B. McCreery, T. G. H. Yuen and L. A. Bullara, Chronic microstimulation in the feline ventral cochlear nucleus: Physiologic and histologic effects, *Hear. Res.* **149** (2000) 223–238.

58. D. B. McCreery, T. G. H. Yuen, W. F. Agnew and L. A. Bullara, A characterization of the effects on neuronal excitability resulting from prolonged microstimulation with chronically implanted microelectrodes, *IEEE Trans. Biomed. Eng.* **44** (1997) 931–939.

59. D. B. McCreery, R. V. Shannon, J. K. Moore and M. Chatterjee, Accessing the tonotopic organization of the ventral cochlear nucleus by intranuclear microstimulation, *IEEE Trans. Rehab. Eng.* **6** (1998) 391–399.

60. D. A. Evans, J. K. Niparko, R. A. Alschuler, K. A. Frey and J. A. Miller, Demonstration of prosthetic activation of central auditory pathways using [14C]-2-deoxyglucose, *Laryngoscope* **100** (1990) 128–135.

61. H. K. El-Kashlan, J. K. Niparko, R. A. Altschuler and J. M. Miller, Direct electrical stimulation of the cochlear nucleus, Surface vs. penetrating stimulation, *Otolaryngol. Head Neck Surg.* **105** (1991) 533–543.

62. H. K. El-Kashlan, Multichannel cochlear nucleus stimulation, *Otolaryngol. Head Neck Surg.* **121** (1999) 169–175.

63. S. K. Rosahl, G. Mark, M. Herzog, C. Pantazis, F. Gharabaghi, C. Matthies, T. Brinker and M. Samii, Far-field responses to stimulation of the cochlear nucleus by microsurgically placed penetrating and surface electrodes in the cat, *J. Neurosurg.* **95** (2001) 845–852.

64. X. Liu, G. McPhee, H. L. Seldon and G. M. Clark, Histological and physiological effects of the central auditory prosthesis, Surface versus penetrating electrode, *Hear. Res.* **114** (1997) 264–274.

65. H. Takagi, H. Saito, S. Nagase and M. Suzuki, Distribution of Fos-like immunoreactivity in the auditory pathway evoked by bipolar electrical brainstem stimulation, *Acta Oto-Laryngol.* **124** (2004) 907–913.

66. N. B. Cant and K. C. Gaston, Pathways connecting the right and left cochlear nuclei, *J. Comp. Neurol.* **212** (1982) 313–326.

67. B. Bernard, M. C. Jean, A. Paul and B. Pierre, Functional anatomy of auditory brainstem nuclei: Application to the anatomical basis of brainstem auditory evoked potentials, *Auris Nasus Larynx* **28** (2001) 85–94.

68. H. Takahashi, M. Nakao and K. Kaga, Accessing ampli-tonotopic organization of rat auditory cortex by microstimulation of cochlear nucleus, *IEEE Trans. Biomed. Eng.* **52** (2005) 1333–1344.

69. H. Takahashi, M. Nakao and K. Kaga, Interfield differences in intensity and frequency representation of evoked potentials in rat auditory cortex, *Hear. Res.* **210** (2005) 9–23.

70. H. Takahashi, T. Ejiri, M. Nakao, N. Nakamura, K. Kaga and T. Hervé, Microelectrode array on folding polyimide ribbon for epidural mapping of functional evoked potentials, *IEEE Trans. Biomed. Eng.* **50** (2003) 510–516.

71. H. Takahashi, J. Suzurikawa, M. Nakao, F. Mase and K. Kaga, Easy-to-prepare assembly array of tungsten microelectrodes, *IEEE Trans. Biomed. Eng.* **52** (2005) 952–956.
72. J. H. Kaas, T. A. Hackett and M. J. Tramo, Auditory processing in primate cerebral cortex, *Curr. Opin. Neurobiol.* **9** (1999) 164–170.
73. H. A. Patterson, *An Antrograde Degeneration and Retrograde Axonal Transport Study of the Cortical Projections of the Rat Medial Geniculate Body* (Boston University Press, Boston, MA, 1976).
74. W. J. S. Kreig, Connections of the cerebral cortex. I. The albino rat. A. The topography of the cortical areas, *J. Comp. Neurol.* **84** (1946) 221–275.
75. W. J. S. Kreig, Connections of the cerebral cortex. I. The albino rat. B. The structure of the cortical areas, *J. Comp. Neurol.* **84** (1946) 277–323.
76. K. Zilles, *The Cortex of the Rat. A Stereotaxic Atlas* (Springer-Verlag, Berlin, 1995).
77. L. M. Romanski and J. E. LeDoux, Organization of rodent auditory cortex: Aterograde transport of PHA-L from MGv to temporal neocortex, *Cereb. Cortex* **3** (1993) 499–514.
78. C. J. Shi and M. D. Cassell, Cortical thalamic and amygdaloid projections of rat temporal cortex, *J. Comp. Neurol.* **382** (1997) 153–175.
79. J. A. Winer, S. L. Sally, D. T. Larue and J. B. Kelly, Origins of medial geniculate body projections to physiologically defined zones of rat primary auditory cortex, *Hear. Res.* **130** (1999) 42–61.
80. S. Di and D. S. Barth, The functional anatomy of middle-latency auditory evoked potentials, Thalamocortical connections, *J. Neurophysiol.* **68** (1992) 425–431.
81. D. S. Barth and S. Di, The functional anatomy of middle latency auditory evoked potentials, *Brain Res.* **565** (1991) 109–115.
82. S. A. Azizi, R. A. Burne and D. J. Woodward, The auditory corticopontocerebellar projection in the rat: Inputs to the paraflocculus and midvermis. An anatomical and physiological study, *Exp. Brain Res.* **59** (1985) 36–49.
83. S. L. Sally and J. B. Kelly, Organization of auditory cortex in the albino rat: Sound frequency, *J. Neurophysiol.* **59** (1988) 1627–1638.
84. J. Horikawa, S. Ito, Y. Hosokawa, T. Homma and K. Murata, Tonotopic representation in the rat auditory cortex, *Proc. Jpn. Acad. B* **64** (1988) 260–263.
85. R. G. Rutkowski, A. A. Miasnikov and N. M. Weinberger, Characterisation of multiple physiological fields within the anatomical core of rat auditory cortex: *Hear. Res.* **181** (2003) 116–130.
86. N. T. Doron, J. E. LeDoux and M. N. Semple, Redefining the tonotopic core of rat auditory cortex: Physiological evidence for a posterior field, *J. Comp. Neurol.* **453** (2002) 345–360.
87. C. E. Schreiner and J. V. Urbas, Representation of amplitude modulation in the auditory cortex of the cat. I. The anterior auditory field (AAF), *Hear. Res.* **21** (1986) 227–241.
88. P. Heil, R. Rajan and D. R. F. Irvine, Topographic representation of tone intensity along the isofrequency axis of cat primary auditory cortex, *Hear. Res.* **76** (1994) 188–202.
89. C. E. Schreiner, J. R. Mendelson and M. L. Sutter, Functional topography of cat primary auditory cortex: Representation of tone intensity, *Exp. Brain Res.* **92** (1992) 105–122.
90. D. P. Phillips, M. N. Semple, M. B. Calford and L. M. Kitzes, Level-dependent representation of stimulus frequency in cat primary auditory cortex, *Exp. Brain Res.* **102** (1994) 210–226.

91. D. P. Phillips, M. N. Semple and L. M. Kitzes, Factors shaping the tone level sensitivity of single neurons in posterior field of cat auditory cortex, *J. Neurophysiol.* **73** (1995) 674–686.

92. J. C. Clarey, P. Barone and T. J. Imig, Functional organization of sound direction and sound pressure level in primary auditory cortex of the cat, *J. Neurophysiol.* **72** (1994) 2383–2405.

93. N. Suga and T. Manabe, Neural basis of amplitude-spectrum representation in auditory cortex of the mustached bat, *J. Neurophysiol.* **47** (1982) 225–255.

94. I. Taniguchi and M. Nasu, Spatio-temporal representation of sound intensity in the guinea pig auditory cortex observed by optical recording, *Neurosci. Lett.* **151** (1993) 178–181.

95. A. R. Tuntri, A difference in the representation of auditory signals for the left and right ears in the iso-frequency contours of the right middle ectosylvian auditory cortex of the dog, *Am. J. Physiol.* **168** (1952) 712–727.

96. H. Takahashi, M. Nakao and K. Kaga, Distributed representation of sound intensity in the rat auditory cortex, *NeuroReport* **15** (2004) 2061–2065.

97. K. Kaga, R. F. Hink, Y. Shinoda and J. Suzuki, Evidence for a primary cortical origin of the middle latency auditory evoked potential in cats, *Electroencephalogr. Clin. Neurophysiol.* **50** (1980) 254–266.

98. M. Steinschneider, C. E. Tenke, C. E. Schroeder, D. C. Javitt, G. V. Simpson, J. C. Arezzo and H. G. Vaughan Jr, Cellular generators of the cortical auditory evoked potential initial component, *Electroencephalogr. Clin. Neurophysiol.* **84** (1992) 196–200.

99. D. S. Barth and S. Di, Three-dimensional analysis of auditory-evoked potentials in rat neocortex, *J. Neurophysiol.* **64** (1990) 1527–1536.

100. F. W. Ohl, H. Scheich and W. J. Freeman, Tonotopic analysis of epidural pure-tone-evoked potentials in gerbil auditory cortex, *J. Neurophysiol.* **83** (2000) 3123–3132.

101. H. Takahashi, M. Nakao and K. Kaga, Cortical mapping of auditory-evoked offset responses in rats, *NeuroReport* **15** (2004) 1565–1569.

102. H. Takahashi, M. Nakao and K. Kaga, Spatial and temporal strategy to analyze steady-state sound intensity in cortex, *NeuroReport* **16** (2005) 137–140.

103. C. M. Gray, P. E. Maldonado, M. Wilson and B. McNaughton, Tetrodes markedly improve the reliability and yield of multiple single-unit isolation from multi-unit recordings in cat striate cortex, *J. Neurosci. Meth.* **63** (1995) 43–54.

104. A. Frien and R. Eckhorn, Functional coupling shows stronger stimulus dependency for fast oscillations than for low-frequency components in striate cortex of awake monkey, *Eur. J. Neurosci.* **12** (2000) 1466–1478.

105. A. Norena and J. J. Eggermont, Comparison between local field potentials and unit cluster activity in primary auditory cortex and anterior auditory field in the cat, *Hear. Res.* **166** (2002) 202–213.

106. J. J. Eggarmont, How homogeneous is cat primary auditory cortex? Evidence from simultaneous single-unit recordings, *Audit. Neurosci.* **2** (1996) 79–182.

107. A. L. Owens, T. J. Denison, H. Versnel, M. Rebbert, M. Pecherar and S. A. Shamma, Multi-electrode array for measuring evoked potentials from surface of feret primary auditory cortex, *J. Neurosci. Meth.* **58** (1995) 209–220.

108. T. Stieglitz, Flexible biomedical microdevices with double-sided electrode arrangements for neural applications, *Sensor. Actuat. A* **90** (2001) 203–211.

109. C. Gonzales and M. Rodriguez, A flexible perforated microelectrode array for action potential recording in nerve and muscle tissues, *J. Neurosci. Meth.* **72** (1997) 189–195.

110. S. Boppart, B. C. Wheeler and C. Wallace, A flexible, perforated microelectrode array for extended neural recording, *IEEE Trans. Biomed Eng.* **39** (1992) 37–42.

111. S. A. Shamma, G. A. May, N. E. Cotter, R. L. White and F. B. Simmons, Thin-film multielectrode arrays for a cochlear prosthesis, *IEEE Trans. Biomed. Eng.* **33** (1986) 223–229.

112. R. S. Pickard, A. J. Collins, P. L. Joseph and R. C. J. Hicks, Flexible printed-circuit probe for electrophysiology, *Med. Biol. Eng. Comput.* **17** (1979) 261–267.

113. J. C. Drummond, Monitoring depth of anesthesia: With emphasis on the application of the bispectral index and the middle latency auditory evoked response to the prevention of recall, *Anesthesiology* **93** (2000) 876–882.

114. F. G. Zeng and R. V. Shannon, Loudness balance between electrical and acoustic stimulation, *Hear. Res.* **60** (1992) 231–235.

115. D. Oertel and E. D. Young, What's a cerebellar circuit doing in the auditory system? *Trends Neurosci.* **27** (2004) 104–110.

116. D. P. Sutherland, K. K. Glendenning and R. B. Masterton, Role of acoustic striae in hearing: Discrimination of sound-source elevation, *Hear. Res.* **120** (1998) 86–108.

117. R. B. Masterton, E. M. Granger and K. K. Glendenning, Role of acoustic striae in hearing: Mechanism for enhancement of sound detection in cats, *Hear. Res.* **73** (1994) 209–222.

# CHAPTER 7

# SPECTRAL ANALYSIS TECHNIQUES IN THE DETECTION OF CORONARY ARTERY STENOSIS

ELİF DERYA ÜBEYLİ*

*Department of Electrical and Electronics Engineering,
Faculty of Engineering, TOBB Ekonomi ve Teknoloji Üniversitesi,
06530 Söğütözü, Ankara, Turkey*
*edubeyli@etu.edu.tr*

İNAN GÜLER

*Department of Electronics and Computer Education,
Faculty of Technical Education, Gazi University,
06500 Teknikokullar, Ankara, Turkey*
*iguler@gazi.edu.tr*

This chapter intends to study an integrated view of the spectral analysis techniques in the detection of coronary artery stenosis. The chapter includes illustrative and detailed information about medical decision support systems and feature extraction/selection from signals recorded from coronary arteries. In this respect, the chapter satisfies the automated diagnostic systems, which includes the spectral analysis techniques, feature extraction and/or selection methods, and decision support systems. The objective of the chapter is coherent with the objective of the book, which includes techniques in the detection of coronary artery stenosis, experiments for implementation of decision support systems, and measuring performance of decision support systems. The major objective of the chapter is to guide readers who want to develop an automated decision support system for detection of coronary artery stenosis. Toward achieving this objective, this chapter will present the techniques which should be considered in developing decision support systems. The authors suggest that the content of the chapter will assist the people in gaining a better understanding of the techniques in the detection of coronary artery stenosis.

*Keywords*: Spectral analysis techniques; automated diagnostic systems; feature extraction/selection; coronary artery stenosis.

## 1. Introduction

Spectral analysis considers the problem of determining the spectral content (distribution of power over frequency) of a time series from a finite set of measurements, by means of various spectral analysis techniques. Spectral analysis finds applications in many diverse fields. In different fields, the spectral analysis may reveal "hidden periodicities" in the studied data, which are to be associated with cyclic behavior or recurring processes.[1-4] Spectral analysis techniques have

---

*Corresponding author.

traditionally been based on Fourier transform and filtering theory. Within the last decade there has been a flurry of research activity into formulating and comparing alternative means of spectral estimation. The impetus has been the promise of high resolution. Since a primary motivation for the recent interest in alternative methods is improved performance, the important but difficult case of short data records is stressed. For longer data records Fourier methods prove to be adequate. It is natural to attempt a definitive comparison of the various spectral estimation methods. However, no judgments have been rendered since the merits of a particular approach tend to be application-dependent, the performance critically dependent on the data type.[1-4] Spectral analysis techniques can be found at the heart of many biomedical signal processing systems designed to extract information. In medicine, spectral analysis of various signals recorded from a subject, such as electrocardiograms (ECGs), electroencephalograms (EEGs), ultrasound signals, can provide useful information for diagnosis.[5-14] In this chapter, the characteristics of each spectral estimate have been presented. It is hoped that this chapter will serve as a guide in helping the reader to make intelligent choices for analysis of signals recorded from coronary arteries of healthy subjects (control group) and subjects suffering from stenosis.

The power spectrum has a shape similar to the histogram of the blood velocities within the sample volume (in the arteries) and thus spectral analysis of the signal produces information concerning the velocity distribution in the artery.[5-14] The estimation of the power spectral density (PSD) of the signal is performed by applying spectral analysis methods. The classical methods (nonparametric or fast Fourier transform-based methods), model-based methods (autoregressive, moving average, and autoregressive moving average methods), time-frequency methods (short-time Fourier transform, Wigner–Ville distribution, wavelet transform), eigenvector methods (Pisarenko, multiple signal classification, Minimum-Norm) can be used to obtain PSD estimates of the signals under study.[5-14] The obtained PSD estimates provide the features which are well defining the signals. These extracted features are then used as inputs for the automated diagnostic systems. Therefore, spectral analysis of the signals are important in representing, interpreting, and discriminating the signals.

Automated diagnostic systems are important applications of pattern recognition, aiming at assisting doctors in making diagnostic decisions. Automated diagnostic systems have been applied to and are of interest for a variety of medical data, such as ECGs, EEGs, ultrasound signals/images, X-rays, and computed tomographic images.[15-37] Conventional methods of monitoring and diagnosing the diseases rely on detecting the presence of particular signal features by a human observer. Due to large number of patients in intensive care units and the need for continuous observation of such conditions, several techniques for automated diagnostic systems have been developed in the past 10 years in an attempt to solve this problem. Such techniques work by transforming the mostly qualitative

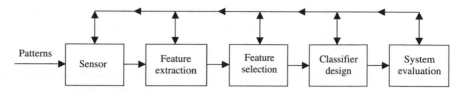

Fig. 1. The basic stages involved in the design of a classification system.

diagnostic criteria into a more objective quantitative signal feature classification problem.[14,38,39] Figure 1 shows the various stages followed for the design of a classification system. As it is apparent from the feedback arrows, these stages are not independent. On the contrary, they are interrelated and, depending on the results, one may go back to redesign earlier stages in order to improve the overall performance.

Medical diagnostic decision support systems have become an established component of medical technology. The main concept of the medical technology is an inductive engine that learns the decision characteristics of the diseases and can then be used to diagnose future patients with uncertain disease states. A number of quantitative models including multilayer perceptron neural networks (MLPNNs), combined neural networks (CNNs), mixture of experts (MEs), modified mixture of experts (MMEs), probabilistic neural networks (PNNs), recurrent neural networks (RNNs), and support vector machines (SVMs) are being used in medical diagnostic support systems to assist human decision-makers in disease diagnosis.[38,39] Artificial neural networks (ANNs) have been used in a great number of medical diagnostic decision support system applications because of the belief that they have greater predictive power. Unfortunately, there is no theory available to guide an intelligent choice of model based on the complexity of the diagnostic task. In most situations, developers are simply picking a single model that yields satisfactory results, or they are benchmarking a small subset of models with cross validation estimates on test sets.[14,38–41]

ANNs are computational architectures composed of interconnected units (neurons). Its name reflects its initial inspiration from biological neural systems, though the functioning of today's ANNs may be quite different from that of the biological ones. Sometimes the term neural network also refers to the corresponding mathematical model, but properly speaking a network is an architecture. It is difficult to give a clear definition of ANNs, due to their variety. However, at least the following two particularities distinguish them from other computational architectures or mathematical models.

*Neural networks are naturally massively parallel:* This is the structural similarity of ANNs to biological ones. Though in some cases neural network models are implemented in software on ordinary digital computers, they are naturally suitable for parallel implementations.

*Neural networks are adaptive:* A neural network is composed of "living" units or neurons. It can learn or memorize information from data. Learning is the most fascinating feature of neural networks.[42–44]

ANNs are computational modeling tools that have recently emerged and found extensive acceptance in many disciplines for modeling complex real-world problems. ANN-based models are empirical in nature, however they can provide practically accurate solutions for precisely or imprecisely formulated problems and for phenomena that are only understood through experimental data and field observations. ANNs produce complicated nonlinear models relating the inputs (the independent variables of a system) to the outputs (the dependent predictive variables). ANNs have been widely used for various tasks, such as pattern classification, time series prediction, nonlinear control, function approximation, and telecommunications. ANNs are desirable because (i) nonlinearity allows better fit to the data, (ii) noise-insensitivity provides accurate prediction in the presence of uncertain data and measurement errors, (iii) high parallelism implies fast processing and hardware failure-tolerance, (iv) learning and adaptivity allow the system to modify its internal structure in response to changing environment, and (v) generalization enables application of the model to unlearned data. Neural networks can be trained to recognize patterns. Also the nonlinear models developed during training allow neural networks to generalize their conclusions and to make application to patterns not previously encountered.[42–44]

On analyzing recent developments, it becomes clear that the trend is to develop new methods for computer decision-making in medicine and to evaluate critically these methods in clinical practice. Diagnosis of diseases may be considered as a pattern classification task. If the inputs are ambiguous and possess variability, the conventional pattern classification system may not work. Two patients may not have similar signs and symptoms resulting in the same disease. The diseases of the patients cannot be classified into a single class unless some more measurements and tests are made to resolve the ambiguity. ANN is capable of classifying patterns under variability and ambiguity.[38–41]

Data acquisition from coronary arteries, spectral analysis techniques, medical decision support systems, feature extraction/selection, review of different decision support systems, experiments for implementation of decision support systems, measuring performance of decision support systems are presented in the sections of this chapter. The requirement of having a more accurate diagnostic tool, the advantages/disadvantages and/or strengths/weaknesses of the presented methods, the further studies, and the potential applications of the methods are explained. The extended conclusions and the discussion of the obtained results in the light of existing literature are presented. These conclusions will assist the readers in gaining intuition about the medical diagnostic decision support systems. The readers will understand that a potential application of automated diagnostic systems is predicting medical outcomes such as coronary artery stenosis.

## 2. Data Acquisition from Coronary Arteries

The cardiovascular system is one of the major systems of the human body. The main purpose of the cardiovascular system is to provide blood to the tissues in human body. Quantitative measurements of blood flow by ultrasonic means have considerable importance in clinical measurement. Doppler ultrasound has become indispensable as a noninvasive tool for the diagnosis and measurement of cardiovascular disease. As with many rapidly expanding technologies there have been a considerable number of types of instruments developed. The majority of Doppler devices presently in wide use may be classified into one (or sometimes more) of the groups: velocity detecting systems, duplex systems, profile detecting systems, and velocity imaging systems.[6] In this section, the mostly used continuous wave (CW) Doppler and pulsed wave (PW) Doppler devices are presented.

Doppler ultrasound provides a noninvasive assessment of the hemodynamic flow condition within arteries including coronary arteries. Diagnostic information is extracted from the Doppler blood flow signal which results from the backscattering of the ultrasound beam by moving red blood cells. Doppler devices work by detecting the change in frequency of a beam of ultrasound that is scattered from targets that are moving with respect to the ultrasound transducer. The Doppler shift frequency $f_D$ is proportional to the speed of the moving targets:

$$f_D = \frac{2vf \cos \theta}{c}, \tag{1}$$

where $v$ is the magnitude of the velocity of target, $f$ is the frequency of transmitted ultrasound, $c$ is the magnitude of the velocity of ultrasound in blood, and $\theta$ is the angle between ultrasonic beam and direction of motion.[6]

Since flow in arteries is pulsatile and the red blood cells have a random spatial distribution, the Doppler signals are highly nonstationary. The stationarity of the signal is further reduced if the flow pattern is disturbed as a result of an obstructed artery. If the blood flow over the cardiac cycle is to be observed, it is necessary to use time frames that are no longer than the length of time that the signal can be considered stationary. If longer time frames are used, the frequency spectra will be smeared and the consecutive frames will not provide a detailed indication of how the velocities within the artery are changing with respect to time. The Doppler power spectrum has a shape similar to the histogram of the blood velocities within the sample volume and thus spectral analysis of the Doppler signal produces information concerning the velocity distribution in the artery.[6,14]

### 2.1. *Continuous wave Doppler*

The simplest Doppler instrument is the CW Doppler shift detector. CW Doppler units both transmit and receive ultrasound continuously, and because of this they usually have no range resolution except in the sense that signals from a large distance

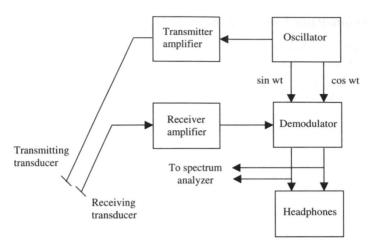

Fig. 2.   The continuous wave Doppler system. Signals from the receiving transducer are compared in frequency to those transmitted, using a scheme known as coherent demodulation. The output of the demodulator is the audible Doppler shift signal.

from the transducer are much more attenuated than those from short distances. A block circuit diagram of a simple CW Doppler unit is shown in Fig. 2.[6] The transducer assembly houses two elements, one to transmit, the other to receive. Their beams are arranged to overlap so as to form a sensitive volume defined by their spatial product. The oscillator produces an electrical voltage varying at the resonant frequency of the transducer (because the transmitter is operating continuously, a narrow band transducer is used, perhaps with only air backing, which has the effect of increasing the overall sensitivity of the system). A continuous stream of echoes arrives at the receiving transducer, whose output is amplified and fed to the demodulator. The function of the demodulator is to compare the frequency of the received echoes to that of the oscillator and to derive a signal whose frequency is equal to their difference — this is the Doppler shift signal. Stationary interfaces give rise to echoes whose frequency is identical to that of the oscillator: these are rejected by the demodulator. Most demodulators employ a technique known as phase quadrature detection, which is capable of distinguishing between signals whose frequency is higher and those whose frequency is lower than that of the transmitted signal, corresponding to Doppler shifts toward or away from the transducer. Such a directional demodulator produces two outputs that, after filtering, have a phase relationship determined by the direction of flow. Further, minor processing can be used to produce a stereo audio signal to feed to the headphones, where the sounds in one ear are the Doppler shifts corresponding to motion toward the transducer and the sounds in the other corresponding to shifts away from the transducer. The frequency of Doppler system depends on the depth of interest since ultrasound attenuation is highly dependent on frequency. Thus 7–10 MHz systems are often used for the examination of the superficial vessels. The continuous wave method is also capable of very high sensitivity to weak signals, so it is preferred for the examination of smaller vessels.[6]

## 2.2. *Pulsed wave Doppler*

Pulsed Doppler ultrasound combines the velocity detection of a CW Doppler with the range discrimination of a pulse-echo system. Short bursts of ultrasound are transmitted at regular intervals and the echoes are demodulated as they return. If the pulses are received in sufficiently rapid succession, the output of the demodulator (which compares the phase of the received pulse with that of the oscillator) consists of a sequence of samples from which the Doppler signal can be synthesized. The same transducer is generally used for transmitting and receiving. The range in tissue at which Doppler signals are detected can be controlled simply by changing the length of time the system waits after sending a pulse before opening the gate that allows it to receive. The axial length of the sensitive volume thus produced is determined by the length of time for which the gate is open. Figure 3 shows that this electronic gate is generally placed after the demodulator and is governed by these two delays, which are under the control of the operator.[6,45]

A master clock ensures synchrony between the emission of pulses and the operation of the delays and gates. Quadrature detection produces directional Doppler signals as the output of the system. In practice, although the range of the sample volume from the transducer is under the control of the operator, the form of the sensitive volume itself is influenced by a variety of factors. The length of time for which the received gate is open determines its axial extent, which may be varied between about 1.5 and 15 mm. However, the lateral dimensions depend on the ultrasound beam width and are consequently affected by the position of the sample volume in the beam as well as the transducer frequency and design. Some scanners using electronic beam focusing are capable of adjusting the focus of the beam to coincide with the location of the sample volume, thus influencing its lateral extent.

The great advantage of the pulsed systems is that it is possible to time gate, i.e. range gate the pulses so that the displayed signal originated from a known depth in the tissues. Thus, the most serious limitation of the CW systems, which is the absence of depth resolution, is overcome. There are important limitations of pulsed systems. One fundamental shortcoming of the pulsed Doppler system arises from the way in which the audible Doppler shift signal is in fact made from a large number of discrete samples, one of which is created each time an ultrasound pulse is received by the transducer. Samples that are created rapidly when compared with the rate of variation of the Doppler shift signal itself have no problems. In fact, sampling theory shows that a signal can be reconstructed unambiguously from a sequence of samples as long as the frequency of the signal is no greater than half the sampling rate (this is known as the Nyquist limit). However, the depth of the target being interrogated for motion imposes a limit on the pulse repetition frequency: an ultrasound pulse cannot

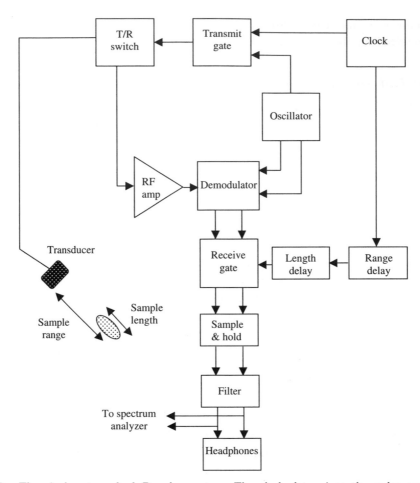

Fig. 3. The single-gate pulsed Doppler system. The clock determines the pulse repetition frequency, which might typically be 5 kHz. The clock initiates the release of a burst of ultrasound produced by the oscillator by opening the transmit gate. Echoes received by the transducer are amplified and demodulated to detect change in phase due to the Doppler effect. As they emerge from the demodulator the receive gate opens so as to accept only those echoes from the range of interest. The output of successive pulses is deposited in a sample and hold circuit, thus forming the Doppler signal.

normally be emitted before the last echo caused by the preceding pulse has been received. Thus, occasions arise when the Doppler shift frequency of the moving blood is above the Nyquist limit for that depth. The result is that the system produces an incorrect, or aliased, Doppler shift frequency which shows an ambiguous relationship between velocity of motion and the displayed Doppler shift frequency.[6,45] Various methods are available for overcoming this problem. One is to simply increase the pulse repetition rate above the limit imposed by the transit time of the ultrasonic pulse to the target and back. This may overcome the aliasing of the Doppler signal but creates a new ambiguity as to the location of echoes received when the gate is open. Other, more straightforward, solutions to the problem of aliasing are to lower the ultrasound frequency (hence lowering the Doppler shift frequencies themselves) or to resort to continuous wave Doppler, which does not suffer from the aliasing limitation. The signal-to-noise ratio of a pulsed system is inherently poorer than that of a continuous wave system because of its higher bandwidth. Narrowing this range improves signal-to-noise performance but degrades spatial resolution.

## 3. Spectral Analysis Techniques

The basic problem that we consider in this chapter is the estimation of the PSD of a signal from the observation of the signal over a finite time interval. The signals recorded from coronary artery is conventionally interpreted by analyzing its spectral content. Diagnosis and disease monitoring are assessed by analysis of spectral shape and parameters.[6,14] In order to determine the degree of coronary artery stenosis, coronary arterial signals are processed by spectral analysis methods to achieve PSD estimates.

In order to obtain PSD estimates which represent the changes in frequency with respect to time, the classical methods (nonparametric or fast Fourier transform-based methods), model-based methods (autoregressive, moving average, and autoregressive moving average methods), time-frequency methods (short-time Fourier transform, Wigner–Ville distribution, wavelet transform), eigenvector methods (Pisarenko, multiple signal classification, Minimum-Norm) are presented in the following sections.

### 3.1. *Nonparametric methods*

The nonparametric methods of spectral estimation rely entirely on the definitions of Eqs. (2) and (3) of PSD to provide spectral estimates. These methods constitute the "classical means" for PSD estimation. We first introduce two common spectral estimators, the periodogram and the correlogram derived directly from Eqs. (2) and (3), respectively,

$$P(f) = \lim_{N \to \infty} E \left\{ \frac{1}{N} \left| \sum_{n=1}^{N} x(n)e^{-j2\pi f} \right|^2 \right\}, \tag{2}$$

$$P(f) = \sum_{k=-\infty}^{\infty} r(k)e^{-j2\pi fk}, \tag{3}$$

where $P(f)$ is power spectral density and $r(k)$ is autocorrelation function of the signal under study.

These methods are equivalent under weak conditions. The periodogram and correlogram methods provide reasonably high resolution for sufficiently long data lengths, but are poor spectral estimators because their variance is high and does not decrease with increasing data length. The high variance of the periodogram and correlogram methods motivates the development of modified methods that have lower variance, at a cost of reduced resolution. The modified power spectrum estimation methods described in this section are developed by Bartlett (1948), Blackman and Tukey (1958), and Welch (1967).[1-4] These methods make no assumption about how the data were generated and hence are called nonparametric. The spectral estimates are expressed as a function of the continuous frequency variable $f$, in practice, the estimates are computed at discrete frequencies via the fast Fourier transform (FFT) algorithm.

### 3.1.1. Periodogram method

The periodogram method relies on the definition of Eq. (2) of the PSD. Neglecting the expectation and the limit operation in Eq. (2), which cannot be performed when the only available information on the signal consists of the samples $\{x(n)\}_{n=1}^{N}$ , we obtain the periodogram PSD estimate,[1-4]

$$\hat{P}_P(f) = \frac{1}{N} \left| \sum_{n=1}^{N} x(n) e^{-j2\pi fn} \right|^2 . \tag{4}$$

### 3.1.2. Correlogram method

The correlation-based definition of Eq. (3) of the PSD leads to the correlogram spectral estimator,

$$\hat{P}_C(f) = \sum_{k=-(N-1)}^{N-1} \hat{r}(k) e^{-j2\pi fk}, \tag{5}$$

where $\hat{r}(k)$ denotes an estimate of the autocorrelation lag $r(k)$ obtained from the available sample $\{x(1), x(2), \ldots, x(N)\}$.[1-4]

### 3.1.3. Blackman–Tukey method

The main problem with the periodogram is the high statistical variability of this spectral estimator, even for very large sample lengths. The poor statistical quality of the periodogram PSD estimator has been intuitively explained as arising from both the poor accuracy of $\hat{r}(k)$ in $\hat{P}_C(f)$ for extreme lags ($|k| \cong N$) and the large number of (even if small) covariance estimation errors that are cumulatively summed up in $\hat{P}_C(f)$. Both these effects may be reduced by truncating the sum in the definition formula of $\hat{P}_C(f)$ given by Eq. (5). Following this idea leads to the Blackman–Tukey estimator, which is given by

$$\hat{P}_{\mathrm{BT}}(f) = \sum_{k=-(M-1)}^{M-1} w(k) \hat{r}(k) e^{-j2\pi fk}, \tag{6}$$

where $\{w(k)\}$ weights the lags of the sample covariance sequence, and it is called a lag window.[1-4]

### 3.1.4. *Bartlett method*

The basic idea of the Bartlett method is to reduce the large fluctuations of the periodogram, split up the available sample of $N$ observations into $L = N/M$ subsamples of $M$ observations each, and then average the periodograms obtained from the subsamples. $\{x_l(n)\}$, $l = 1, \ldots, K$ are signal intervals and each interval's length is equal to $M$. The Bartlett spectral estimator is defined as

$$\hat{P}_l(f) = \frac{1}{M} \left| \sum_{n=1}^{N} x_l(n) e^{-j2\pi fn} \right|^2 \quad \text{and} \quad \hat{P}_B(f) = \frac{1}{K} \sum_{l=1}^{K} \hat{P}_l(f), \tag{7}$$

where $\hat{P}_l(f)$ is the periodogram estimate of each signal interval.[1-4]

### 3.1.5. *Welch method*

Welch spectral estimator can be efficiently computed via FFT and is one of the most frequently used PSD estimation methods. In the Welch method, signals are divided into overlapping segments, each data segment is windowed, periodograms are calculated, and then the average of periodograms is found. $\{x_l(n)\}$, $l = 1, \ldots, K$ are signal intervals and each interval's length equals to $M$. The Welch spectral estimator is defined as

$$\hat{P}_l(f) = \frac{1}{M} \frac{1}{P} \left| \sum_{n=1}^{M} v(n) x_l(n) e^{-j2\pi fn} \right|^2 \quad \text{and} \quad \hat{P}_W(f) = \frac{1}{K} \sum_{l=1}^{K} \hat{P}_l(f), \tag{8}$$

where $\hat{P}_l(f)$ is the periodogram estimate of each signal interval, $v(n)$ is the data window, $P$ is the average of $v(n)$ given as $P = \frac{1}{M} \sum_{n=1}^{M} |v(n)|^2$.[1-4]

## 3.2. *Parametric methods*

The parametric or model-based methods of spectral estimation assume that the signal satisfies a generating model with known functional form, and then proceed by estimating the parameters in the assumed model. The signal's spectral characteristics of interest are then derived from the estimated model. The models to be discussed are the time series or rational transfer function models. They are the autoregressive (AR) model, the moving average (MA) model, and the autoregressive–moving average (ARMA) model. The AR model is suitable for representing spectra with narrow peaks. The MA model provides a good approximation for those spectra which are characterized by broad peaks and sharp nulls. Such spectra are encountered less frequently in applications than narrowband spectra, so there is a somewhat limited interest in using the MA model for spectral estimation. For this reason, our discussion of the MA spectral estimation will be brief. Spectra with both sharp peaks and deep nulls can be modeled by ARMA model. However, the great initial promise of ARMA spectral estimation diminishes to some extent because there is yet no well-established algorithm, from both theoretical and practical standpoints, for ARMA parameter estimation. The theoretically optimal ARMA estimators are based on iterative procedures whose global convergence is not guaranteed. The practical ARMA estimators are computationally simple and often quite reliable, but their statistical accuracy may be poor in some cases.[1-4]

### 3.2.1. AR method

AR method is the most frequently used parametric method because estimation of the AR parameters can be done easily by solving linear equations. In the AR method, data can be modeled as output of a causal, all-pole, discrete filter whose input is white noise. The AR method of order $p$ is expressed by the following equation:

$$x(n) = -\sum_{k=1}^{p} a(k)x(n-k) + w(n),\tag{9}$$

where $a(k)$ are the AR coefficients and $w(n)$ is white noise of variance equal to $\sigma^2$. The AR($p$) model can be characterized by the AR parameters $\{a[1], a[2], \ldots, a[p], \sigma^2\}$. The PSD is

$$P_{AR}(f) = \frac{\sigma^2}{|A(f)|^2},\tag{10}$$

where $A(f) = 1 + a_1 e^{-j2\pi f} + \cdots + a_p e^{-j2\pi fp}$.

To obtain stable and high performance AR method, some factors must be taken into consideration such as selection of the optimum estimation method, selection of the model order, the length of the signal which will be modeled, and the level of stationary of the data.[1-4]

Because of the good performance of the AR spectral estimation methods as well as the computational efficiency, many of the estimation methods to be described are widely used in practice and given in the following. The AR spectral estimation methods are based on estimation of either the AR parameters or the reflection coefficients. Except the maximum likelihood estimation, the techniques estimate the parameters by minimizing an estimate of the prediction error power. The maximum likelihood estimation method is based on maximizing the likelihood function.[1-4]

### 3.2.1.1. Yule–Walker method

It is assumed that the data $\{x(0), x(1), \ldots, x(N-1)\}$ are observed. In the Yule–Walker method, or the autocorrelation method as it is sometimes referred to, the AR parameters are estimated by minimizing an estimate of prediction error power.

In matrix form the set of equations in terms of autocorrelation function estimates becomes,

$$
\begin{bmatrix} \hat{r}(1) \\ \vdots \\ \hat{r}(p) \end{bmatrix} + \begin{bmatrix} \hat{r}(0) & \cdots & \hat{r}(-p+1) \\ \vdots & \ddots & \vdots \\ \hat{r}(p-1) & \cdots & \hat{r}(0) \end{bmatrix} \begin{bmatrix} \hat{a}(1) \\ \vdots \\ \hat{a}(p) \end{bmatrix} = \begin{bmatrix} 0 \\ \vdots \\ 0 \end{bmatrix}
$$

or

$$
\hat{r}_p + \hat{R}_p \hat{a} = 0. \tag{11}
$$

From Eq. (11) the AR parameter estimates are found as

$$
\hat{a} = -\hat{R}_p^{-1} \hat{r}_p. \tag{12}
$$

The estimate of the white noise variance $\sigma^2$ is found as

$$
\hat{\sigma}^2 = \hat{r}(0) + \sum_{k=1}^{p} \hat{a}(k)\hat{r}(-k). \tag{13}
$$

From the estimates of the AR parameters, PSD estimation is formed as[1-4]

$$
\hat{P}_{\text{YW}}(f) = \frac{\hat{\sigma}^2}{\left|1 + \sum_{k=1}^{p} \hat{a}(k)e^{-j2\pi fk}\right|^2}. \tag{14}
$$

### 3.2.1.2. Covariance method

The only difference between the covariance method and the autocorrelation method is the range of summation in the prediction error power estimate. In the covariance method all the data points needed to compute the prediction error power estimate. No zeroing of the data is necessary. The AR parameter estimates as the solution of the equations can be written as

$$
\begin{bmatrix} c(1,0) \\ \vdots \\ c(p,0) \end{bmatrix} + \begin{bmatrix} c(1,1) & \cdots & c(1,p) \\ \vdots & \ddots & \vdots \\ c(p,1) & \cdots & c(p,p) \end{bmatrix} \begin{bmatrix} \hat{a}(1) \\ \vdots \\ \hat{a}(p) \end{bmatrix} = \begin{bmatrix} 0 \\ \vdots \\ 0 \end{bmatrix}
$$

or

$$
c_p + C_p \hat{a} = 0, \tag{15}
$$

where

$$
c(j,k) = \frac{1}{N-p} \sum_{n=p}^{N-1} x^*(n-j)x(n-k).
$$

From Eq. (15) the AR parameter estimates are found as

$$
\hat{a} = -C_p^{-1} c_p. \tag{16}
$$

The white noise variance is estimated as

$$\hat{\sigma}^2 = c(0,0) + \sum_{k=1}^{p} \hat{a}(k)c(0,k). \tag{17}$$

From the estimates of the AR parameters, PSD estimation is formed as[1-4]

$$\hat{P}_{COV}(f) = \frac{\hat{\sigma}^2}{\left|1 + \sum_{k=1}^{p} \hat{a}(k)e^{-j2\pi fk}\right|^2}. \tag{18}$$

### 3.2.1.3. Modified covariance method

The modified covariance method estimates the AR parameters by minimizing the average of the estimated forward and backward prediction error powers.

The AR parameter estimates can be written in the matrix form,

$$\begin{bmatrix} c(1,0) \\ \vdots \\ c(p,0) \end{bmatrix} + \begin{bmatrix} c(1,1) & \cdots & c(1,p) \\ \vdots & \ddots & \vdots \\ c(p,1) & \cdots & c(p,p) \end{bmatrix} \begin{bmatrix} \hat{a}(1) \\ \vdots \\ \hat{a}(p) \end{bmatrix} = \begin{bmatrix} 0 \\ \vdots \\ 0 \end{bmatrix}$$

or

$$c_p + C_p\hat{a} = 0, \tag{19}$$

where

$$c(j,k) = \frac{1}{2(N-p)} \left( \sum_{n=p}^{N-1} x^*(n-j)x(n-k) + \sum_{n=0}^{N-1-p} x(n+j)x^*(n+k) \right).$$

From Eq. (19) the AR parameter estimates are found as

$$\hat{a} = -C_p^{-1}c_p. \tag{20}$$

The estimate of the white noise variance is

$$\hat{\sigma}^2 = c(0,0) + \sum_{k=1}^{p} \hat{a}(k)c(0,k). \tag{21}$$

It is observed that the modified covariance method is identical to the covariance except for the definition of $c(j,k)$, the autocorrelation estimator. From the estimates of the AR parameters, PSD estimation is formed as[1-4]:

$$\hat{P}_{MCOV}(f) = \frac{\hat{\sigma}^2}{\left|1 + \sum_{k=1}^{p} \hat{a}(k)e^{-j2\pi fk}\right|^2}. \tag{22}$$

### 3.2.1.4. Burg method

The Burg method is based on the minimization of the forward and backward prediction errors and on the estimation of the reflection coefficient. The forward and backward prediction errors for a $p$th-order model are defined as

$$\hat{e}_{f,p}(n) = x(n) + \sum_{i=1}^{p} \hat{a}_{p,i} x(n-i), \quad n = p+1, \ldots, N, \tag{23}$$

$$\hat{e}_{b,p}(n) = x(n-p) + \sum_{i=1}^{p} \hat{a}_{p,i}^{*} x(n-p+i), \quad n = p+1, \ldots, N. \tag{24}$$

The AR parameters are related to the reflection coefficient $\hat{k}_p$ by

$$\hat{a}_{p,i} = \begin{cases} \hat{a}_{p-1,i} + \hat{k}_p \hat{a}_{p-1,p-i}^{*}, & i = 1, \ldots, p-1 \\ \hat{k}_p, & i = p \end{cases} . \tag{25}$$

The Burg method considers the recursive-in-order estimation of $\hat{k}_p$ given that the AR coefficients for order $p - 1$ have been computed. The reflection coefficient estimate is given by

$$\hat{k}_p = \frac{-2 \sum_{n=p+1}^{N} \hat{e}_{f,p-1}(n) \hat{e}_{b,p-1}^{*}(n-1)}{\sum_{n=p+1}^{N} \left[ |\hat{e}_{f,p-1}(n)|^2 + |\hat{e}_{b,p-1}(n-1)|^2 \right]}. \tag{26}$$

From the estimates of the AR parameters, PSD estimation is formed as

$$\hat{P}_{\text{Burg}}(f) = \frac{\hat{e}_p}{|1 + \sum_{k=1}^{p} \hat{a}_p(k) e^{-j2\pi fk}|^2}, \tag{27}$$

where $\hat{e}_p = \hat{e}_{f,p} + \hat{e}_{b,p}$ is the total least squares error.[1-4]

### 3.2.1.5. Least squares method

Linear prediction of the AR method is to predict the unobserved data sample $x(n)$ based on the observed data samples $\{x(n-1), x(n-2), \ldots, x(n-p)\}$,

$$\hat{x}(n) = -\sum_{k=1}^{p} \alpha_k x(n-k); \tag{28}$$

the prediction coefficients $\{\alpha_1, \alpha_2, \ldots, \alpha_p\}$ are chosen to minimize the power of the prediction error $e(n)$:

$$\rho = E\{|e(n)|^2\} = E\{|x(n) - \hat{x}(n)|^2\}. \tag{29}$$

For minimizing $\rho$ the orthogonality principle is used,

$$r(k) = -\sum_{l=1}^{p} \alpha_l r(k-l) \quad k = 1, 2 \ldots, p, \tag{30}$$

$$\rho_{\min} = r(0) + \sum_{k=1}^{p} \alpha_k r(-k), \tag{31}$$

where $\alpha_k = a[k]$ for $k = 1, 2, \ldots, p$ and $\rho_{\min} = \sigma^2$.

Given a finite set of data samples $\{x(n)\}_{n=1}^{N}$ minimum of $E\{|e(n)|^2\}$ is calculated with respect to $\alpha_k$ $(k = 1, 2, \ldots, p)$.

$$f(\alpha) = E\{|e(n)|^2\} = \sum_{n=N_1}^{N_2} |e(n)|^2$$

$$= \sum_{n=N_1}^{N_2} \left| x(n) + \sum_{k=1}^{p} \alpha[k] x(n-k) \right|^2, \quad k = 1, 2, \ldots, p$$

$$= \left\| \begin{bmatrix} x(N_1) \\ x(N_1+1) \\ \vdots \\ x(N_2) \end{bmatrix} + \begin{bmatrix} x(N_1-1) & \cdots\cdots & x(N_1-p) \\ x(N_1) & \cdots\cdots & x(N_1+1-p) \\ \vdots & & \vdots \\ x(N_2-1) & \cdots\cdots & x(N_2-p) \end{bmatrix} \alpha \right\|^2$$

$$= \|x + X\alpha\|^2. \tag{32}$$

The vector $\alpha$ that minimizes $f(\alpha)$ is given by

$$\hat{\alpha} = -(X^*X)^{-1}(X^*x). \tag{33}$$

By substituting autocorrelation function estimates $\{\hat{r}(k)\}_{k=0}^{p}$ and $\hat{\alpha}$ in Eq. (31), $\hat{\rho}_{\min}$ is obtained,

$$\hat{\rho}_{\min} = \hat{r}(0) + \sum_{k=1}^{p} \hat{\alpha}\hat{r}(-k). \tag{34}$$

From the estimates of the AR parameters, PSD estimation is formed as[1-4]:

$$\hat{P}_{LS}(f) = \frac{\hat{\rho}_{\min}}{|1 + \sum_{k=1}^{p} \hat{a}_p(k)e^{-j2\pi fk}|^2}. \tag{35}$$

### 3.2.1.6. Maximum likelihood estimation method

If the maximum likelihood estimation (MLE) of a parameter exists under regular condition, it is consistent, asymptotically unbiased, efficient, and normally distributed. Likelihood function of $\{x \sim N(0, C(\theta))\}$ Gaussian random process is expressed as

$$p(x; \theta) = \frac{1}{(2\pi)^{N/2} \det^{1/2}(C(\theta))} \exp\left[-\frac{1}{2}x^T C^{-1}(\theta)x\right]. \tag{36}$$

The logarithm of Eq. (36) equals log-likelihood function,

$$\ln p(x; \theta) = -\frac{N}{2}\ln 2\pi - \frac{N}{2}\int_{-1/2}^{1/2}\left[\ln P(f) + \frac{I(f)}{P(f)}\right]df, \tag{37}$$

where $I(f)$ is periodogram of the data,

$$I(f) = \frac{1}{N}\left|\sum_{n=0}^{N-1} x(n)\exp(-j2\pi fn)\right|^2.$$

The MLE of $\theta$ is obtained by calculating the maximum of Eq. (37). The set of equations to be solved for the MLE of AR parameters,

$$\sum_{l=1}^{p} \hat{a}(l)\hat{r}(k-l) = -\hat{r}(k), \quad k = 1, 2, \ldots, p,$$

or in matrix form

$$\begin{bmatrix} \hat{r}(0) & \hat{r}(1) & \cdots & \hat{r}(p-1) \\ \hat{r}(1) & \hat{r}(0) & \cdots & \hat{r}(p-2) \\ \vdots & \vdots & \ddots & \vdots \\ \hat{r}(p-1) & \hat{r}(p-2) & \cdots & \hat{r}(0) \end{bmatrix} \begin{bmatrix} \hat{a}(1) \\ \hat{a}(2) \\ \vdots \\ \hat{a}(p) \end{bmatrix} = - \begin{bmatrix} \hat{r}(1) \\ \hat{r}(2) \\ \vdots \\ \hat{r}(p) \end{bmatrix}. \tag{38}$$

Equation (38) is equal to the estimated Yule–Walker equations and the MLE of AR parameters are calculated from this equation. Then the MLE of $\sigma^2$ is found as

$$\hat{\sigma}^2 = \hat{r}(0) + \sum_{k=1}^{p} \hat{a}(k)\hat{r}(k). \tag{39}$$

These estimated parameters are used to compute the AR PSD as[1–4]

$$\hat{P}_{\text{MLE}}(f) = \frac{\hat{\sigma}^2}{|1 + \sum_{k=1}^{p} \hat{a}(k)e^{-j2\pi fk}|^2}. \tag{40}$$

### 3.2.2. *MA method*

MA method is one of the model-based methods in which the signal is obtained by filtering white noise with an all-zero filter. Estimation of the MA spectrum can be done by the reparameterization of the PSD in terms of the autocorrelation function. The $q$th-order MA PSD estimation is[1-4]

$$\hat{P}_{MA}(f) = \sum_{k=-q}^{q} \hat{r}(k)e^{-j2\pi fk}. \tag{41}$$

### 3.2.3. ARMA method

The spectral factorization problem associated with a rational PSD has multiple solutions, with the stable and minimum phase ARMA model being one of the model-based methods. A reliable method is to construct a set of linear equations and to use the method of least squares on the set of equations. Suppose that for an ARMA of order $p, q$ the autocorrelation sequence can be accurately estimated up to lag $M$, where $M > p + q$. Then the following set of linear equations can be written:

$$\begin{bmatrix} r(q) & r(q-1) & \cdots & r(q-p+1) \\ r(q+1) & r(q) & \cdots & r(q-p+2) \\ \vdots & \vdots & & \\ r(M-1) & r(M-2) & & r(M-p) \end{bmatrix} \begin{bmatrix} a_1 \\ a_2 \\ \vdots \\ a_p \end{bmatrix} = - \begin{bmatrix} r(q+1) \\ r(q+2) \\ \vdots \\ r(M) \end{bmatrix}, \tag{42}$$

or equivalently,

$$Ra = -r. \tag{43}$$

Since dimension of $R$ is $(M - q)xp$ and $M - q > p$ the least squares criterion can be used to solve for the parameter vector $a$. The result of this minimization is

$$\hat{a} = - (R^*R)^{-1}(R^*r). \tag{44}$$

Finally the estimated ARMA power spectrum is[1-4]

$$\hat{P}_{ARMA}(f) = \frac{\hat{P}_{MA}(f)}{|1 + \sum_{k=1}^{p} \hat{a}(k)e^{-j2\pi fk}|^2}, \tag{45}$$

where $\hat{P}_{MA}(f)$ is the estimate of MA PSD and is given in Eq. (41).

### 3.2.4. Selection of AR, MA, and ARMA model orders

One of the most important aspects of the use in model-based methods is the selection of the model order. Much work has been done by various investigators on this problem and many experimental results have been given in the literature.[1-4] One of the better known criteria for selecting the model order proposed by Akaike (1974),[46] called the Akaike information criterion (AIC), is based on selecting the order that minimizes Eq. (46) for the AR method, Eq. (47) for the MA method, and Eq. (48)

for the ARMA method:

$$\text{AIC}(p) = \ln \hat{\sigma}^2 + 2p/N, \tag{46}$$

$$\text{AIC}(q) = \ln \hat{\sigma}^2 + 2q/N, \tag{47}$$

$$\text{AIC}(p, q) = \ln \hat{\sigma}^2 + 2(p + q)/N, \tag{48}$$

where $\hat{\sigma}^2$ is the estimated variance of the linear prediction error.

### 3.3. *Time–frequency methods*

Mappings between the time and the frequency domains have been widely used in signal analysis and processing. Since Fourier methods may not be appropriate to nonstationary signals, or signals with short-lived components, alternative approaches have been sought. Among the early works in this area, one can cite Gabor's development of the short-time Fourier transform (STFT), a procedure in which a window function is passed through a signal, with the assumption that inside the window the signal is stationary. Another approach is the Wigner–Ville distribution. In this case, a quadratic distribution of the time and the frequency characteristics of the signal was derived. The major drawback of this representation was in its interpretation. Namely, the representation not only contained the signal components but also interference terms generated by the interaction of those signal components with each other. The wavelet transform (WT) provides a representation of the signal in a lattice of "building blocks" which have good frequency and time localization. The wavelet representation, in its continuous and discrete versions, as well as in terms of a multiresolution approximation is presented.[5]

#### 3.3.1. *Short-time Fourier transform*

Spectral analysis of the signal is performed using STFT, in which the signal is divided into small sequential or overlapping data frames and FFT applied to each one. The output of successive STFTs can provide a time–frequency representation of the signal. To accomplish this the signal is truncated into short data frames by multiplying it by a window so that the modified signal is zero outside the data frame. In order to analyze the whole signal, the window is translated in time and then reapplied to the signal.[5,12]

In STFT analysis, the signal is multiplied by a window function $w(t)$ and the spectrum of this signal frame is calculated using the Fourier transform. Thus

$$\text{STFT}(t, f) = \left| \int_{-\infty}^{+\infty} x(\tau)w(\tau - t)e^{-j2\pi f \tau} d\tau \right|^2, \tag{49}$$

where $x(t)$ represents the analyzed signal.

The problem with STFT is, choosing a short analysis window may cause poor frequency resolution. On the other hand, while a long analysis window may improve frequency resolution, it compromises the assumption of stationarity within the window. A more flexible approach would be to use a scalable window: a compressed window for analyzing high frequency detail and a dilated window for uncovering low frequency trends within the signal.[5,12]

### 3.3.2. Wigner–Ville distribution

The direct use of the Wigner–Ville distribution as

$$\text{WD}(t, f) = \int x(t + \tau/2)x^*(t - \tau/2)e^{-j2\pi f\tau}d\tau \qquad (50)$$

is rarely encountered for biomedical applications, where the interference terms have classically no meaning in terms of physiological or clinical interpretations.[5]

### 3.3.3. Wavelet transform

WT is designed to address the problem of nonstationary signals. It involves representing a time function in terms of simple, fixed building blocks, termed wavelets. These building blocks are actually a family of functions which are derived from a single generating function called the mother wavelet by translation and dilation operations. Dilation, also known as scaling, compresses or stretches the mother wavelet and translation shifts it along the time axis.[5,12,47,48]

WT can be categorized into continuous and discrete. Continuous wavelet transform (CWT) is defined by

$$\text{CWT}(a, b) = \int\limits_{-\infty}^{+\infty} x(t)\psi_{a,b}^*(t)dt, \qquad (51)$$

where $x(t)$ represents the analyzed signal, $a$ and $b$ represent the scaling factor (dilatation/compression coefficient) and translation along the time axis (shifting coefficient), respectively, and the superscript asterisk denotes the complex conjugation. $\psi_{a,b}(\cdot)$ is obtained by scaling the wavelet at time $b$ and scale $a$:

$$\psi_{a,b}(t) = \frac{1}{\sqrt{|a|}}\psi\left(\frac{t - b}{a}\right), \qquad (52)$$

where $\psi(t)$ represents the wavelet.[5,47]

Continuous, in the context of WT, implies that the scaling and translation parameters $a$ and $b$ change continuously. However, calculating wavelet coefficients for every possible scale can represent a considerable effort and result in a vast amount of data. Therefore, discrete wavelet transform (DWT) is often used. WT can be thought of as an extension of the classic Fourier transform, except that, instead of working on a single scale (time or frequency), it works on a multi-scale basis. This multi-scale feature of WT allows the decomposition of a signal into a number of scales, each scale representing a particular coarseness of the signal under study. In the procedure of multi-resolution decomposition of a signal $x[n]$, each stage consists of two digital filters and two downsamplers by 2. The first filter $g[\cdot]$ is the discrete mother wavelet, high-pass in nature, and the second, $h[\cdot]$ is its mirror version, low-pass in nature. The downsampled outputs of the first high-pass and low-pass filters provide the detail, $D_1$ and the approximation, $A_1$, respectively. The first approximation, $A_1$ is further decomposed and this process is continued.

All wavelet transforms can be specified in terms of a low-pass filter $h$, which satisfies the standard quadrature mirror filter condition:

$$H(z)H(z^{-1}) + H(-z)H(-z^{-1}) = 1, \tag{53}$$

where $H(z)$ denotes the $z$-transform of the filter $h$. Its complementary high-pass filter can be defined as

$$G(z) = zH(-z^{-1}). \tag{54}$$

A sequence of filters with increasing length (indexed by $i$) can be obtained:

$$\begin{aligned} H_{i+1}(z) &= H(z^{2^i})H_i(z) \\ G_{i+1}(z) &= G(z^{2^i})H_i(z), \quad i = 0, \ldots, I-1, \end{aligned} \tag{55}$$

with the initial condition $H_0(z) = 1$. It is expressed as a two-scale relation in time domain

$$\begin{aligned} h_{i+1}(k) &= [h]_{\uparrow 2^i} * h_i(k) \\ g_{i+1}(k) &= [g]_{\uparrow 2^i} * h_i(k), \end{aligned} \tag{56}$$

where the subscript $[\cdot]_{\uparrow m}$ indicates the up-sampling by a factor of $m$ and $k$ is the equally sampled discrete time.

The normalized wavelet and scale basis functions $\varphi_{i,l}(k)$, $\psi_{i,l}(k)$ can be defined as

$$\begin{aligned} \varphi_{i,l}(k) &= 2^{i/2} h_i(k - 2^i l), \\ \psi_{i,l}(k) &= 2^{i/2} g_i(k - 2^i l), \end{aligned} \tag{57}$$

where the factor $2^{i/2}$ is an inner product normalization, $i$ and $l$ are the scale parameter and the translation parameter, respectively. The DWT decomposition can be described as

$$\begin{aligned} a_{(i)}(l) &= x(k) * \varphi_{i,l}(k) \\ d_{(i)}(l) &= x(k) * \psi_{i,l}(k), \end{aligned} \tag{58}$$

where $a_{(i)}(l)$ and $d_i(l)$ are the approximation coefficients and the detail coefficients at resolution $i$, respectively.

The concept of being able to decompose a signal totally and then perfectly reconstruct the signal again is practical, but it is not particularly useful by itself. In order to make use of this tool it is necessary to manipulate the wavelet coefficients to identify characteristics of the signal that were not apparent from the original time domain signal.[5,12,47,48]

## 3.4. Eigenvector methods

Eigenvector methods are used for estimating frequencies and powers of signals from noise–corrupted measurements. These methods are based on an eigen-decomposition of the correlation matrix of the noise–corrupted signal. Even when the signal-to-noise ratio (SNR) is low, the eigenvector methods produce frequency spectra of high resolution. The eigenvector methods (Pisarenko, multiple signal classification, and Minimum-Norm) are best suited to signals that can be assumed to be composed of several specific sinusoids buried in noise.[2,3,10,49]

### 3.4.1. Pisarenko method

The Pisarenko method is particularly useful for estimating PSD which contains sharp peaks at the expected frequencies. The polynomial $A(f)$ which contains zeros on the unit circle can then be used to estimate PSD.

$$A(f) = \sum_{k=0}^{m} a_k e^{-j2\pi fk}, \tag{59}$$

where $A(f)$ represents the desired polynomial, $a_k$ represents coefficients of the desired polynomial, and $m$ represents the order of the eigenfilter, $A(f)$.

The polynomial can also be expressed in terms of the autocorrelation matrix $R$ of the input signal. Assuming that the noise is white:

$$R = E\{x(n)^* \cdot x(n)^T\} = SPS^{\#} + \sigma\nu^2 I, \tag{60}$$

where $x(n)$ is the observed signal, $S$ represents the signal direction matrix of dimension $(m+1) \times L$, and $L$ is the dimension of the signal subspace, $R$ is the autocorrelation matrix of dimension $(m+1) \times (m+1)$, $P$ is the signal power matrix of dimension $(L) \times (L)$, $\sigma\nu^2$ represents the noise power, $*$ represents the complex conjugate, $I$ is the identity matrix, $\#$ represents the complex conjugate transposed, and $T$ shows the matrix transposed. $S$, the signal direction matrix is expressed as

$$S = [Sw_1 \ Sw_2 \ \cdots \ Sw_L],$$

where $w_1, w_2, \ldots, w_L$ represent the signal frequencies:

$$Sw_i = [1 e^{jwi} e^{j2wi} \cdots e^{jmwi}]^T \quad i = 1, 2, \ldots, L.$$

In practical applications, it is common to construct the estimated autocorrelation matrix $\hat{R}$ from the autocorrelation lags:

$$\hat{R}(k) = \frac{1}{N} \sum_{n=0}^{N-1-k} x(n+k) \cdot x(n) \quad k = 0, 1, \cdots, m, \tag{61}$$

where $k$ is the autocorrelation lag index and $N$ is the number of the signal samples.

Then, the estimated autocorrelation matrix becomes

$$\hat{R}(k) = \begin{bmatrix} \hat{R}(0) & \hat{R}(1) & \hat{R}(2) & \cdots & \hat{R}(m) \\ \hat{R}(1) & \hat{R}(0) & \hat{R}(1) & \cdots & \hat{R}(m-1) \\ \hat{R}(2) & \hat{R}(1) & \hat{R}(0) & \cdots & \hat{R}(m-2) \\ \vdots & \vdots & \vdots & \ddots & \vdots \\ \hat{R}(m) & \hat{R}(m-1) & \cdots & \cdots & \hat{R}(0) \end{bmatrix}. \tag{62}$$

Multiplying by the eigenvector of the autocorrelation matrix $a$, Eq. (60) can be rewritten as

$$\hat{R}a = SPS^{\#}a + \sigma v^2 a, \tag{63}$$

where $a$ represents the eigenvector of the estimated autocorrelation matrix $\hat{R}$ and $a$ is expressed as $[a_0, a_1, \ldots, a_m]^T$.

The Pisarenko method uses only the eigenvector corresponding to the minimum eigenvalue to construct the desired polynomial (59) and to calculate the spectrum. Thus, the Pisarenko method determines $a$ such that $S^{\#}a = 0$. The eigenvector $a$ can then be considered to lie in the noise subspace, and Eq. (63) reduces to

$$\hat{R}a = \sigma v^2 a \tag{64}$$

under the constraint $a^{\#}a = 1$, where $\sigma v^2$ is the noise power which in the Pisarenko method is the same as the minimum eigenvalue corresponding to the eigenvector $a$.

In principle, under the assumption of white noise all noise subspace eigenvalues should be equal,

$$\lambda_1 = \lambda_2 = \cdots = \lambda_K = \sigma v^2,$$

where $\lambda_i$ represents the noise subspace eigenvalues, $i = 1, 2, \ldots, K$ and $K$ represents the dimension of the noise subspace.

From the eigenvector corresponding to the minimum eigenvalue, the Pisarenko method determines the signal PSD from the desired polynomial:

$$P_{\text{Pisarenko}}(f) = \frac{1}{|A(f)|^2}. \tag{65}$$

The order $m$ of the autocorrelation matrix $\hat{R}$ should be greater than, or equal to, the number of sinusoids $L$ contained in the signal. However, this method, employing only the eigenvector corresponding to the minimum eigenvalue, may produce spurious zeros.[2,3,10,49]

### 3.4.2. *MUSIC method*

The multiple signal classification (MUSIC) method is also a noise subspace frequency estimator. The MUSIC method eliminates the effects of spurious zeros by using the averaged spectra of all of the eigenvectors corresponding to the noise subspace. The resultant PSD is determined from

$$P_{\text{MUSIC}}(f) = \frac{1}{\dfrac{1}{K}\displaystyle\sum_{i=0}^{K-1}|A_i(f)|^2},$$

(66)

where $K$ represents the dimension of noise subspace, $A_i(f)$ represents the desired polynomial that corresponds to all the eigenvectors of the noise subspace.[2,3,10,49]

### 3.4.3. *Minimum-norm method*

In addition to the Pisarenko and MUSIC methods, the Minimum-Norm method was investigated. In order to differentiate spurious zeros from real zeros, the Minimum-Norm method forces spurious zeros inside the unit circle and calculates a desired noise subspace vector $a$ from either the noise or signal subspace eigenvectors. Thus, while the Pisarenko method uses only the noise subspace eigenvector corresponding to the minimum eigenvalue, the Minimum-Norm method uses a linear combination of all the noise subspace eigenvectors. Using the Minimum-Norm method, the polynomial $A(f)$ is written as

$$A(f) = A_1(f)A_2(f),$$

(67)

where

$$A_1(f) = \sum_{k=0}^{L} b_k e^{-j2\pi fk} \quad b_0 = 1$$

(68)

$$A_2(f) = \sum_{k=0}^{m-L} c_k z^{-k} \quad c_0 = 1,$$

(69)

where $b_k$ and $c_k$ are the coefficients of the two polynomial components of $A(f)$.

The polynomial $A_1(f)$ has $L$ desired zeros on the unit circle while $A_2(f)$ has $m - L$ spurious zeros. In order to force the zeros of $A_2(f)$ into the unit circle, $A_2(f)$ must be a minimum phase polynomial. The primary motivation behind the Minimum-Norm method is to construct $A_2(f)$ such that the value $Q$, defined below, will be minimum. This can be achieved by constructing $A_2(f)$ as a linear predictive filter:

$$Q = \sum_{k=0}^{M} |a_k|^2 \quad a_0 = 1.$$

(70)

The polynomial $A(f)$ can be estimated from either the signal subspace eigenvectors $E_s$ or from the noise subspace eigenvectors $E_n$. These eigenvectors can be expressed as

$$E_s = \begin{bmatrix} s^T \\ E_s' \end{bmatrix} \tag{71}$$

$$E_n = \begin{bmatrix} n^T \\ E_n' \end{bmatrix}, \tag{72}$$

where $s$ and $n$ vectors consist of the first element of the signal and the noise subspace eigenvectors. $E_s'$ and $E_n'$ have the same elements of $E_s$ and $E_n$, respectively, but with the first row deleted.

The desired eigenvector $a$ can be constructed from either signal subspace eigenvectors or noise subspace eigenvectors:

$$a = \begin{bmatrix} a_0 \\ E_s' s^* / (1 - s^\# s) \end{bmatrix} \quad a_0 = 1, \tag{73}$$

$$a = \begin{bmatrix} a_0 \\ E_n' n^* / n^* n \end{bmatrix} \quad a_0 = 1. \tag{74}$$

The resulting eigenvector $a$ has the desired zeros on the unit circle and the spurious zeros inside the unit circle:

$$a = [a_0, a_1, \ldots, a_m]^T. \tag{75}$$

The Minimum-Norm PSD can be estimated from $a$ as follows:

$$P_{\mathrm{MIN}}(f, K) = \frac{1}{|A(f)|^2}, \tag{76}$$

where $K$ represents the dimension of the noise subspace.

In order to calculate the MUSIC and Minimum-Norm PSD, the dimension of the noise subspace $K$ must be determined by a technique such as the AIC or minimum description length (MDL) criteria. MDL criterion gives a consistent estimate of the number of signals while the AIC criterion gives an inconsistent estimate that tends to overestimate the number of signals asymptotically. Since MDL criterion gives consistent estimates, the dimension of the noise subspace $K$ can be calculated according to the MDL criterion. This criterion is defined as

$$\mathrm{MDL}(k) = -N \cdot k \cdot \phi(k) + 1/2(m+1-k) \cdot (m+1+k) \cdot \log(N), \quad k = 1, 2, \ldots, m+1, \tag{77}$$

where $m$ is the maximum number of lags in the autocorrelation matrix as well as the order of the eigenfilter as defined by Eq. (59), $N$ is the number of signal samples, $\phi(k)$ is the likelihood function which can be expressed as

$$\phi(k) = \log \left[ \frac{\prod_{i=0}^{k-1} (\lambda_i)^{1/k}}{\sum_{i=0}^{k-1} \lambda_i / k} \right]. \tag{78}$$

The dimension of the noise subspace $K$ is the value that minimizes $\mathrm{MDL}(k)$.[2,3,10,49]

## 4. Medical Decision Support Systems

Medical decision support aims at providing healthcare professionals with therapy guidelines directly at the point of care. This should enhance the quality of clinical care, since the guidelines sort out high value practices from those that have little or no value. The goal of decision support is to supply the best recommendation under all circumstances. This goal may be achieved by the following measures:

- Standardization of care leading to a reduction of intra- and inter-individual variance of care.
- Development of standards and guidelines following rational principles.
- Development of explicit, standardized treatment protocols.
- Continuous control and validation of standards and guidelines against new scientific evidence and against actual patient data.

The foundation for any medical decision support is the medical knowledge base which contains the necessary rules and facts. This knowledge needs to be acquired from information and data in the fields of interest, such as medicine. Three general methodologies to acquire this knowledge can be distinguished:

- Traditional expert systems.
- Evidence-based methods.
- Statistical and artificial intelligence methods.

The medical decision support system consisting of differential diagnosis, computer-assisted instruction, consultation components and subsystems is given in Fig. 4. The computer-assisted instruction component consists of the differential diagnosis. The differential diagnosis component contains three subsystems: ANN model, time series analysis, and medical image analysis. Time series analysis is based on the extraction of information from medical signal data. Medical image analysis can be used for medical decision-making.[50-52]

ANN models are computational modeling tools that have recently emerged and found extensive acceptance in many disciplines for modeling complex real-world problems. ANNs produce complicated nonlinear models relating the inputs (the independent variables of a system) to the outputs (the dependent predictive variables). ANNs are valuable tools in the medical field for the development of decision support systems. Important tools in modern decision-making, in any field, include those that allow the decision-maker to assign an object to an appropriate group, or classification. Clinical decision-making is a challenging, multifaceted process. Its goals are precision in diagnosis and institution of efficacious treatment. Achieving these objectives involves access to pertinent data and application of previous knowledge to the analysis of new data in order to recognize patterns and relations. Practitioners apply various statistical techniques in processing the data to assist in clinical decision-making and to facilitate the management of patients. As the volume and complexity of data have increased, use of digital computers

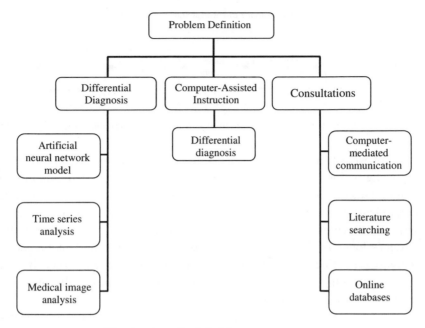

Fig. 4.   A medical decision support system.

to support data analysis has become a necessity. In addition to computerization of standard statistical analysis, several other techniques for computer-aided data classification and reduction, generally referred to as ANN, have evolved. The ANN model discussed above has expanded in two directions. First, time series analysis and medical image analysis supply important parameters to medical decision-making process and the parameters can be used as the input of the ANN model. The second direction of expansion includes databases available locally or through internet access.

The consultation component contains three subsystems: computer-mediated communication, literature searching, online databases. The term "computer-mediated communication" is used to refer primarily to the forms of communication that operate through computers and telecommunication networks. Applications of computer-mediated communication that relate specifically to health have been described using the term "interactive health communication." Interactive health communication that uses internet-based technologies has several advantages over earlier health education approaches that are based on the inherent capacities of this communication media. Advantages include flexibility of use, automated data collection, and openness of communication. Access to the internet allows users to receive information from a vast array of sources. Information is accessible on demand and not restricted in terms of time or location. Computer-mediated communication also has the advantage that it can automatically collect data and generate feedback. Participant histories can be generated based on the frequency

Time-varying Biomedical Signals Classifiers

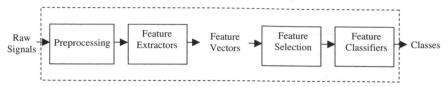

Fig. 5.   General structure of the implemented time-varying biomedical signals classifiers.

and nature of website materials use, as well as on the response options given to questions using online forms. Some evidence suggests that participants interacting with computer-mediated assessments may be less influenced by social conventions and communicate more openly than those responding to face-to-face or telephone interviews. Furthermore, computer-mediated assessments can more rapidly ask follow-up questions, using branching logic based on each respondent's answers.

Literature searching can easily be done with the use of the internet. In addition to literature searching, online information is vital. The best solution would be to have articles available directly online in the form of a digital library and to provide electronic access to high impact clinical journals. Many physicians and participants find access to evidence-based medical information on the internet. A growing number of databases exist on the internet which can be freely accessed, including medical information, archived images representing healthy and diseased conditions. Medical information generally consists of risk factors of diseases and demographic and medical data of subjects.[50–52]

Various methodologies of automated diagnosis have been adopted, however the entire process can generally be subdivided into a number of disjoint processing modules: pre-processing, feature extraction/selection, and classification (Fig. 5).[14,38–41] Signal/image acquisition, artifact removing, averaging, thresholding, signal/image enhancement, and edge detection are the main operations in the course of pre-processing. Feature extraction is the determination of a feature or a feature vector from a pattern vector. The feature vector, which is comprised of the set of all features used to describe a pattern, is a reduced-dimensional representation of that pattern. The module of feature selection is an optional stage, whereby the feature vector is reduced in size including only, from the classification viewpoint, what may be considered as the most relevant features required for discrimination. The classification module is the final stage in automated diagnosis. It examines the input feature vector and based on its algorithmic nature, produces a suggestive hypothesis.[14,38–41]

## 5. Feature Extraction/Selection

Feature is a distinctive (sets it apart) or characteristic (its makeup) measurement, transform, structural component made on a segment of a pattern. Features are used to represent patterns with minimal loss of important information. The feature vector, which is comprised of the set of all features used to describe a pattern, is a reduced-dimensional representation of that pattern. This, in effect, means that the set of all features that could be used to describe a given pattern (large and in fact infinite infinitesimal changes in some parameter are allowed to separate different features) is limited to those actually stated in the feature vector. One purpose of the dimensionality reduction is to meet engineering constraints in software and hardware complexity, the computing cost, and the desirability of compressing pattern information. In addition, classification is often more accurate when the pattern is simplified through representation by important features or properties only (Fig. 6).[14,38-41]

Feature extraction is the determination of a feature or a feature vector from a pattern vector. For pattern processing problems to be tractable requires the conversion of patterns to features, which are condensed representations of patterns, ideally containing only salient information. Feature extraction methods are subdivided into: (1) statistical characteristics and (2) syntactic descriptions. Spectral analysis techniques can be used for extraction of features characterizing the signals under study.[14,38-41]

Feature selection provides a means for choosing the features which are best for classification, based on various criteria. The feature selection process is performed on a set of pre-determined features. Features are selected based on either (1) best representation of a given class of signals, or (2) best distinction between classes.

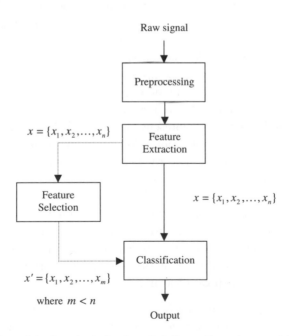

Fig. 6.   Functional modules in a typical automated diagnostic system used for arterial diseases.

Therefore, feature selection plays an important role in classifying systems such as neural networks. For the purpose of classification problems, the classifying system has usually been implemented with rules using if–then clauses, which state the conditions of certain attributes and resulting rules. However, it has proven to be a difficult and time-consuming method. From the viewpoint of managing large quantities of data, it would still be most useful if irrelevant or redundant attributes could be segregated from relevant and important ones, although the exact governing rules may not be known. In this case, the process of extracting useful information from a large dataset can be greatly facilitated.[14,39]

High-dimension of feature vectors increased computational complexity and therefore, in order to reduce the dimensionality of the extracted feature vectors, statistics over the set of the features can be used. The following statistical features can be used to represent the segments of signals:

1.  Maximum of the computed features in each segment.
2.  Mean of the computed features in each segment.
3.  Minimum of the computed features in each segment.
4.  Standard deviation of the computed features in each segment.

There are numerous methods to represent patterns as a grouping of features. The choice of methods appropriate for a given pattern analysis task is rarely obvious. At each level (feature extraction, feature selection, classification) many methods exist. Since the architecture of the decision support system can be compatible with different types of features, it is necessary to know how to fuse different types of features. Fusion of features for some types of decision support systems can increase the accuracy of the system. In this respect, this section is important in dealing with the accuracy of the developed decision support system.[33,40,41] In the following, a brief explanation about diverse and composite features is presented.

In the feature extraction stage, numerous different methods can be used so that several diverse features can be extracted from the same raw data. To a large extent, each feature can independently represent the original data, but none of them is totally perfect for practical applications. Moreover, there seems to be no simple way to measure relevance of the features for a pattern classification task. For this kind of pattern classification tasks, diverse features often need to be jointly used in order to achieve robust performance. This kind of pattern classification tasks is called as classification with diverse features. In order to perform a classification, two different methods are used. One is the use of a composite feature formed by lumping diverse features together and the other is combination of multiple classifiers that have been already trained on diverse feature sets. Several problems given as follows occur with the usage of composite feature:

• Its dimension is higher than that of any component feature and it is well known that high-dimension vectors will not only increase computational complexity but will also produce implementation problems and accuracy problems.

- It is difficult to lump several features together due to their diversified forms, e.g. they may be continuous variables, binary values, discrete labels, structural primitives.
- Those component features are usually not independent.

In general, therefore, the use of a composite feature does not provide a significantly improved performance. However, the combination of multiple classifiers is a good solution for the problem involving a variety of features.[53-55]

## 6. Review of Different Decision Support Systems

ANNs are massively parallel, highly connected structures consisting of a number of simple, nonlinear processing elements; because of their massively parallel structure, they can perform computations at a very high rate if implemented on a dedicated hardware; because of their adaptive nature, they can learn the characteristics of input signals and adapt to changes in the data; because of their nonlinear nature they can perform functional approximation and signal filtering operations which are beyond optimal linear techniques.[42-44] Feedforward neural networks are a basic type of neural networks capable of approximating generic classes of functions, including continuous and integrable ones. An important class of feedforward neural networks is MLPNNs. MLPNNs, which have features such as the ability to learn and generalize, smaller training set requirements, fast operation, and ease of implementation and therefore most commonly used neural network architectures, have been adapted for the automated diagnostic systems.[42-44] An appropriate structure would help to achieve higher model accuracy.

### 6.1. *Multilayer perceptron neural networks*

MLPNN (Fig. 7) is a nonparametric technique for performing a wide variety of detection and estimation tasks.[42-44] Suppose the total number of hidden layers is $L$. The input layer is considered as layer 0. Let the number of neurons in hidden layer $l$ be $N_l$, $l = 1, 2, \ldots, L$. Let $w_{ij}^l$ represent the weight of the link between the $j$th neuron of the $l - 1$th hidden layer and $i$th neuron of the $l$th hidden layer, and $\theta_i^l$ be the bias parameter of $i$th neuron of the $l$th hidden layer. Let $x_i$ represent the $i$th input parameter to the MLPNN. Let $\bar{y}_i^l$ be the output of $i$th neuron of the $l$th hidden layer, which can be computed according to the standard MLPNN formulas as,

$$\bar{y}_i^l = f\left(\sum_{j=1}^{N_{l-1}} w_{ij}^l \cdot \bar{y}_j^{l-1} + \theta_i^l\right), \quad i = 1, \ldots, N_l, \ l = 1, \ldots, L, \tag{79}$$

$$\bar{y}_i^0 = x_i, \quad i = 1, \ldots, N_x, \ N_x = N_0, \tag{80}$$

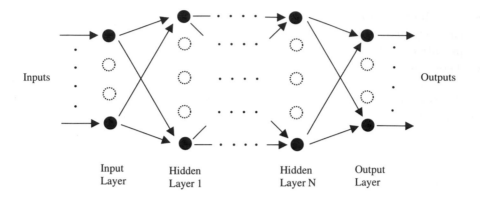

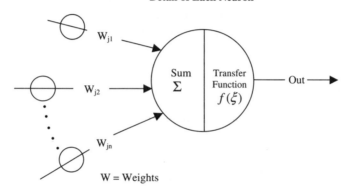

Fig. 7. Multilayer perceptron neural network architecture.

where $f(\cdot)$ is the activation function. Let $v_{ki}$ represent the weight of the link between the $i$th neuron of the $L$th hidden layer and the $k$th neuron of the output layer, and $\beta_k$ be the bias parameter of the $k$th output neuron. The outputs of MLPNN can be computed as,

$$y_k = \sum_{i=1}^{N_L} v_{ki} \cdot \bar{y}_i^L + \beta_k, \quad k = 1, \ldots, N_y. \tag{81}$$

Training algorithms are an integral part of ANN model development. An appropriate topology may still fail to give a better model, unless trained by a suitable training algorithm. A good training algorithm will shorten the training time, while achieving a better accuracy. Therefore, training process is an important characteristic of the ANNs, whereby representative examples of the knowledge are iteratively presented to the network, so that it can integrate this knowledge within its structure. There are a number of training algorithms used to train a MLPNN and a frequently used one is called the backpropagation training algorithm.[42–44]

The backpropagation algorithm, which is based on searching an error surface using gradient descent for points with minimum error, is relatively easy to implement. However, backpropagation has some problems for many applications. The algorithm is not guaranteed to find the global minimum of the error function since gradient descent may get stuck in local minima, where it may remain indefinitely. In addition to this, long training sessions are often required in order to find an acceptable weight solution because of the well-known difficulties inherent in gradient descent optimization. Therefore, a lot of variations to improve the convergence of the backpropagation were proposed. Optimization methods such as second order methods (conjugate gradient, quasi-Newton, Levenberg–Marquardt) have also been used for ANN training in recent years. The Levenberg–Marquardt algorithm combines the best features of the Gauss–Newton technique and the steepest-descent algorithm, but avoids many of their limitations. In particular, it generally does not suffer from the problem of slow convergence.[56,57] Therefore, the Levenberg–Marquardt algorithm is presented below.

**Levenberg–Marquardt algorithm**     ANN training is usually formulated as a nonlinear least-squares problem. Essentially, the Levenberg–Marquardt algorithm is a least-squares estimation algorithm based on the maximum neighborhood idea. Let $E(\mathbf{w})$ be an objective error function made up of $m$ individual error terms $e_i^2(\mathbf{w})$ as follows:

$$E(\mathbf{w}) = \sum_{i=1}^{m} e_i^2(\mathbf{w}) = \|f(\mathbf{w})\|^2 , \tag{82}$$

where $e_i^2(\mathbf{w}) = (\mathbf{y}_{di} - \mathbf{y}_i)^2$ and $\mathbf{y}_{di}$ is the desired value of output neuron $i$, $\mathbf{y}_i$ is the actual output of that neuron.

It is assumed that function $f(\cdot)$ and its Jacobian $J$ are known at point $\mathbf{w}$. The aim of the Levenberg–Marquardt algorithm is to compute the weight vector $\mathbf{w}$ such that $E(\mathbf{w})$ is minimum. Using the Levenberg–Marquardt algorithm, a new weight vector $\mathbf{w}_{k+1}$ can be obtained from the previous weight vector $\mathbf{w}_k$ as follows:

$$\mathbf{w}_{k+1} = \mathbf{w}_k + \delta\mathbf{w}_k, \tag{83}$$

where $\delta\mathbf{w}_k$ is defined as

$$\delta\mathbf{w}_k = -(J_k^T f(\mathbf{w}_k))(J_k^T J_k + \lambda\mathbf{I})^{-1}. \tag{84}$$

In Eq. (84), $J_k$ is the Jacobian of $f$ evaluated at $\mathbf{w}_k$, $\lambda$ is the Marquardt parameter, $\mathbf{I}$ is the identity matrix.[56,57]

### 6.2. *Combined neural network models*

The CNN models often result in a prediction accuracy that is higher than that of the individual models. This construction is based on a straightforward approach

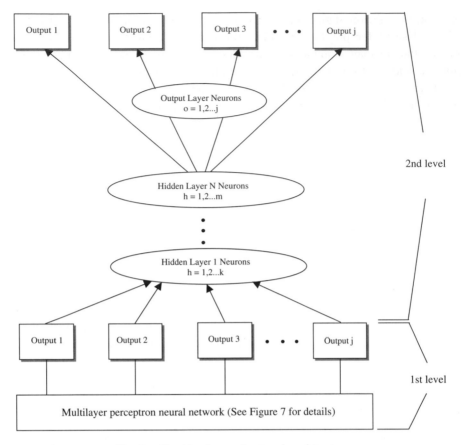

Fig. 8.   Combined neural network architecture.

that has been termed stacked generalization (Fig. 8). Training data that are difficult to learn usually demonstrate high dispersion in the search space due to the inability of the low-level measurement attributes to describe the concept concisely. Because of the complex interactions among variables and the high degree of noise and fluctuations, a significant number of data used for applications are naturally available in representations that are difficult to learn. The degree of difficulty in training a neural network is inherent in the given set of training examples. By developing a technique for measuring this learning difficulty, a feature construction methodology is devised that transforms the training data and attempts to improve both the classification accuracy and computational times of ANN algorithms. The fundamental notion is to organize data by intelligent pre-processing, so that learning is facilitated.[24,27,58] The stacked generalization concepts formalized by Wolpert[58] predate these ideas and refer to schemes for feeding information from one set of generalizers to another before forming the final predicted value (output). The unique contribution of stacked generalization is that the information fed into the net of generalizers comes from multiple partitionings of the original learning set. The stacked generalization scheme can be viewed as a more sophisticated version of cross validation and has been shown experimentally to effectively improve generalization ability of ANN models over using individual neural networks. The MLPNNs can be used at the first level and second level for the implementation of the CNN.

The Levenberg–Marquardt algorithm employing the cross-entropy error function as cost function can be used to train the CNNs and MLPNNs.[59] The error function is

$$E(\mathbf{w}) = -\sum_{n=1}^{N}\sum_{i=1}^{C} \mathbf{t}_i^n \ln(y_i(\mathbf{w}, \mathbf{x}^n)), \qquad (85)$$

where $N$ is the number of training data, $C$ is the number of classes, $\{\mathbf{x}^n, \mathbf{t}^n\}$ is the set of training input–output pairs, and $\mathbf{t}^n$, the expected output, is given by:

$$\mathbf{t}_k^n = \begin{cases} 1 & \text{if } \mathbf{x}^n \in C_k \\ 0 & \text{otherwise,} \end{cases} \qquad (86)$$

where $k = 1, \ldots, C$ and $C_k$ is the set of patterns in the class $k$.

## 6.3. *Mixture of experts*

The ME architecture is composed of a gating network and several expert networks (Fig. 9). The gating network receives the vector $\mathbf{x}$ as input and produces scalar outputs that are partitions of unity at each point in the input space. Each expert network produces an output vector for an input vector. The gating network provides

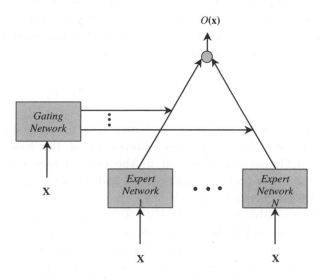

Fig. 9.   Architecture of the mixture of experts.

linear combination coefficients as veridical probabilities for expert networks and, therefore, the final output of the ME architecture is a convex weighted sum of all the output vectors produced by expert networks. Suppose that there are $N$ expert networks in the ME architecture. All the expert networks are linear with a single output nonlinearity that is also referred to as "generalized linear." The $i$th expert network produces its output $o_i(\mathbf{x})$ as a generalized linear function of the input $\mathbf{x}$[60–62]:

$$o_i(\mathbf{x}) = f(\mathbf{W}_i\mathbf{x}), \tag{87}$$

where $\mathbf{W}_i$ is a weight matrix and $f(\cdot)$ is a fixed continuous nonlinearity. The gating network is also a generalized linear function, and its $i$th output, $g(\mathbf{x}, \mathbf{v}_i)$, is the multinomial logit or softmax function of intermediate variables $\xi_i$:

$$g(\mathbf{x}, \mathbf{v}_i) = \frac{e^{\xi_i}}{\sum_{k=1}^{N} e^{\xi_k}}, \tag{88}$$

where $\xi_i = \mathbf{v}_i^T\mathbf{x}$ and $\mathbf{v}_i$ is a weight vector. The overall output $o(\mathbf{x})$ of the ME architecture is

$$o(\mathbf{x}) = \sum_{k=1}^{N} g(\mathbf{x}, \mathbf{v}_k)o_k(\mathbf{x}). \tag{89}$$

The ME architecture can be given a probabilistic interpretation. For an input–output pair $(\mathbf{x}, \mathbf{y})$, the values of $g(\mathbf{v}_i, \mathbf{x})$ are interpreted as the multinomial probabilities associated with the decision that terminates in a regressive process that maps $\mathbf{x}$ to $\mathbf{y}$. Once the decision has been made, resulting in a choice of regressive process $i$, the output $\mathbf{y}$ is then chosen from a probability density $P(\mathbf{y}|\mathbf{x}, \mathbf{W}_i)$, where $\mathbf{W}_i$ denotes the set of parameters or weight matrix of the $i$th expert network in the model. Therefore, the total probability of generating $\mathbf{y}$ from $\mathbf{x}$ is the mixture of the probabilities of generating $\mathbf{y}$ from each component densities, where the mixing proportions are multinomial probabilities:

$$P(\mathbf{y}|\mathbf{x}, \Phi) = \sum_{k=1}^{N} g(\mathbf{x}, \mathbf{v}_k)P(\mathbf{y}|\mathbf{x}, \mathbf{W}_k), \tag{90}$$

where $\Phi$ is the set of all the parameters including both expert and gating network parameters. Moreover, the probabilistic component of the model is generally assumed to be a Gaussian distribution in the case of regression, a Bernoulli distribution in the case of binary classification, and a multinomial distribution in the case of multiclass classification.[38–41]

Based on the probabilistic model in Eq. (90), learning in the ME architecture is treated as a maximum likelihood problem. Jordan and Jacobs[63] have proposed an expectation–maximization (EM) algorithm for adjusting the parameters of the architecture. Suppose that the training set is given as $\chi = \{(\mathbf{x}_t, \mathbf{y}_t)\}_{t=1}^{T}$. The EM algorithm consists of two steps. For the $s$th epoch, the posterior probabilities $h_i^{(t)}$ ($i =$

$1, \ldots, N$), which can be interpreted as the probabilities $P(i | \mathbf{x}_t, \mathbf{y}_t)$, are computed in the E-step as

$$h_i^{(t)} = \frac{g(\mathbf{x}_t, \mathbf{v}_i^{(s)}) P(\mathbf{y}_t | \mathbf{x}_t, \mathbf{W}_i^{(s)})}{\sum_{k=1}^{N} g(\mathbf{x}_t, \mathbf{v}_k^{(s)}) P(\mathbf{y}_t | \mathbf{x}_t, \mathbf{W}_k^{(s)})}. \tag{91}$$

The M-step solves the following maximization problems:

$$\mathbf{W}_i^{(s+1)} = \arg\max_{\mathbf{W}_i} \sum_{t=1}^{T} h_i^{(t)} \log P(\mathbf{y}_t | \mathbf{x}_t, \mathbf{W}_i), \tag{92}$$

and

$$V^{(s+1)} = \arg\max_{V} \sum_{t=1}^{T} \sum_{k=1}^{N} h_k^{(t)} \log g(\mathbf{x}_t, \mathbf{v}_k), \tag{93}$$

where $V$ is the set of all the parameters in the gating network. Therefore, the EM algorithm is summarized as:

1. For each data pair $(\mathbf{x}_t, \mathbf{y}_t)$, compute the posterior probabilities $h_i^{(t)}$ using the current values of the parameters.
2. For each expert network $i$, solve the maximization problem in Eq. (92) with observations $\{(\mathbf{x}_t, \mathbf{y}_t)\}_{t=1}^{T}$ and observation weights $\{h_i^{(t)}\}_{t=1}^{T}$.
3. For the gating network, solve the maximization problem in Eq. (93) with observations $\{(x_t, h_k^{(t)})\}_{t=1}^{T}$.
4. Iterate by using the updated parameter values.

In this framework a number of relatively small expert networks can be used together with a gating network designed to divide the global classification task into simpler subtasks (Fig. 9).[29,61,62] Both the gating and expert networks can be MLPNNs consisting of neurons arranged in contiguous layers. This configuration occurred on the theory that MLPNN has features such as the ability to learn and generalize, smaller training set requirements, fast operation, and ease of implementation.

## 6.4. *Modified mixture of experts*

The MME architecture is composed of $N$ expert networks and a gate-bank (Fig. 10). The ensemble of expert networks is divided into $K$ groups in terms of $K$ diverse features, and there are $N_i$ expert networks in the $i$th group subject to $\sum_{i=1}^{K} N_i = N$. Expert networks in the same group receive the same feature vector, while any two expert networks in different groups receive different feature vectors. For an input sample, each expert network produces an output vector in terms of a specific feature. In the gate-bank, there are $K$ gating networks and $K$ different feature vectors are input to these networks, respectively. Each gating network produces an

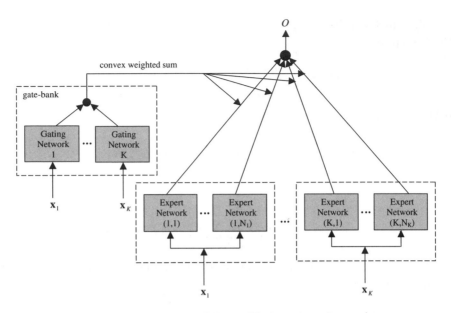

Fig. 10.    Architecture of the modified mixture of experts.

output vector in terms of a specific input feature. The output vector consists of $N$ components, where each component corresponds to an expert network. The overall output of the gate-bank is a convex weighted sum of outputs produced by all the gating networks and can be interpreted as a partition of unity at each point in the input space based on diverse features. As a result, the overall output of the MME architecture is a linear combination of outputs of all $N$ expert networks weighted by the output of the gate-bank. There are two soft competition mechanisms in the MME architecture; on the basis of the supervised error, expert networks compete for the right to learn the training data, while gating networks associated with diverse features compete for the right to select an appropriate expert network as the winner for generating the output. Parameter estimation in the MME architecture is a maximum likelihood learning problem.[53] The EM algorithm can be used to solve the problem. Both the gating and expert networks can be MLPNNs consisting of neurons arranged in contiguous layers.[33]

## 6.5. *Probabilistic neural network*

The PNN was first proposed by Specht.[64] A single PNN is capable of handling multiclass problem. This is opposite to the so-called one-against-the rest or one-per-class approach taken by some classifiers, such as the SVM, which decompose a multiclass classification problem into dichotomies and each chotomizer has to separate a single class from all others. The architecture of a typical PNN is as shown in Fig. 11. The PNN architecture is composed of many interconnected

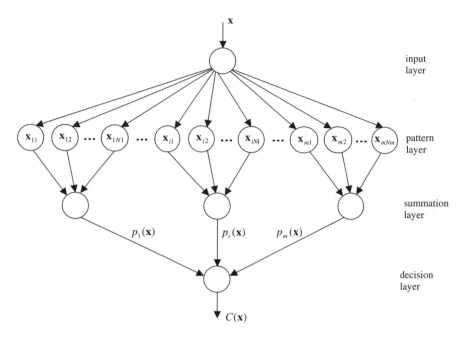

Fig. 11.   Architecture of the probabilistic neural network.

processing units or neurons organized in successive layers. The input layer unit does not perform any computation and simply distributes the input to the neurons in the pattern layer. On receiving a pattern $\mathbf{x}$ from the input layer, the neuron $\mathbf{x}_{ij}$ of the pattern layer computes its output

$$\phi_{ij}(\mathbf{x}) = \frac{1}{(2\pi)^{d/2}\sigma^d} \exp\left[-\frac{(\mathbf{x} - \mathbf{x}_{ij})^T(\mathbf{x} - \mathbf{x}_{ij})}{2\sigma^2}\right], \tag{94}$$

where $d$ denotes the dimension of the pattern vector $\mathbf{x}$, $\sigma$ is the smoothing parameter, and $\mathbf{x}_{ij}$ is the neuron vector.

The summation layer neurons compute the maximum likelihood of pattern $\mathbf{x}$ being classified into $C_i$ by summarizing and averaging the output of all neurons that belong to the same class

$$p_i(\mathbf{x}) = \frac{1}{(2\pi)^{d/2}\sigma^d} \frac{1}{N_i} \sum_{j=1}^{N_i} \exp\left[-\frac{(\mathbf{x} - \mathbf{x}_{ij})^T(\mathbf{x} - \mathbf{x}_{ij})}{2\sigma^2}\right], \tag{95}$$

where $N_i$ denotes the total number of samples in class $C_i$. If the *a priori* probabilities for each class and the losses associated with making an incorrect decision for each class are the same, the decision layer unit classifies the pattern $\mathbf{x}$ in accordance with the Bayess' decision rule based on the output of all the summation layer neurons

$$\hat{C}(\mathbf{x}) = \arg\max\{p_i(\mathbf{x})\}, \quad i = 1, 2, \ldots, m, \tag{96}$$

where $\hat{C}(\mathbf{x})$ denotes the estimated class of the pattern $\mathbf{x}$ and $m$ is the total number of classes in the training samples.[64,65]

## 6.6. *Recurrent neural networks*

A particular architecture of the neural models is the multilayered architecture. Multilayered networks can be classified as feedforward and feedback networks, with respect to the direction of their connections.[42–44] RNNs can perform highly nonlinear dynamic mappings and thus have temporally extended applications, whereas multilayer feedforward networks are confined to performing static mappings.[66–68] RNNs have been used in a number of interesting applications including associative memories, spatiotemporal pattern classification, control, optimization, forecasting, and generalization of pattern sequences.[31,69,70]

Fully recurrent networks use unconstrained fully interconnected architectures and learning algorithms that can deal with time-varying input and/or output in nontrivial ways. In spite of several modifications of learning algorithms to reduce the computational expense, fully recurrent networks are still complicated when dealing with complex problems. Therefore, we introduce the partially recurrent networks, whose connections are mainly feedforward, but they include a carefully chosen set of feedback connections. The recurrence allows the network to remember cues from the past without complicating the learning excessively. The structure proposed by Elman[68] is an illustration of this kind of architecture. In the following, the Elman RNN is presented.

An Elman RNN is a network which in principle is set up as a regular feedforward network. This means that all neurons in one layer are connected with all neurons in the next layer. An exception is the so-called context layer which is a special case of a hidden layer. Figure 12 shows the architecture of an Elman RNN. The neurons in the context layer (context neurons) hold a copy of the output of the hidden neurons. The output of each hidden neuron is copied into a specific neuron in the context layer. The value of the context neuron is used as an extra input signal for all the neurons in the hidden layer one time step later. Therefore, the Elman network has an explicit memory of one time lag.[68]

Similar to a regular feedforward neural network, the strength of all connections between neurons are indicated with a weight. Initially, all weight values are chosen randomly and are optimized during the stage of training. In an Elman network, the weights from the hidden layer to the context layer are set to one and are fixed because the values of the context neurons have to be copied exactly. Furthermore, the initial output weights of the context neurons are equal to half the output range of the other neurons in the network. The Elman network can be trained with gradient descent backpropagation and optimization methods, similar to regular feedforward neural networks.[71] The backpropagation has some problems for many applications. The algorithm is not guaranteed to find the global minimum of the error function

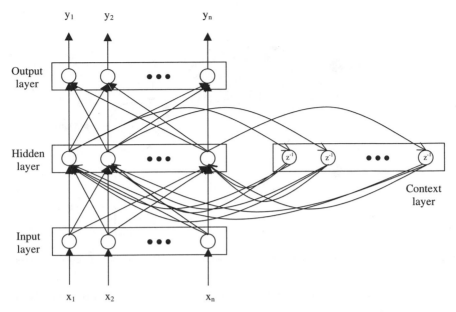

Fig. 12. A schematic representation of an Elman recurrent neural network. $z^{-1}$ represents a one-time step delay unit.

since gradient descent may get stuck in local minima, where it may remain indefinitely. In addition to this, long training sessions are often required in order to find an acceptable weight solution because of the well-known difficulties inherent in gradient descent optimization.[42-44] Therefore, the Levenberg–Marquardt algorithm can yield a good cost function compared with the other training algorithms.[31]

### 6.7. *Support vector machine*

SVM proposed by Vapnik[72] has been studied extensively for classification, regression, and density estimation. Figure 13 shows the architecture of the SVM. SVM maps the input patterns into a higher dimensional feature space through some nonlinear mapping chosen *a priori*. A linear decision surface is then constructed in this high-dimensional feature space. Thus, SVM is a linear classifier in the parameter space, but it becomes a nonlinear classifier as a result of the nonlinear mapping of the space of the input patterns into the high-dimensional feature space. Training SVM is a quadratic optimization problem. The construction of a hyperplane $\mathbf{w}^T\mathbf{x}+b = 0$ ($\mathbf{w}$ is the vector of hyperplane coefficients, $b$ is a bias term) so that the margin between the hyperplane and the nearest point is maximized can be posed as the quadratic optimization problem. SVM has been shown to provide high generalization ability. For a two-class problem, assuming the optimal hyperplane in the feature space is

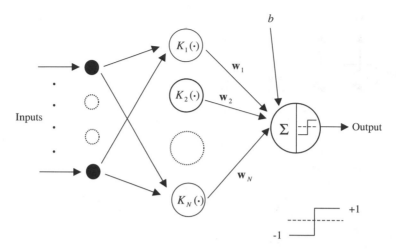

Fig. 13.   Architecture of the support vector machine ($N$ is the number of support vectors).

generated, the classification decision of an unknown pattern $\mathbf{y}$ will be made based on

$$f(\mathbf{y}) = \text{sgn}\left(\sum_{i=1}^{N} \alpha_i y_i K(\mathbf{x}_i, \mathbf{y}) + b\right), \qquad (97)$$

where $\alpha_i \geq 0$, $i = 1, 2, \ldots, N$ are nonnegative Lagrange multipliers that satisfy $\sum_{i=1}^{N} \alpha_i y_i = 0$, $\{y_i | y_i \in \{-1, +1\}.\}_{i=1}^{N}$ are class labels of training patterns $\{\mathbf{x}_i | \mathbf{x}_i \in R^N.\}_{i=1}^{N}$, and $K(\mathbf{x}_i, \mathbf{y})$ for $i = 1, 2, \ldots, N$ represents a symmetric positive definite kernel function that defines an inner product in the feature space. This shows that $f(\mathbf{y})$ is a linear combination of the inner products or kernels. The kernel function enables the operations to be carried out in the input space rather than in the high-dimensional feature space. Some typical examples of kernel functions are $K(\mathbf{u}, \mathbf{v}) = \mathbf{v}^T \mathbf{u}$ (linear SVM); $K(\mathbf{u}, \mathbf{v}) = (\mathbf{v}^T \mathbf{u} + 1)^n$ (polynomial SVM of degree $n$); $K(\mathbf{u}, \mathbf{v}) = \exp(-\|\mathbf{u} - \mathbf{v}\|^2 / 2\sigma^2)$ (radial basis function — RBF SVM); $K(\mathbf{u}, \mathbf{v}) = \tanh(\kappa \mathbf{v}^T \mathbf{y} + \theta)$ (two layer neural SVM), where $\sigma$, $\kappa$, $\theta$ are constants.[72,73] However, a proper kernel function for a certain problem is dependent on the specific data and till now there is no good method on how to choose a kernel function. The choice of the kernel functions is studied empirically and optimal results can be achieved with different kernel functions depending on the classification problem.

SVM is a binary classifier which can be extended by fusing several of its kind into a multiclass classifier. In this study, we fuse SVM decisions using the error correcting output codes (ECOC) approach, adopted from the digital communication theory.[74] In the ECOC approach, up to $2^{n-1} - 1$ (where $n$ is the number of classes) SVMs are trained, each of them aimed at separating a different combination of classes. For three classes (A, B, and C) we need three classifiers; one SVM classifies A from B and C, a second SVM classifies B from A and C, and a third SVM classifies C from A and B. The multiclass classifier output code for a pattern is a combination of targets of all the separate SVMs. That is, in our example, vectors from classes A, B, and C have codes $(1, -1, -1)$, $(-1, 1, -1)$, and $(-1, -1, 1)$, respectively. If each of the separate SVMs classifies a pattern correctly, the multiclass classifier target code is met and the ECOC approach reports no error for that pattern. However, if at least one of the SVMs misclassifies the pattern, the class selected for this pattern is the one its target code closest in the Hamming distance sense to the actual output code and this may be an erroneous decision.

## 7. Experiments for Implementation of Decision Support Systems

The key design decisions for the neural networks used in classification are the architecture and the training process. The architectures of the MLPNN, CNN, ME, MME, PNN, RNN, SVM used for classification of the signals are shown in Figs. 7–13, respectively. The adequate functioning of neural networks depends on the sizes of the training set and test set. To comparatively evaluate the performance of the classifiers, all the classifiers can be trained by the same training dataset and tested with the evaluation dataset. The explanations about the training algorithms of the classifiers are presented in Sec. 6 with the related references for further reading.

The EM algorithm[63] can be used to train the MME and ME classifiers and the Levenberg–Marquardt algorithm[56,57] employing the cross-entropy error function as cost function can be used to train the RNNs, CNNs, and MLPNNs. The cross-entropy error function is used as it is a more suitable error function for classification problems. In the MME and ME classifiers, the classification problem is divided into simpler problems and then each solution is combined. In addition to this, the training algorithm of the MME and ME classifiers is a general technique for maximum likelihood estimation that fits well with the modular structure and enables a significant speed up over the other training algorithms. Thus, the convergence rates of the MME and ME classifiers are significantly higher than that of the CNNs and MLPNNs.

Training algorithm of the SVM, based on quadratic programming, incorporates several optimization techniques such as decomposition and caching. The quadratic programming problem in the SVM was solved by using the MATLAB optimization toolbox. The SVMs and the ECOC algorithm can be used to classify the signals. As mentioned earlier, each of the SVMs of the classifier can use different kernel functions. For the implementation of the SVMs with the RBF kernel functions, one has to assume a value for $\sigma$. The optimal $\sigma$ can only be found by systematically varying its value in the different training sessions. To do this, the support vectors are extracted from the training data file with an assumed $\sigma$ value. The generalization ability of the SVM is controlled by two different factors: the training error rate and the capacity of the learning machine measured by its Vapnik–Chervonenkis (VC) dimension.[72] The smaller the VC dimension of the function set of the learning machine, the larger the value of training error rate. We can control the trade-off between the complexity of decision rule and training error rate by changing the

Table 1.   Network parameters of the classifiers.

| Classifier (features) | Dataset |
|---|---|
| SVM (composite feature) | 41·9·3[a] |
| RNN (composite feature) | 34·30r·25r·4[b], 600[c] |
| PNN (composite feature) | 41·21·3·1[d] |
| MME (diverse features) | 5·25·3[e], 4·25·3[e], 28·25·3[e], 4·25·3[e], 5·25·3[f], 4·25·3[f], 28·25·3[f], 4·25·3[f], 500[c] |
| ME (composite feature) | 41·25·3[e], 41·25·3[g], 700[c] |
| CNN (composite feature) | 41·25·9[h], 9·30·3[i], 1200[c] |
| MLPNN (composite feature) | 41·25·3[j], 1900[c] |

[a]Design of SVMs: Number of input neurons · support vectors · output neurons, respectively.
[b]Design of RNNs: Number of input neurons · recurrent neurons in the first hidden layer recurrent neurons in the second hidden layer · output neurons, respectively.
[c]Number of training epochs.
[d]Design of PNNs: Number of input neurons · pattern layer neurons · summation layer neurons · output layer neurons, respectively.
[e]Design of expert networks: Number of input · hidden · output neurons, respectively.
[f]Design of gating networks in gate-bank: Number of input · hidden · output neurons, respectively.
[g]Design of gating network: Number of input · hidden · output neurons, respectively.
[h]Design of first level network: Number of input · hidden · output neurons, respectively.
[i]Design of second level network: Number of input · hidden · output neurons, respectively.
[j]Design of neural network: Number of input · hidden · output neurons, respectively.

parameter $C$[73] in the SVM. The SVMs are trained for different $C$ values until we get the best result.[72–74]

There is an outstanding issue associated with the PNN concerning network structure determination, that is determining the network size, the locations of pattern layer neurons as well as the value of the smoothing parameter. The objective is to select representative pattern layer neurons from the training samples. The output of a summation layer neuron becomes a linear combination of the outputs of pattern layer neurons. Subsequently, an orthogonal algorithm was used to select pattern layer neurons. As in the SVM training, the smoothing parameter $\sigma$ can be determined based on the minimum misclassification rate computed from the partial evaluation dataset.[64,65]

Different experiments are performed during implementation of these classifiers and the number of support vectors in the SVMs, pattern layer neurons in the PNNs, expert networks in the MEs and MMEs, recurrent neurons in the RNNs, hidden layers and hidden neurons in the MLPNNs are determined by taking into consideration the classification accuracies. In the hidden layers and the output layers, sigmoid, tan-sigmoid, linear functions can be used as the activation functions. The sigmoidal function with the range between zero and one introduces two important properties. First, the sigmoid is nonlinear, allowing the network to perform complex mappings of input to output vector spaces, and secondly it is continuous and differentiable, which allows the gradient of the error to be used in updating the weights. Table 1 defines the examples of the network parameters of the classifiers.

## 8. Measuring Performance of Decision Support Systems

Given a random set of initial weights, the outputs of the network will be very different from the desired classifications. As the network is trained, the weights of the system are continually adjusted to reduce the difference between the output of the system and the desired response. The difference is referred to as the error and can be measured in different ways. The most common measurement is the mean square error (MSE). The MSE is the average of the squares of the difference between each output and the desired output. In addition to MSE, normalized mean squared error (NMSE), mean absolute error (MAE), minimum absolute error, and maximum absolute error can be used for measuring the error of the neural network.[42–44,59]

The training holds the key to an accurate solution, so the criterion to stop training must be very well described. In general, it is known that a network with enough weights will always learn the training set better as the number of iterations is increased. However, neural network researchers have found that this decrease in the training set error was not always coupled to better performance in the test. When the network is trained too much, the network memorizes the training patterns and does not generalize well. The aim of the stop criterion is to maximize the network's generalization.[42–44,59]

The size of MSE can be used to determine how well the network output fits the desired output, but it may not reflect whether the two sets of data move in the same direction. The correlation coefficient $(r)$ solves this problem. The correlation coefficient is limited with the range $[-1, 1]$. When $r = 1$ there is a perfect positive linear correlation between network output and desired output, which means that they vary by the same amount. When $r = -1$ there is a perfectly linear negative correlation between network output and desired output, that means they vary in opposite ways (when network output increases, desired output decreases by the same amount). When $r = 0$ there is no correlation between network output and desired output (the variables are called uncorrelated). Intermediate values describe partial correlations.[42–44,59]

Neural networks are used for both classification and regression. In classification, the aim is to assign the input patterns to one of several classes, usually represented by outputs restricted to lie in the range from 0 to 1, so that they represent the probability of class membership. While the classification is carried out, a specific pattern is assigned to a specific class according to the characteristic features selected for it. In regression, desired output and actual network output results can be shown on the same graph and the performance of network can be evaluated in this way. Classification results of the classifiers are displayed by a confusion matrix. In a confusion matrix, each cell contains the raw number of exemplars classified for the corresponding combination of desired and actual network outputs.[42–44,59] From the confusion matrices one can tell the frequency with which a signal is misclassified as another. Table 2 shows examples of confusion matrices of the classifiers used for classification of the coronary arterial signals.

Table 2. Confusion matrices of the classifiers used for classification of the coronary arterial signals.

| Classifiers | Desired Result | Output Result | |
|---|---|---|---|
| (features) | | Healthy | Coronary artery stenosis |
| SVM | Healthy | 43 | 0 |
| (composite feature) | Coronary artery stenosis | 0 | 32 |
| RNN | Healthy | 41 | 0 |
| (composite feature) | Coronary artery stenosis | 2 | 32 |
| PNN | Healthy | 41 | 1 |
| (composite feature) | Coronary artery stenosis | 2 | 31 |
| MME | Healthy | 42 | 0 |
| (diverse features) | Coronary artery stenosis | 1 | 32 |
| ME | Healthy | 42 | 1 |
| (composite feature) | Coronary artery stenosis | 1 | 31 |
| CNN | Healthy | 41 | 1 |
| (composite feature) | Coronary artery stenosis | 2 | 31 |
| MLPNN | Healthy | 40 | 2 |
| (composite feature) | Coronary artery stenosis | 3 | 30 |

The test performance of the classifiers can be determined by the computation of specificity, sensitivity, and total classification accuracy. The specificity, sensitivity, and total classification accuracy are defined as:

*Specificity*: number of true negative decisions/number of actually negative cases
*Sensitivity*: number of true positive decisions/number of actually positive cases
*Total classification accuracy*: number of correct decisions/total number of cases

A true negative decision occurs when both the classifier and the physician suggested the absence of a positive detection. A true positive decision occurs when the positive detection of the classifier coincided with a positive detection of the physician.[6]

In order to compare the classifiers used for classification problems, the classification accuracies (specificity, sensitivity, total classification accuracy) on the test sets and the central processing unit (CPU) times of training of the classifiers can be presented. The classification accuracies (specificity, sensitivity, total classification accuracy) on the test sets computed by the usage of the example values shown in Table 2 and the CPU times of training of the classifiers are presented in Table 3.

Receiver operating characteristic (ROC) plots provide a view of the whole spectrum of sensitivities and specificities because all possible sensitivity/specificity pairs for a particular test are graphed. The performance of a test can be evaluated by plotting a ROC curve for the test and therefore, ROC curves are used to describe the performance of the classifiers.[6,75] A good test is one for which sensitivity rises rapidly and 1-specificity hardly increases at all until sensitivity becomes high (Fig. 14).

Table 3. The classification accuracies and the CPU times of training of the classifiers used for classification of the coronary arterial signals.

| Classifier | Classification Accuracies (%) | | | CPU time |
|---|---|---|---|---|
| (features) | Specificity | Sensitivity (Coronary artery stenosis) | Total classification accuracy | (min:s) |
| SVM (composite feature) | 100.00 | 100.00 | 100.00 | 7:55 |
| RNN (composite feature) | 95.35 | 100.00 | 97.33 | 12:17 |
| PNN (composite feature) | 95.35 | 96.88 | 96.00 | 11:09 |
| MME (diverse features) | 97.67 | 100.00 | 98.67 | 7:06 |
| ME (composite feature) | 97.67 | 96.88 | 97.33 | 9:05 |
| CNN (composite feature) | 95.35 | 96.88 | 96.00 | 12:41 |
| MLPNN (composite feature) | 93.02 | 93.75 | 93.33 | 14:16 |

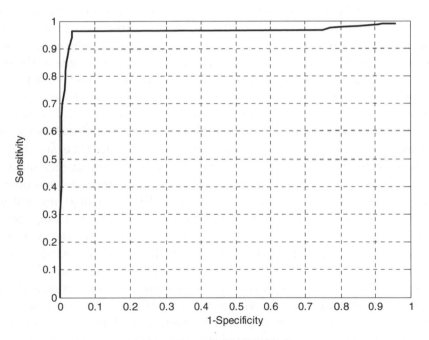

Fig. 14. ROC curve of the classifier.

## 9. Discussion and Analysis

The FFT-based methods are based on a finite record of data and their frequency resolution are limited by the data record duration, independent of the characteristics of the data. These methods suffer from spectral leakage effects, due to windowing that are inherent in finite-length data records. Furthermore, the principal effect of windowing that occurs when processing with the FFT-based methods is to smear or smooth the estimated spectrum. The basic limitation of the FFT-based methods is the inherent assumption that the autocorrelation estimate is zero outside the window. From another viewpoint, the inherent assumption in the FFT-based methods is that the data are periodic. Neither one of these assumptions is realistic.[1–4,9,11]

The model-based methods do not require such assumptions. The modeling approach eliminates the need for window functions and the assumption that the autocorrelation sequence is zero outside the window. The model-based methods spectra have better statistical stability for short segments of signal and have better spectral resolution and the resolution is less dependent on the length of the record. The model-based methods have better temporal resolution and produce continuous spectra. The disadvantages of the model-based methods compared to the FFT-based methods are: the FFT-based methods are more widely available and are the traditional engineering approach to spectrum analysis; the model-based spectra are slower to compute; the model-based methods are not reversible; the model-based methods are slightly more complicated to code; the model-based methods are more sensitive to round-off errors, and finally, the orders of the model-based methods depend on the characteristics of the signal and the current objective methods for model order determination are not satisfactory. Based on the results of the studies existing in the literature, performance characteristics of the AR and ARMA methods were found extremely valuable for spectral analysis of biomedical signals.[1–4,9,11]

There is a distinct qualitative improvement in spectral analysis of nonstationary signals using the time–frequency analysis methods over the classical and model-based methods. The problem with the STFT is that both time and frequency resolutions of the transform are fixed over the entire time–frequency plane. The STFT involves the implicit assumption that the data are quasi-stationary for the duration of each analyzed segment. Taking the FFT of a short segment of the Doppler signal leads to a distortion of the spectral estimate and leakage of signal energy into spurious side lobes due to the sharp truncation of the signal. To reduce this distortion it is common practice to multiply the signal by a window function which reduces the amplitude of the analyzed signal toward the beginning and end of the data segment. Using longer data segments reduces the distortion and leakage of the spectral estimates but may violate the nonstationarity assumption. There is an obvious trade-off when using the STFT between the distortion and poor spectral resolution introduced by short data windows and the spectral broadening that arises from nonstationary characteristics of the signal when using longer data windows. A more flexible approach would be to use a scalable window: a compressed window for analyzing high frequency detail and a dilated window for uncovering low frequency trends within the signal. The WT addresses the problem of fixed resolution by using base functions that can be scaled. The wavelets act in a similar way to the windowed complex exponentials that are used in the STFT, except that with the

WT the length of signal being analyzed is not fixed. It is known that wavelets are better suited to analyzing nonstationary signals, since they are well localized in time and frequency. The property of time and frequency localization is known as compact support and is one of the most attractive features of the WT. The WT of a signal is the decomposition of the signal over a set of functions obtained after dilatation and translation of an analyzing wavelet. The main advantage of the WT is that it has a varying window size, being broad at low frequencies and narrow at high frequencies, thus leading to an optimal time–frequency resolution in all frequency ranges. Furthermore, owing to the fact that windows are adapted to the transients of each scale, wavelets lack the requirement of stationarity.[5,12]

The eigenvector methods provide sufficient resolution to estimate the sinusoids from the data. Hence, to gain some noise immunity it is reasonable to retain only the principal eigenvector components in the estimation of the autocorrelation matrix.[2,3,10,49] Spectral analysis of the signals under study and implementation of the classifiers can be performed by the usage of MATLAB software package.[34]

Each of the classifiers and their respective results give insights into the diverse and composite features of the signals under study. The results of the experience in signal analysis and classifiers are highlighted as follows:

1.  The SVM training algorithm aims to extract support vectors near the decision boundary to construct a hyperplane based on the principle of structural risk minimization. During SVM training, most of the computational effort is spent on solving the quadratic programming problem in order to find the support vectors. The SVM maps the features to higher dimensional space and then uses an optimal hyperplane in the mapped space. This implies that though the original features carry adequate information for good classification, mapping to a higher dimensional feature space could potentially provide better discriminatory clues that are not present in the original feature space. The selection of suitable kernel function appears to be a trial-and-error process. One would not know the suitability of a kernel function and performance of the SVM until one has tried and tested with the representative data. For training the SVMs with RBF kernel functions, one has to pre-determine the $\sigma$ values. The optimal or near-optimal $\sigma$ values can only be ascertained after trying out several, or even many values. Beside this, the choice of $C$ parameter in the SVM is very critical in order to have a properly trained SVM. The SVM has to be trained for different $C$ values until we get the best result.[72–74]

2.  The PNN training is to build prototype vectors that act as cluster centers among the training patterns. As a matter of fact, the pattern layer of a PNN often consists of all training samples of which many could be redundant. Including redundant samples can potentially lead to a large network structure, which in turn induces two problems. First, it would result in higher computational overhead simply because the amount of computation necessary to classify an unknown pattern is proportional to the size of the network. Second, a

consequence of a large network structure is that the classifier tends to be oversensitive to the training data and is likely to exhibit poor generalization capabilities to the unseen data. On the other hand, the smoothing parameter also plays a crucial role in the PNN classifier, and an appropriate smoothing parameter is often data-dependent.[64,65]

3. The EM algorithm can be used to train the MME and ME classifiers and the Levenberg–Marquardt algorithm can be used to train the RNNs, CNNs, and MLPNNs. In the MME and ME classifiers, the classification problem is divided into simpler problems and then each solution is combined. In addition to this, the training algorithm of the MME and ME classifiers is a general technique for maximum likelihood estimation that fits well with the modular structure and enables a significant speed up over the other training algorithms. Thus, the convergence rates of the MME and ME classifiers are significantly higher than that of the RNNs, CNNs, and MLPNNs.[24,25,27,29,31,42]

4. The MME trained on diverse features converged sooner than the other neural network models and therefore required less computation to train the network. High-dimension of composite feature vector increases computational complexity and the neural networks trained on composite feature (MLPNN, CNN, ME, PNN, RNN) produce lower accuracy.[33,53]

5. In the CNN, the first level networks are implemented for the diagnosis of disorders using the composite features as inputs. To improve diagnostic accuracy, the second level networks are trained using the outputs of the first level networks as input data. The CNN models achieve accuracy rates which are higher than that of the MLPNNs.[24,27]

6. Doppler ultrasonography is a noninvasive method that is known to be useful in evaluating blood flow velocities in arteries. It has been hypothesized that each artery in the human body has its own characteristic — a unique Doppler profile which can identify the artery and which may also be modified by the presence of a disease. To test this hypothesis ANN was trained to recognize three groups of maximum frequency envelopes derived from Doppler ultrasound spectrograms; these were the common carotid, common femoral, and popliteal arteries.[17] In the study presented by Wright *et al.*[17] the maximum frequency envelopes were used to create sets of training and testing vectors for a backpropagation ANN. The ANN demonstrated classification accuracy, 100% for the carotid, 92% for the femoral, and 96% for the popliteal artery. The study presented by Wright and Gough[18] indicated the results of a backpropagation ANN, which was trained and tested with the features derived from maximum frequency envelopes of common femoral artery. The ANN correctly classified 80% of "no significant disease" data and 85% of "occlusion" data. The results of these two studies[17,18] demonstrated that ANNs may offer a potentially superior method of Doppler signal analysis to the spectral analysis methods. In contrast to the conventional spectral analysis methods, ANNs not only model the signal, but also make a decision as to the class of the signal. Another advantage of ANN analysis over existing methods of

Doppler waveform analysis is that, after an ANN has trained satisfactorily and the values of the weights and biases have been stored, testing and subsequent implementation is rapid. Beside this, the authors mentioned that interpretation of the Doppler waveform may be regarded as a process of pattern recognition, whereby salient features are extracted from the Doppler spectrogram to produce a "feature vector" to represent the data to be classified. The performance of the classifier depends on the features, which are used as inputs of the classifier. In this chapter, in order to obtain the features, which are well representing the signals under study, we present different feature extraction methods. This study found that it is possible to some extent to determine the best classifier for the signals by the usage of the diverse and composite features.

7. The results of the studies existing in the literature indicated excellent performance of the SVMs and MMEs on the classification of the signals.[33,53,72,73]

## 10. Conclusion

The automated diagnostic systems trained on diverse or composite features for classification of the signals are presented. The signals classification is considered as a typical problem of classification with diverse features since the methods used for feature extraction have different performance and no unique robust feature has been found. The inputs (diverse or composite features) of the automated diagnostic systems are obtained by pre-processing of the signals with various spectral analysis methods. The superiorities of the WT and eigenvector methods will make them useful in spectral analysis of the signals recorded from coronary arteries. In order to compare the used classifiers, the classification accuracies, the CPU times of training, and ROC curves of the classifiers can be considered. According to the presented results, the SVM classifiers show a great performance since it maps the features to a higher dimensional space. Beside this, the MME classifiers provided encouraging results which could be originated from training of the MMEs on diverse features. The performance of the ME, RNN, PNN, CNN, and MLPNN are not as high as the SVM and MME. This may be attributed to several factors including the training algorithms, estimation of the network parameters, and the scattered and mixed nature of the features. The behavior of each classifier provides valuable insights to the properties of the feature space and from these insights it may be possible to implement a classification model that will give perfect classification results on the data. Based on the drawn conclusions, the SVM and MME trained on the features extracted by especially the WT and eigenvector methods can be useful in the detection of coronary artery stenosis.

## References

1. S. M. Kay, *Modern Spectral Estimation: Theory and Application* (Prentice Hall, New Jersey, 1988).

2. J. G. Proakis and D. G. Manolakis, *Digital Signal Processing Principles, Algorithms, and Applications* (Prentice Hall, New Jersey, 1996).
3. P. Stoica and R. Moses, *Introduction to Spectral Analysis* (Prentice Hall, New Jersey, 1997).
4. S. M. Kay and S. L. Marple, Spectrum analysis — A modern perspective, in *Proc. IEEE* **69** (1981) 1380–1419.
5. M. Akay, *Time Frequency and Wavelets in Biomedical Signal Processing* (Institute of Electrical and Electronics Engineers, Inc., New York, 1998).
6. D. H. Evans, W. N. McDicken, R. Skidmore and J. P. Woodcock, *Doppler Ultrasound: Physics, Instrumentation and Clinical Applications* (Wiley, Chichester, 1989).
7. J. Y. David, S. A. Jones and D. P. Giddens, Modern spectral analysis techniques for blood flow velocity and spectral measurements with pulsed Doppler ultrasound, *IEEE Trans. Biomed. Eng.* **38** (1991) 589–596.
8. İ. Güler, F. Hardalaç and E. D. Übeyli, Determination of Behcet disease with the application of FFT and AR methods, *Comp. Biol. Med.* **32**(6) (2002) 419–434.
9. İ. Güler and E. D. Übeyli, Application of classical and model-based spectral methods to ophthalmic arterial Doppler signals with uveitis disease, *Comp. Biol. Med.* **33**(6) (2003) 455–471.
10. E. D. Übeyli and İ. Güler, Comparison of eigenvector methods with classical and model-based methods in analysis of internal carotid arterial Doppler signals, *Comp. Biol. Med.* **33**(6) (2003) 473–493.
11. E. D. Übeyli and İ. Güler, Spectral analysis of internal carotid arterial Doppler signals using FFT, AR, MA, and ARMA methods, *Comp. Biol. Med.* **34**(4) (2004) 293–306.
12. E. D. Übeyli and İ. Güler, Spectral broadening of ophthalmic arterial Doppler signals using STFT and wavelet transform, *Comp. Biol. Med.* **34**(4) (2004) 345–354.
13. E. D. Übeyli and İ. Güler, Selection of optimal AR spectral estimation method for internal carotid arterial Doppler signals using Cramer-Rao bound, *Comp. Elec. Eng.* **30**(7) (2004) 491–508.
14. E. D. Übeyli and İ. Güler, Feature extraction from Doppler ultrasound signals for automated diagnostic systems, *Comp. Biol. Med.* **35**(9) (2005) 735–764.
15. A. S. Miller, B. H. Blott and T. K. Hames, Review of neural network applications in medical imaging and signal processing, *Med. Biol. Eng. Comput.* **30** (1992) 449–464.
16. B. A. Mobley, E. Schechter, W. E. Moore, P. A. McKee and J. E. Eichner, Predictions of coronary artery stenosis by artificial neural network, *Artif. Intell. Med.* **18** (2000) 187–203.
17. I. A. Wright, N. A. J. Gough, F. Rakebrandt, M. Wahab and J. P. Woodcock, Neural network analysis of Doppler ultrasound blood flow signals: A pilot study, *Ultrasound Med. Biol.* **23**(5) (1997) 683–690.
18. I. A. Wright and N. A. J. Gough, Artificial neural network analysis of common femoral artery Doppler shift signals: Classification of proximal disease, *Ultrasound Med. Biol.* **24**(5) (1999) 735–743.
19. İ. Güler and E. D. Übeyli, Detection of ophthalmic artery stenosis by least-mean squares backpropagation neural network, *Comp. Biol. Med.* **33**(4) (2003) 333–343.
20. E. D. Übeyli and İ. Güler, Neural network analysis of internal carotid arterial Doppler signals: Predictions of stenosis and occlusion, *Expert Sys. Appl.* **25**(1) (2003) 1–13.
21. N. F. Güler and E. D. Übeyli, Wavelet-based neural network analysis of ophthalmic artery Doppler signals, *Comp. Biol. Med.* **34**(7) (2004) 601–613.
22. İ. Güler and E. D. Übeyli, Application of adaptive neuro-fuzzy inference system for detection of electrocardiographic changes in patients with partial epilepsy using feature extraction, *Expert Sys. Appl.* **27**(3) (2004) 323–330.

23. E. D. Übeyli and İ. Güler, Detection of electrocardiographic changes in partial epileptic patients using Lyapunov exponents with multilayer perceptron neural networks, *Eng. Appl. Artif. Intell.* **17**(6) (2004) 567–576.

24. İ. Güler and E. D. Übeyli, ECG beat classifier designed by combined neural network model, *Patt. Recog.* **38**(2) (2005) 199–208.

25. İ. Güler and E. D. Übeyli, Detection of ophthalmic arterial Doppler signals with Behcet disease using multilayer perceptron neural network, *Comp. Biol. Med.* **35**(2) (2005) 121–132.

26. İ. Güler and E. D. Übeyli, Feature saliency using signal-to-noise ratios in automated diagnostic systems developed for ECG beats, *Expert Sys. Appl.* **28**(2) (2005) 295–304.

27. E. D. Übeyli and İ. Güler, Improving medical diagnostic accuracy of ultrasound Doppler signals by combining neural network models, *Comp. Biol. Med.* **35**(6) (2005) 533–554.

28. İ. Güler and E. D. Übeyli, An expert system for detection of electrocardiographic changes in patients with partial epilepsy using wavelet-based neural networks, *Expert Sys.* **22**(2) (2005) 62–71.

29. İ. Güler and E. D. Übeyli, A mixture of experts network structure for modelling Doppler ultrasound blood flow signals, *Comp. Biol. Med.* **35**(7) (2005) 565–582.

30. İ. Güler and E. D. Übeyli, Automatic detection of ophthalmic artery stenosis using adaptive neuro-fuzzy inference system, *Eng. Appl. Artif. Intell.* **18**(4) (2005) 413–422.

31. N. F. Güler, E. D. Übeyli and İ. Güler, Recurrent neural networks employing Lyapunov exponents for EEG signals classification, *Expert Sys. Appl.* **29**(3) (2005) 506–514.

32. E. D. Übeyli and İ. Güler, Adaptive neuro-fuzzy inference systems for analysis of internal carotid arterial Doppler signals, *Comp. Biol. Med.* **35**(8) (2005) 687–702.

33. İ. Güler and E. D. Übeyli, A modified mixture of experts network structure for ECG beats classification with diverse features, *Eng. Appl. Artif. Intell.* **18**(7) (2005) 845–856.

34. E. D. Übeyli and İ. Güler, Teaching automated diagnostic systems for Doppler ultrasound blood flow signals to biomedical engineering students using MATLAB, *Int. J. Eng. Edu.* **21**(4) (2005) 649–667.

35. İ. Güler and E. D. Übeyli, Adaptive neuro-fuzzy inference system for classification of EEG signals using wavelet coefficients, *J. Neurosci. Meth.* **148**(2) (2005) 113–121.

36. İ. Güler and E. D. Übeyli, Neural network analysis of ophthalmic arterial Doppler signals with uveitis disease, *Neural Comput. Appl.* **14**(4) (2005) 353–360.

37. İ. Güler and E. D. Übeyli, Feature saliency using signal-to-noise ratios in automated diagnostic systems developed for Doppler ultrasound signals, *Eng. Appl. Artif. Intell.* **19**(1) (2006) 53–63.

38. H. Kordylewski, D. Graupe and K. Liu, A novel large-memory neural network as an aid in medical diagnosis applications, *IEEE Trans. Inform. Technol. Biomed.* **5**(3) (2001) 202–209.

39. N. Kwak and C.-H. Choi, Input feature selection for classification problems, *IEEE Trans. Neural Networks* **13**(1) (2002) 143–159.

40. D. West and V. West, Model selection for a medical diagnostic decision support system: A breast cancer detection case, *Artif. Intell. Med.* **20**(3) (2000) 183–204.

41. D. West and V. West, Improving diagnostic accuracy using a hierarchical neural network to model decision subtasks, *Int. J. Med. Informatics* **57**(1) (2000) 41–55.

42. S. Haykin, *Neural Networks: A Comprehensive Foundation* (Macmillan, New York, 1994).

43. I. A. Basheer and M. Hajmeer, Artificial neural networks: Fundamentals, computing, design, and application, *J. Microbiol. Meth.* **43**(1) (2000) 3–31.

44. B. B. Chaudhuri and U. Bhattacharya, Efficient training and improved performance of multilayer perceptron in pattern classification, *Neurocomputing* **34** (2000) 11–27.

45. İ. Güler and Y. Savaş, Design parameters of pulsed wave ultrasonic Doppler blood flowmeter, *J. Med. Sys.* **22**(4) (1998) 273–278.

46. H. Akaike, A new look at the statistical model identification, *IEEE Trans. Automatic Contr.* AC **19** (1974) 716–723.

47. I. Daubechies, The wavelet transform, time–frequency localization and signal analysis, *IEEE Trans. Inform. Theory* **36**(5) (1990) 961–1005.

48. M. Akay, Wavelet applications in medicine, *IEEE Spectrum* **34**(5) (1997) 50–56.

49. M. Akay, J. L. Semmlow, W. Welkowitz, M. D. Bauer and J. B. Kostis, Noninvasive detection of coronary stenoses before and after angioplasty using eigenvector methods, *IEEE Trans. Biomed. Eng.* **37**(11) (1990) 1095–1104.

50. A. M. Thornett, Computer decision support systems in general practice, *Int. J. Inform. Management* **21** (2001) 39–47.

51. B. D. Bliven, S. E. Kaufman and J. A. Spertus, Electronic collection of health-related quality of life data: Validity, time, benefits, and patient preference, *Qual. Life Res.* **10** (2001) 15–22.

52. E. R. Carson, Decision support systems in diabetes: A systems perspective, *Comp. Meth. Prog. Biomed.* **56** (1998) 77–91.

53. K. Chen, A connectionist method for pattern classification with diverse features, *Patt. Recog. Lett.* **19**(7) (1998) 545–558.

54. L. Xu, A. Krzyzak and C. Y. Suen, Methods of combining multiple classifiers and their applications to handwriting recognition, *IEEE Trans. Sys., Man, Cybernet.* **22**(3) (1992) 418–435.

55. K. Chen, L. Wang and H. Chi, Methods of combining multiple classifiers with different features and their applications to text-independent speaker identification, *Int. J. Patt. Recog. Artif. Intell.* **11**(3) (1997) 417–445.

56. M. T. Hagan and M. B. Menhaj, Training feedforward networks with the Marquardt algorithm, *IEEE Trans. Neural Networks* **5**(6) (1994) 989–993.

57. R. Battiti, First- and second-order methods for learning: Between steepest descent and Newton's method, *Neural Comput.* **4** (1992) 141–166.

58. D. H. Wolpert, Stacked generalization, *Neural Networks* **5** (1992) 241–259.

59. C. M. Bishop, *Neural Networks for Pattern Recognition* (Oxford University Press, New York, 2003).

60. R. A. Jacobs, M. I. Jordan, S. J. Nowlan and G. E. Hinton, Adaptive mixtures of local experts, *Neural Comput.* **3**(1) (1991) 79–87.

61. K. Chen, L. Xu and H. Chi, Improved learning algorithms for mixture of experts in multiclass classification, *Neural Networks* **12**(9) (1999) 1229–1252.

62. X. Hong and C. J. Harris, A mixture of experts network structure construction algorithm for modelling and control, *Appl. Intell.* **16**(1) (2002) 59–69.

63. M. I. Jordan and R. A. Jacobs, Hierarchical mixture of experts and the EM algorithm, *Neural Comput.* **6**(2) (1994) 181–214.

64. D. F. Specht, Probabilistic neural networks, *Neural Networks* **3**(1) (1990) 109–118.

65. P. Burrascano, Learning vector quantization for the probabilistic neural network, *IEEE Trans. Neural Networks* **2**(4) (1991) 458–461.

66. E. W. Saad, D. V. Prokhorov and D. C. Wunsch II, Comparative study of stock trend prediction using time delay, recurrent and probabilistic neural networks, *IEEE Trans. Neural Networks* **9**(6) (1998) 1456–1470.

67. L. Gupta, M. McAvoy and J. Phegley, Classification of temporal sequences via prediction using the simple recurrent neural network, *Patt. Recog.* **33**(10) (2000) 1759–1770.

68. J. L. Elman, Finding structure in time, *Cognitive Sci.* **14**(2) (1990) 179–211.

69. A. Petrosian, D. Prokhorov, R. Homan, R. Dasheiff and D. Wunsch II, Recurrent neural network based prediction of epileptic seizures in intra- and extracranial EEG, *Neurocomputing* **30** (2000) 201–218.

70. J.-S. Shieh, C.-F. Chou, S.-J. Huang and M.-C. Kao, Intracranial pressure model in intensive care unit using a simple recurrent neural network through time, *Neurocomputing* **57** (2004) 239–256.

71. F. J. Pineda, Generalization of back-propagation to recurrent neural networks, *Phys. Rev. Lett.* **59**(9) (1987) 2229–2232.

72. V. Vapnik, *The Nature of Statistical Learning Theory* (Springer-Verlag, New York, 1995).

73. C. Cortes and V. Vapnik, Support vector networks, *Mach. Learn.* **20**(3) (1995) 273–297.

74. T. G. Dietterich and G. Bakiri, Solving multiclass learning problems via error-correcting output codes, *J. Artif. Intell. Res.* **2** (1995) 263–286.

75. M. H. Zweig and G. Campbell, Receiver-operating characteristic (ROC) plots: A fundamental evaluation tool in clinical medicine, *Clin. Chem.* **39**(4) (1993) 561–577.

# CHAPTER 8

# TECHNIQUES IN THE CONTOUR DETECTION OF KIDNEYS AND THEIR APPLICATIONS

M. MARTIN-FERNANDEZ*, L. CORDERO-GRANDE, E. MUNOZ-MORENO
and C. ALBEROLA-LOPEZ
*Valladolid University, ETSI Telecommunication
Cra. Cementerio s/n, Valladolid 47011, Spain
*marcma@tel.uva.es

## 1. Introduction

Renal volume is an important parameter in clinical settings for the adult,[4] newborns and fetuses. On the former, evaluation and follow-up of patients with urinary tract infections, renal vessels stenosis, and others are done in terms of both the length and the volume within the organ. In newborns and fetuses, the *neonatal hydronephrosis* is detected by means of abnormal large volumes enclosed by the organ.

The usual procedure to calculate the volume within the organ is to apply the ellipsoid method to ultrasound (US) images. The physician either looks for three orthogonal planes to calculate the main axes kidney lengths (one of the planes is shown in Fig. 1(a)), and then uses the ellipsoid volume formula, or alternatively, manually adjusts — with help of cursors — an ellipse to the guessed external boundary of the kidney (as shown in Fig. 1(b)), and the system approximates the kidney volume as the volume of the ellipsoid generated by rotating the sketched ellipse about its main axis. The pelvis volume is determined similarly (inner contour in Fig. 1(b)). The ellipsoid method, however, is known to underestimate the kidney volume up to a 25% error.[4] Actually, it has been experimentally tested[3] that the volume determination of an *in vitro* kidney after a totally manual segmentation (the volume calculation is a simple voxel counting procedure) is much more accurate than the one obtained through the ellipsoid method. This improvement has also been reported for the kidney of a fetus when it is manually segmented from a series of *in vivo* echographical slices.[55] Magnetic resonance imaging (MRI) gives accurate results for this calculation,[4,23] but this imaging modality has longer acquisition times and it is not as affordable as US equipment is. Nowadays, a two dimensional (2D) US probe equipped with a magnetic positioning device suffices to get US volume data reconstructed with accurate results.[46,47,49] Such volumes calculated out of 3D US data are reliable, and they can serve at least to carry out screening

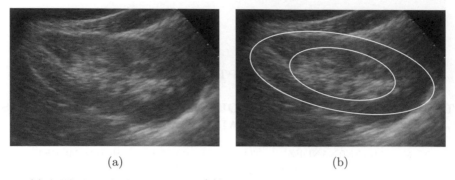

(a)         (b)

Fig. 1. (a) A US slice of a human kidney. (b) Manual adjustments of the ellipses for the kidney and pelvis.

operations with inexpensive imaging modalities; for this to be clinically deployed, a piece of equipment needs to be provided with accurate segmentation tools so that results can be obtained within short time periods and with a small manual interaction.

Semiautomatic methods for *in vitro* organ segmentation have been reported in the past,[49] and specifically, for the case of a kidney.[41] However, it is important to highlight the fact that the organ is segmented *in vitro* (i.e. submerged in a liquid, therefore, with a clear echographical transition between the liquid and the organ) is not directly applicable to a clinical situation, in which, obviously, the patient's kidney is *in vivo*. Therefore, robust methods that as automatically as possible provide renal volume information with a high accuracy and speed are needed. Classical segmentation methods[27] are fast and useful only in very simple or very controlled situations. In the problem that we describe in this chapter, the situation is far from being so, since US images are fairly noisy and the signal to noise ratio is, generally speaking, poor. It is therefore necessary to resort to more robust methods that make use of prior information to compensate for the inherent difficulties that arise with such an imaging modality.[44]

This chapter will be organized as follows. Section 2 reviews the operations needed to deal with contours and, specifically, with discrete contours. In particular, some expressions to obtain several measurements from a given contour are presented which, together with affine transformations, will allow contour fitting. Other topics covered along this section will be contour reparameterization and template adjustment for which the complex representation of a contour will be used. This section provides background material for the forthcoming sections and it is included here to make the chapter self-contained. Then we focus on techniques for contour detection, and we will concentrate on two contributions; the first of them is the one in Sec. 3, in which we describe a solution based on shape priors.[54] The second solution is the one proposed by Martin-Fernandez and Alberola-Lopez,[39] which will be reviewed in Sec. 4, and it is extended here also. It is worth mentioning that these two solutions were released simultaneously in two different journals in the same month of year 2005. Finally, Sec. 5 will summarize the chapter and will also include some concluding remarks.

## 2. Contour Operations

Image analysis algorithms deal with extracting information from images. Segmentation is a common task which involves finding specific objects in the image as well as a suitable description for them. This is, generally speaking, the first step within a more complex image analysis framework, which comprises describing a scene with multiple objects and the interrelation among them. The two most common approaches to describe objects are to describe the region an object occupies, or to define the boundary that separates the object from other structures. The choice of representation is, as a rule, guided by the subsequent processing steps since such a representation has a great influence on what can be done.[37] Although, regional representations in image segmentation are important,[45] contour representation has gained interest after the appearance of a seminal paper,[30] which describes Active Contours (ACs), i.e. contours that can evolve following forces derived from both image and smoothing constraints.[a] Although several approaches can be used to deal with contours, continuous functional descriptions have proved to be one of the most attractive representations as all the mathematical methods developed for functions can be directly applied to contours.[7,31] The curve evolution scheme introduced in Ref. 30 uses a 2D Cartesian representation of the curve. A similar approach, but using a polar description, was later proposed in Ref. 19, reducing the optimization problem from 2D to 1D. The authors also introduced the monotonic phase property, the core of the current section. In this case, the contours that hold this property were referred to as *star-like*. This representation is not only convenient for the optimization problem presented in Ref. 19, but also for the shape analysis concerning kidney contours determined by the methods presented throughout the following sections. This is an important topic which we address here systematically; to that end, we begin with a continuous formulation and then introduce its discrete counterpart by means of the finite difference method. In Ref. 31, aspects related to our work were pointed out, but not fully developed as the complex representation for the contour or the ambiguity of choosing a proper contour center. Here, we will analyze the application of novel representations for affine transformation problems that can also be applied to contour fitting, more generally known as shape matching.[51] In connection with kidney contour segmentation, two important topics will be covered. The first one deals with contour reparameterizations. The constant arclength parameterization has been proposed in the literature[52] as one of the most interesting parameterizations whenever point

---

[a]In this chapter we will assume that the topology of the object sought is roughly known. Therefore *topological changes* will not be an issue for us. This is the reason why we concentrate on parametric deformable models, and particularly, on ACs, leaving geometric deformable models[8,38] aside.

homogeneity is important. Here we reformulate the problem proposing a new iterative algorithm that converges to the solution sought. The result is compared to uniform phase and uniform area representations. The second topic is related to template matching[51] and tries to solve a common routine procedure that comes up when dealing with US images in kidney segmentation.[39]

## 2.1. *Continuous contours*

A *continuous contour* is a continuous curve $\mathbf{r}(s)$, which can be defined as a parametric vector function that depends on a continuous parameter $s \in R$. In *Cartesian coordinates* the curve can be described by $\mathbf{r}_c(s) = (x(s), y(s))^T$. If the curve $\mathbf{r}_c(s)$ is closed, $x(s)$ and $y(s)$ are periodic functions in $s$. In this case, let $S$ denote a period of the curve. In *polar coordinates* it can be written as $\mathbf{r}_p(s) = (\rho(s), \theta(s))^T$. If the curve $\mathbf{r}_p(s)$ is closed, $\rho(s)$ and $\theta(s)$ are periodic in $s$. The relationship between the Cartesian and polar coordinates is given by

$$\rho(s) = \sqrt{x^2(s) + y^2(s)}, \quad \theta(s) = \angle(x(s) + iy(s)),$$
$$x(s) = \rho(s)\cos\theta(s), \quad y(s) = \rho(s)\sin\theta(s), \tag{1}$$

where $\angle(\cdot)$ denotes the complex angle in radians in interval $(-\pi, \pi)$. In Fig. 2 we can schematically see the relationship between Cartesian and polar coordinates for a given contour. We will see that the selection of a proper center is an important issue. Figure 3(a) shows a given contour representation. This contour can be described by its parametric functions. Figure 3(b) shows the Cartesian coordinates represented as a function of parameter $s$. As the contour is closed the Cartesian functions are periodic with unity period. For this case $S$ ranges in interval $(0, 1)$. In Fig. 3(c) the polar functions are represented as a function of parameter $s$. The radial coordinate $\rho(s)$ is also periodic with the same period. With respect to the

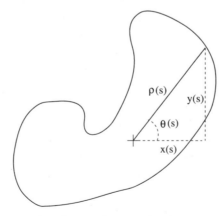

Fig. 2. Parametric representation for continuous closed contours in Cartesian and polar coordinates.

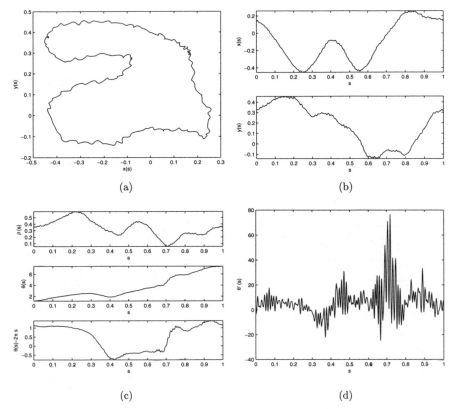

Fig. 3.  (a) Example of a continuous closed contour without the monotonic phase property. (b) Cartesian parameterization of the curve in (a). (c) Polar parameterization of the curve in (a): magnitude function (top), angular (phase) function (middle), and phase function with the linear trend removed (bottom). (d) The derivative of the angular function in (c).

phase function $\theta(s)$, as the center is inside the contour, the phase varies within a $2\pi$ range and tends to increase. In the trivial case of a circular contour the phase is linear.

We are interested in a particular kind of closed contours $r(s)$ for which their phase $\theta(s)$ is *monotonic*[b] in interval $(-\pi, \pi)$. This means that the origin of the coordinate system must be inside the contour and that from this origin one can arrive at any point of the contour without crossing it.[c] This also means that the contour has no loops. Figure 3(d) shows the derivative of the phase function for the contour in Fig. 3(a). This derivative is negative for several ranges of parameter $s$; so the phase is not monotonically increasing, i.e. the monotonic phase property

[b]For closed contours we have periodicity in $s$, and the monotonicity must be considered with respect to only one period $S$.
[c]That is, we say that the from the origin of the coordinate system one can *see* every point of the contour.

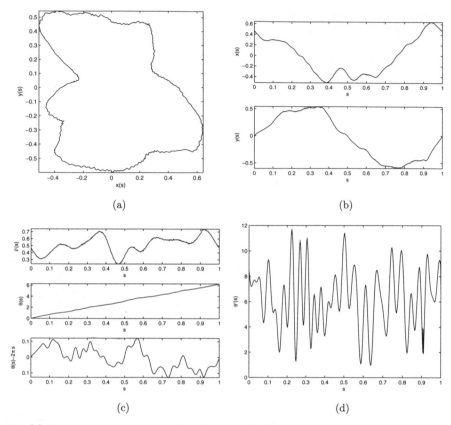

Fig. 4. (a) Example of a continous closed contour holding the monotonic phase property. (b) Cartesian parameterization of the curve in (a). (c) Polar parameterization of the curve in (a): magnitude function (top), angular (phase) function (middle), and phase function with the linear trend removed (bottom). (d) The derivative of the angular function in (c).

is violated. Figure 4(a) shows a second contour. Figures 4(b) and 4(c) show the Cartesian and polar representations, respectively. The middle graph in Fig. 4(c) has a linear component that can be removed to better show the phase variation (see Fig. 4(c) bottom graph). From these graphs it is difficult to see whether the phase is monotonic or not. However, if we calculate the derivative of the phase function (see Fig. 4(d)), we can appreciate that the phase derivative is always positive, and hence the phase function is always increasing, assuring the monotonic phase property hold.

For *period* $S$ in the parameter domain $s$ for which the phase of contour $\theta(s)$ is monotonic in interval $(-\pi, \pi)$, the *inverse function* of phase $\theta(s)$ can be determined. If we call $u = \theta(s)$, then we have $s = \theta^{-1}(u)$, and we can replace parameter $s$ in the contour expressions and consider that now the parameter is $u = \theta(s) = \theta$. We are doing a contour reparameterization.

In doing so we can define a contour with respect to a parameter that represents its own phase. The periodicity of that phase gives rise directly to the periodicity of the parameter of the closed contour. The new parameter $\theta$ takes on values in the $(-\pi, \pi)$ range and is periodic with period $2\pi$. Thus the contour is given by the parametric curve $\mathbf{r}(\theta)$. In Cartesian coordinates the curve can be written as $\mathbf{r}_c(\theta) = (x(\theta), y(\theta))^T$ and in polar coordinates as $\mathbf{r}_p(\theta) = (\rho(\theta), \theta)^T$. In polar coordinates the contour is represented by only one parametric function $\rho(\theta)$. This is very important because it reduces the problem from 2D to 1D. In this case it is more convenient to work in the polar domain whenever possible. Hence the relationship between the Cartesian and polar coordinates is given by

$$\rho(\theta) = \sqrt{x^2(\theta) + y^2(\theta)}, \quad x(\theta) = \rho(\theta)\cos\theta, \quad y(\mathbf{s}) = \rho(\theta)\sin\theta. \tag{2}$$

Since the reparameterization of the curve by $\mathbf{s} = \theta^{-1}(\mathbf{u})$ is not linear, both the Cartesian and the polar representation change. Figure 5 shows this result after reparameterization. This new parameterization has the advantage of being described by only the polar function as the phase is equal to the parameter.

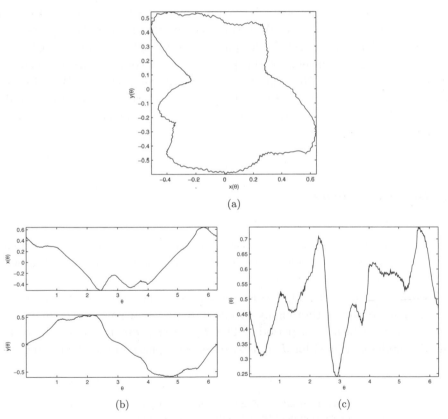

(a)

(b)

(c)

Fig. 5. (a) The contour in Fig. 4(a) reparameterized by its phase $\theta$. (b) New Cartesian functions. (c) New polar function.

We will define the *complex form* of contour $\mathbf{r}(\mathsf{s})$ as $Z_{\mathbf{r}}(\mathsf{s}) = x(\mathsf{s}) + iy(\mathsf{s}) = \rho(\mathsf{s})e^{i\theta(\mathsf{s})}$. This representation will allow us to define *affine transformations* very easily.

When the contour is closed, it is very convenient to work with a coordinate system whose origin is matched to the contour center $Z_c$ (determined either by means of the perimeter or the area method as explained in Sec. 2.2.5). Thus, contour $Z_{\mathbf{r}}(\mathsf{s})$ can be represented by pair $(Z_c, Z_{\mathbf{r}}^N(\mathsf{s}))$. $Z_c$ is the contour center, and $Z_{\mathbf{r}}^N(\mathsf{s})$ is the *normalized contour*, i.e. the contour defined for the coordinate system with origin at $Z_c$. Thus the center of the normalized contour $Z_{\mathbf{r}}^N(\mathsf{s})$ will always be point $(0,0)$, i.e. the origin of the new coordinate system. For determining the normalized contour we have $Z_{\mathbf{r}}^N(\mathsf{s}) = Z_{\mathbf{r}}(\mathsf{s}) - Z_c$.

For contours with monotonic phase the complex form of contour $\mathbf{r}(\theta)$ is $Z_{\mathbf{r}}(\theta) = x(\theta) + iy(\theta) = \rho(\theta)e^{i\theta}$. We can also define a normalized form $(Z_c, Z_{\mathbf{r}}^N(\theta))$ for the contour to represent contour $Z_{\mathbf{r}}(\theta)$. We have that $Z_{\mathbf{r}}^N(\theta) = Z_{\mathbf{r}}(\theta) - Z_c$. After doing that, a contour reparameterization is needed. This is due to the fact that $\psi(\theta) = \angle Z_{\mathbf{r}}^N(\theta) \neq \theta$, and this means that the new contour phase $\psi(\theta)$ is equal to the contour parameter (the old phase) $\theta$ is no longer true. In this case the function $\rho^N(\theta) = |Z_{\mathbf{r}}^N(\theta)|$ alone no longer represents the contour, but it would be necessary to consider the phase function $\psi(\theta)$ as well. With this transformation the polar representation, has increased from 1D to 2D. If the phase function $\psi(\theta)$ is monotonic[d] for $\theta$ in the $(-\pi, \pi)$ range the inverse of the phase function could be determined. If we denote the phase as $\mathsf{u} = \psi(\theta)$, the inverse function is $\theta = \psi^{-1}(\mathsf{u})$. By substituting that expression in contour $Z_{\mathbf{r}}^N(\theta)$, we have reparameterized the contour obtaining $Z_{\mathbf{r}}^N(\psi)$, and $\psi$ represents both the phase and the parameter of the translated contour.

## 2.2. *Discrete contours*

### 2.2.1. *Definition*

In this section we will focus on the discrete version of closed contours that hold the monotonic property. The reader is referred to all the examples presented in Sec. 2.1 concerning the contour in Fig. 5(a).

We will start by describing the discrete version of the monotonic phase defined in Sec. 2.1. This contour is thoroughly specified by the polar parametric function $\rho(\theta)$ for $\theta \in (-\pi, \pi)$, which is $2\pi$-periodic. The *discrete representation* for the contour[e] using $J$ samples is defined for $J$ equispaced phases (phase uniform sampling) in the

---

[d] This occurs whenever the translation of the coordinates origin has not moved that origin too much so as not to *see* all the points of the contour from that origin.
[e]The contour must be smooth enough so as not to have high frequency components that violate the Nyquist theorem.

$(-\pi, \pi)$ range. The $J$ angular positions are given by

$$\theta_j = \frac{(2j - J)\pi}{J} \tag{3}$$

for $1 \leq j \leq J$. Thus, the discrete components that represent that contour in Cartesian coordinates are $x(j) = x(\theta_j)$ and $y(j) = y(\theta_j)$, and in polar coordinates $\rho(j) = \rho(\theta_j)$ and $\theta(j) = \theta_j$. Here it is interesting to highlight that in polar coordinates as $\theta(j) = \theta_j$ are the same for all the contours sampled with $J$ components and given by Eq. (3), components $\rho(j) = \rho(\theta_j)$ uniquely define the contour. We will consequently focus on the polar representation, although for the sake of completeness, we will also include expressions given in Cartesian coordinates.

### 2.2.2. *Interpolation and uniform sampling*

We will address the problem of determining, or at least approximating, the value for that function $\rho(\theta)$ in the $\varphi_1 \leq \theta \leq \varphi_2$ range. We also assume that the value for that function is known at points $\rho_1 = \rho(\varphi_1)$ and $\rho_2 = \rho(\varphi_2)$. By using linear interpolation, we can approximate function $\rho(\theta)$ in the $\varphi_1 \leq \theta \leq \varphi_2$ range by means of the segment that joins points $(\varphi_1, \rho_1)$ and $(\varphi_2, \rho_2)$. That segment will be given by

$$\rho(\theta) \approx a_1\theta + a_0, \tag{4}$$

where $a_1$ and $a_0$ are the unknown parameters. We can write the following system of equations:

$$\begin{aligned} \varphi_1 a_1 + a_0 = \rho_1, \\ \varphi_2 a_1 + a_0 = \rho_2, \end{aligned} \tag{5}$$

the solution of which will give us the values for the unknown parameters. Using these values in Eq. (4) we can determine an approximation for $\rho(\theta)$ for any point in the $\varphi_1 \leq \theta \leq \varphi_2$ range.

The linear interpolation is not a good approximation in general whenever the size of the $\varphi_1 \leq \theta \leq \varphi_2$ range is not small. In this case more sophisticated methods can be applied.[7] One of these is the *cubic interpolation*. In this case the goal is the same: the value, or at least an approximation for it, for function $\rho(\theta)$ in the $\varphi_2 \leq \theta \leq \varphi_3$ range is sought. We suppose that the value for that function is known at points $\rho_2 = \rho(\varphi_2)$ and $\rho_3 = \rho(\varphi_3)$. In this case, for the problem to have a valid solution, the value of that function at two points outside the $\varphi_2 \leq \theta \leq \varphi_3$ range under search is also needed. We assume the value of this function at two other different points $\rho_1 = \rho(\varphi_1)$ and $\rho_4 = \rho(\varphi_4)$ for which $\varphi_1 < \varphi_2 < \varphi_3 < \varphi_4$. The points in the plane $(\varphi_1, \rho_1)$, $(\varphi_2, \rho_2)$, $(\varphi_3, \rho_3)$, and $(\varphi_4, \rho_4)$ will allow us to approximate function $\rho(\theta)$ in the $\varphi_2 \leq \theta \leq \varphi_3$ range by means of the polynomial equation

$$\rho(\theta) \approx a_3\theta^3 + a_2\theta^2 + a_1\theta + a_0, \tag{6}$$

where $a_3$, $a_2$, $a_1$ and $a_0$ are the unknown parameters. We can write the following system of equations:

$$\begin{aligned}
\varphi_1^3 a_3 + \varphi_1^2 a_2 + \varphi_1 a_1 + a_0 &= \rho_1, \\
\varphi_2^3 a_3 + \varphi_2^2 a_2 + \varphi_2 a_1 + a_0 &= \rho_2, \\
\varphi_3^3 a_3 + \varphi_3^2 a_2 + \varphi_3 a_1 + a_0 &= \rho_3, \\
\varphi_4^3 a_3 + \varphi_4^2 a_2 + \varphi_4 a_1 + a_0 &= \rho_4,
\end{aligned} \tag{7}$$

the solution of which will give us the value for the unknown parameters and thus the cubic representation for function $\rho(\theta)$ in the $\varphi_2 \leq \theta \leq \varphi_3$ range.

Let us assume that we know $M$ points $(\rho_1, \ldots, \rho_M)$ on contour $\rho(\theta)$ at phases $(\varphi_1, \ldots, \varphi_M)$. We also assume that these angular positions have been sorted so as to have $\varphi_m < \varphi_{m+1}$ and $-\pi \leq \varphi_m < \pi$. If no restrictions exist on phases $\varphi_m$, we would have a *non-uniform* sampling for contour $\rho(\theta)$. We are going to see how to obtain the discrete contour $\rho(j)$ with $J$ points for $1 \leq j \leq J$ that corresponds to sampling the continuous contour $\rho(\theta)$ by using *uniform samples* for the angular positions $\theta_j$ given by Eq. (3).

If we decide to use linear interpolation, for each $j$, value $m$ for which $\varphi_m < \theta_j < \varphi_{m+1}$ can be first determined. Then, we can write

$$\rho(j) \approx a_1\theta_j + a_0, \tag{8}$$

where $a_1$ and $a_0$ can be calculated by solving the linear system given by Eq. (5) using points $(\varphi_m, \rho_m)$ and $(\varphi_{m+1}, \rho_{m+1})$. As the contour is closed and the phases are $2\pi$-periodic special care should be taken at the end points of the contour.[f]

If we choose cubic interpolation, we can proceed similarly. For each $j$, value $m$ for which $\varphi_{m-1} < \varphi_m < \theta_j < \varphi_{m+1} < \varphi_{m+2}$ can be determined. Thus, we can write

$$\rho(j) \approx a_3\theta_j^3 + a_2\theta_j^2 + a_1\theta_j + a_0, \tag{9}$$

where $a_3$, $a_2$, $a_1$, and $a_0$ can be calculated by solving the linear system given by Eq. (7) using points $(\varphi_{m-1}, \rho_{m-1})$, $(\varphi_m, \rho_m)$, $(\varphi_{m+1}, \rho_{m+1})$, and $(\varphi_{m+2}, \rho_{m+2})$. Here similar care should be taken at the end points of the contour.[g]

---

[f] For the special case $\theta_j < \varphi_1$, points $(\varphi_M - 2\pi, \rho_M)$ and $(\varphi_1, \rho_1)$ can be used, and for the case $\theta_j > \varphi_M$, points $(\varphi_M, \rho_M)$ and $(\varphi_1 + 2\pi, \rho_1)$.

[g] When $\varphi_1 < \theta_j < \varphi_2$, we can use points $(\varphi_M - 2\pi, \rho_M)$, $(\varphi_1, \rho_1)$, $(\varphi_2, \rho_2)$, and $(\varphi_3, \rho_3)$; when $\theta_j < \varphi_1$, points $(\varphi_{M-1} - 2\pi, \rho_{M-1})$, $(\varphi_M - 2\pi, \rho_M)$, $(\varphi_1, \rho_1)$, and $(\varphi_2, \rho_2)$; when $\varphi_{M-1} < \theta_j < \varphi_M$, points $(\varphi_{M-2}, \rho_{M-2})$, $(\varphi_{M-1}, \rho_{M-1})$, $(\varphi_M, \rho_M)$, and $(\varphi_1 + 2\pi, \rho_1)$; and finally when $\varphi_M < \theta_j$, points $(\varphi_{M-1}, \rho_{M-1})$, $(\varphi_M, \rho_M)$, $(\varphi_1 + 2\pi, \rho_1)$, and $(\varphi_2 + 2\pi, \rho_2)$.

## 2.2.3. *Discrete derivatives*

In many cases we are interested in curves which are *smooth*.[30] The modulus of the curve derivative with respect to the parameter gives us a quantitative value of the curve smoothness. Common smoothness constraints are based on the first-order derivative, which is small whenever the curve varies slowly as we change parameter $\theta$, and the second-order derivative to penalize high curvature. In order to be able to derive metric properties of the curve, the curve needs to be expressed in Cartesian coordinates, i.e. $\mathbf{r}_c(\theta)$. We will derive the discrete counterpart of the continuous derivatives. We will address this problem by means of the *finite difference method*.

We can define the *angular increment* as

$$\Delta\theta = \theta_j - \theta_{j-1} = \frac{2\pi}{J}. \tag{10}$$

The first-order derivative in Cartesian coordinates using centered finite differences can be approximated by

$$\left.\frac{dx(\theta)}{d\theta}\right|_{\theta_j} \approx \frac{x(j+1) - x(j-1)}{2\Delta\theta}, \quad \left.\frac{dy(\theta)}{d\theta}\right|_{\theta_j} \approx \frac{y(j+1) - y(j-1)}{2\Delta\theta}, \tag{11}$$

where we have defined $x(0) = x(J)$ and $x(J+1) = x(1)$ for $x(j)$ and $y(0) = y(J)$ and $y(J+1) = y(1)$ for $y(j)$ in order to account for the periodicity of the closed contour. In polar coordinates we have

$$\left.\frac{d\rho(\theta)}{d\theta}\right|_{\theta_j} \approx \frac{\rho(j+1) - \rho(j-1)}{2\Delta\theta}, \tag{12}$$

where we have $\rho(0) = \rho(J)$ and $\rho(J+1) = \rho(1)$ for $\rho(j)$. Hence we can write in Cartesian coordinates

$$\left.\left|\frac{d}{d\theta}\mathbf{r}_c(\theta)\right|\right|_{\theta_j} \approx \frac{1}{2\Delta\theta}\sqrt{\left(x(j+1) - x(j-1)\right)^2 + \left(y(j+1) - y(j-1)\right)^2}, \tag{13}$$

and in polar coordinates

$$\left.\left|\frac{d}{d\theta}\mathbf{r}_c(\theta)\right|\right|_{\theta_j} \approx \frac{1}{2\Delta\theta}\sqrt{\left(\rho(j+1) - \rho(j-1)\right)^2 + \left(2\,\Delta\theta\,\rho(j)\right)^2}. \tag{14}$$

Figure 6 (top) shows the first-order derivative for the contour with the monotonic phase property in Fig. 5(a).

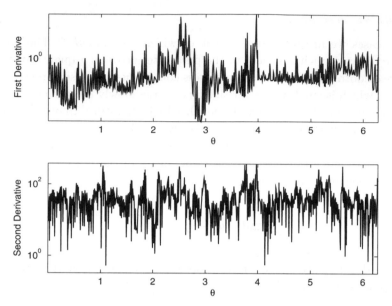

Fig. 6.   First- and second-order derivatives for the continuous closed contour in Fig. 5(a). Notice
how the lower envelope of the first-order derivative (top) follows the polar function in Fig. 5(c).

The second-order derivative in Cartesian coordinates using centered finite
differences can be written as

$$\frac{d^2x(\theta)}{d\theta^2}\bigg|_{\theta_j} \approx \frac{x(j+1)-2x(j)+x(j-1)}{(\Delta\theta)^2},$$

$$\frac{d^2y(\theta)}{d\theta^2}\bigg|_{\theta_j} \approx \frac{y(j+1)-2y(j)+y(j-1)}{(\Delta\theta)^2}, \tag{15}$$

and in polar coordinates

$$\frac{d^2\rho(\theta)}{d\theta^2}\bigg|_{\theta_j} \approx \frac{\rho(j+1)-2\rho(j)+\rho(j-1)}{(\Delta\theta)^2}. \tag{16}$$

We can write in Cartesian coordinates

$$\left|\frac{d^2}{d\theta^2}\mathbf{r}_c(\theta)\right|_{\theta_j} \approx \frac{1}{(\Delta\theta)^2}\sqrt{\Big(x(j+1)-2x(j)+x(j-1)\Big)^2+\Big(y(j+1)-2y(j)+y(j-1)\Big)^2}, \tag{17}$$

and in polar coordinates

$$\left|\frac{d^2}{d\theta^2}\mathbf{r}_c(\theta)\right|_{\theta_j} \approx \frac{1}{(\Delta\theta)^2}\sqrt{A^2(j)+B^2(j)+(\Delta\theta)^2\rho^2(j)-2\Delta\theta\rho(j)A(j)}, \tag{18}$$

where

$$A(j) = \rho(j+1)-2\rho(j)+\rho(j-1), \quad B(j) = \rho(j+1)-\rho(j-1). \tag{19}$$

Figure 6 (bottom) shows the second-order derivative for the contour with the monotonic phase property in Fig. 5(a).

From Eqs. (14) and (18) it is clear that the derivatives of the contour depend on the derivatives of $\rho(\theta)$ and on $\rho(\theta)$ itself. This means that for two equally smooth contours and one enclosing the other, the outermost takes on values of Eqs. (14) and (18) greater than that of the innermost. This is an undesirable effect if one is to measure smoothness. This is due to the fact that, on differentiating the contour in Cartesian coordinates, a metric is implicitly used. This problem can be solved using *angular derivatives* instead. Using the contour in polar coordinates $\mathbf{r}_p(\theta)$, the magnitude of the derivatives is approximately given by

$$\left| \frac{d}{d\theta} \mathbf{r}_p(\theta) \right|_{\theta_j} \approx \frac{1}{2\Delta\theta} \sqrt{\left( \rho(j+1) - \rho(j-1) \right)^2 + 4(\Delta\theta)^2},$$

$$\left| \frac{d^2}{d\theta^2} \mathbf{r}_p(\theta) \right|_{\theta_j} \approx \frac{\left| \rho(j+1) - 2\rho(j) + \rho(j-1) \right|}{(\Delta\theta)^2}. \tag{20}$$

These derivatives can only be used as smoothness constraints of the contour, but not when any kind of measure is involved. In Fig. 6 (top) the dependence of the lower envelop on $\rho(\theta)$ in Fig. 5(c) is clear. If we use the first-order angular derivative, we obtain Fig. 7 (top), which is better for contour regularization purposes.[19,30,39]

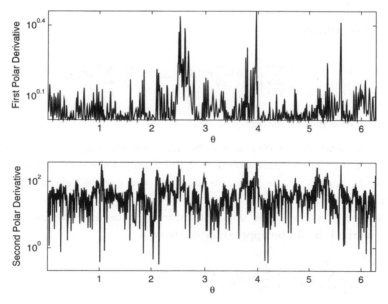

Fig. 7. First- and second-order *angular* derivatives for the continuous closed contour in Fig. 5(a). Notice now that there is no dependence of the first-order derivative on the polar function shown in Fig. 5(c).

### 2.2.4. *Perimeter and area*

Perimeter and area are defined from the contour in Cartesian coordinates $\mathbf{r}_c(\theta)$. These measures are defined for *closed curves* exclusively. The integration must be carried out in only one period of the curves. We will derive the discrete counterpart.

In Cartesian coordinates, the perimeter can be approximated by

$$P_\mathbf{r} \approx \sum_{j=1}^{J} \left| \frac{d}{d\theta} \mathbf{r}_c(\theta) \right|_{\theta_j} \Delta\theta \approx \frac{1}{2} \sum_{j=1}^{J} \sqrt{ \Big( x(j+1) - x(j-1) \Big)^2 + \Big( y(j+1) - y(j-1) \Big)^2 },$$

(21)

and in polar coordinates

$$P_\mathbf{r} \approx \sum_{j=1}^{J} \left| \frac{d}{d\theta} \mathbf{r}_c(\theta) \right|_{\theta_j} \Delta\theta \approx \frac{1}{2} \sum_{j=1}^{J} \sqrt{ \Big( \rho(j+1) - \rho(j-1) \Big)^2 + \Big( 2\Delta\theta\rho(j) \Big)^2 }. \quad (22)$$

In Cartesian coordinates, the area can be approximated by

$$A_\mathbf{r} \approx \frac{1}{2} \sum_{j=1}^{J} \left| \mathbf{r}_c(\theta) \frac{d}{d\theta} \mathbf{r}_c(\theta) \right|_{\theta_j} \Delta\theta$$

$$\approx \frac{1}{4} \sum_{j=1}^{J} \left\{ x(j) \Big( y(j+1) - y(j-1) \Big) - y(j) \Big( x(j+1) - x(j-1) \Big) \right\}, \quad (23)$$

and in polar coordinates

$$A_\mathbf{r} \approx \frac{1}{2} \sum_{j=1}^{J} \left| \mathbf{r}_c(\theta) \frac{d}{d\theta} \mathbf{r}_c(\theta) \right|_{\theta_j} \Delta\theta \approx \frac{\Delta\theta}{2} \sum_{j=1}^{J} \rho^2(j). \quad (24)$$

### 2.2.5. *Center and inertia matrix*

For the *center* and the *inertia matrix* we also use the curve given in Cartesian coordinates $\mathbf{r}_c(\theta)$. These attributes are defined only for closed curves. They are determined by means of the moments method and can be related either to the perimeter or to the area.[7]

The center is a *first-order moment*, and in Cartesian coordinates using the perimeter method, it can be approximated by

$$\mathbf{C}_\mathbf{r}^P \approx \frac{1}{P_\mathbf{r}} \sum_{j=1}^{J} \mathbf{r}_c(\theta_j) \left| \frac{d}{d\theta} \mathbf{r}_c(\theta) \right|_{\theta_j} \Delta\theta$$

$$\approx \frac{1}{2P_\mathbf{r}} \sum_{j=1}^{J} \binom{x(j)}{y(j)} \sqrt{ \Big( x(j+1) - x(j-1) \Big)^2 + \Big( y(j+1) - y(j-1) \Big)^2 }, \quad (25)$$

and in polar coordinates

$$\mathbf{C_r^P} \approx \frac{1}{P_r} \sum_{j=1}^{J} \mathbf{r}_c(\theta_j) \left| \frac{d}{d\theta} \mathbf{r}_c(\theta) \right|_{\theta_j} \Delta\theta$$

$$\approx \frac{1}{2P_r} \sum_{j=1}^{J} \rho(j) \begin{pmatrix} \cos\theta_j \\ \sin\theta_j \end{pmatrix} \sqrt{\left(\rho(j+1) - \rho(j-1)\right)^2 + \left(2\,\Delta\theta\,\rho(j)\right)^2}. \qquad (26)$$

In Cartesian coordinates, the center by means of the area method, can be approximated by

$$\mathbf{C_r^A} \approx \frac{1}{3A_r} \sum_{j=1}^{J} \mathbf{r}_c(\theta_j) \left| \mathbf{r}_c(\theta) \frac{d}{d\theta} \mathbf{r}_c(\theta) \right|_{\theta_j} \Delta\theta$$

$$\approx \frac{1}{6A_r} \sum_{j=1}^{J} \begin{pmatrix} x(j) \\ y(j) \end{pmatrix} \left\{ x(j)\left(y(j+1) - y(j-1)\right) - y(j)\left(x(j+1) - x(j-1)\right) \right\}, \qquad (27)$$

and in polar coordinates

$$\mathbf{C_r^A} \approx \frac{1}{3A_r} \sum_{j=1}^{J} \mathbf{r}_c(\theta_j) \left| \mathbf{r}_c(\theta) \frac{d}{d\theta} \mathbf{r}_c(\theta) \right|_{\theta_j} \Delta\theta \approx \frac{\Delta\theta}{3A_r} \sum_{j=1}^{J} \rho^3(j) \begin{pmatrix} \cos\theta_j \\ \sin\theta_j \end{pmatrix}. \qquad (28)$$

The inertia matrix is the array of the *second-order centered moments*. By means of the perimeter method, it can be approximated by

$$\mathbf{I_r^P} \approx \frac{1}{P_r} \sum_{j=1}^{J} \left(\mathbf{r}_c(\theta_j) - \mathbf{C_r^P}\right)\left(\mathbf{r}_c(\theta_j) - \mathbf{C_r^P}\right)^T \left| \frac{d}{d\theta} \mathbf{r}_c(\theta) \right|_{\theta_j} \Delta\theta$$

$$= \frac{1}{P_r} \sum_{j=1}^{J} \mathbf{r}_c(\theta_j)\mathbf{r}_c^T(\theta_j) \left| \frac{d}{d\theta} \mathbf{r}_c(\theta) \right|_{\theta_j} \Delta\theta - \begin{pmatrix} \left(Cx_r^P\right)^2 & Cx_r^P Cy_r^P \\ Cx_r^P Cy_r^P & \left(Cy_r^P\right)^2 \end{pmatrix}, \qquad (29)$$

where in Cartesian coordinates, we can obtain

$$\sum_{j=1}^{J} \mathbf{r}_c(\theta_j)\mathbf{r}_c^T(\theta_j) \left| \frac{d}{d\theta} \mathbf{r}_c(\theta) \right|_{\theta_j} \Delta\theta$$

$$\approx \frac{1}{2} \sum_{j=1}^{J} \begin{pmatrix} x^2(j) & x(j)y(j) \\ x(j)y(j) & y^2(j) \end{pmatrix} \sqrt{\left(x(j+1) - x(j-1)\right)^2 + \left(y(j+1) - y(j-1)\right)^2}$$

$$\qquad (30)$$

and in polar coordinates

$$\sum_{j=1}^{J} \mathbf{r}_c(\theta_j)\mathbf{r}_c^T(\theta_j) \left| \frac{d}{d\theta}\mathbf{r}_c(\theta) \right|_{\theta_j} \Delta\theta$$

$$\approx \frac{1}{2}\sum_{j=1}^{J} \rho^2(j) \begin{pmatrix} \cos^2\theta_j & \cos\theta_j\sin\theta_j \\ \cos\theta_j\sin\theta_j & \sin^2\theta_j \end{pmatrix} \sqrt{\Big(\rho(j+1)-\rho(j-1)\Big)^2 + \Big(2\Delta\theta\rho(j)\Big)^2}.$$

$$(31)$$

The inertia matrix by means of the area method can be approximated by

$$\mathbf{I}_{\mathbf{r}}^A \approx \frac{1}{3A_{\mathbf{r}}} \sum_{j=1}^{J} \Big(\mathbf{r}_c(\theta_j)-\mathbf{C}_{\mathbf{r}}^P\Big)\Big(\mathbf{r}_c(\theta_j)-\mathbf{C}_{\mathbf{r}}^P\Big)^T \left| \mathbf{r}_c(\theta)\frac{d}{d\theta}\mathbf{r}_c(\theta) \right|_{\theta_j} \Delta\theta$$

$$= \frac{1}{3A_{\mathbf{r}}} \sum_{j=1}^{J} \mathbf{r}_c(\theta_j)\mathbf{r}_c^T(\theta_j) \left| \mathbf{r}_c(\theta)\frac{d}{d\theta}\mathbf{r}_c(\theta) \right|_{\theta_j} \Delta\theta - \frac{4}{3} \begin{pmatrix} \big(Cx_{\mathbf{r}}^A\big)^2 & Cx_{\mathbf{r}}^A Cy_{\mathbf{r}}^A \\ Cx_{\mathbf{r}}^A Cy_{\mathbf{r}}^A & \big(Cy_{\mathbf{r}}^A\big)^2 \end{pmatrix}, \quad (32)$$

where in Cartesian coordinates, we can obtain

$$\sum_{j=1}^{J} \mathbf{r}_c(\theta_j)\mathbf{r}_c^T(\theta_j) \left| \mathbf{r}_c(\theta)\frac{d}{d\theta}\mathbf{r}_c(\theta) \right|_{\theta_j} \Delta\theta$$

$$\approx \frac{1}{2}\sum_{j=1}^{J} \begin{pmatrix} x^2(j) & x(j)y(j) \\ x(j)y(j) & y^2(j) \end{pmatrix} \{x(j)(y(j+1)-y(j-1))-y(j)(x(j+1)-x(j-1))\},$$

$$(33)$$

and in polar coordinates

$$\sum_{j=1}^{J} \mathbf{r}_c(\theta_j)\mathbf{r}_c^T(\theta_j) \left| \mathbf{r}_c(\theta)\frac{d}{d\theta}\mathbf{r}_c(\theta) \right|_{\theta_j} \Delta\theta$$

$$\approx \Delta\theta \sum_{j=1}^{J} \rho^4(j) \begin{pmatrix} \cos^2\theta(j) & \cos\theta(j)\sin\theta(j) \\ \cos\theta(j)\sin\theta(j) & \sin^2\theta(j) \end{pmatrix}. \quad (34)$$

Let $\lambda_1$ and $\lambda_2$ be the *eigenvalues* of the inertia matrix (either using the perimeter or the area methods) such that $\lambda_1 \geq \lambda_2$, and let $\mathbf{v}_1$ and $\mathbf{v}_2$ be the corresponding eigenvectors. The length of the major semiaxis of the curve is given by $d_1 = \sqrt{2\lambda_1}$ and the length of the minor semiaxis $d_2 = \sqrt{2\lambda_2}$, in the case of the perimeter method. For the area method, the corresponding minor and major semiaxes are given by $d_1 = \sqrt{3\lambda_1}$ and $d_2 = \sqrt{3\lambda_2}$, respectively. The steering of the major semiaxis is given by $\phi = \angle(v_{11} + iv_{12})$, where $\mathbf{v}_1 = (v_{11}, v_{12})^T$. Angle $\phi$ has an ambiguity of $\pi$ radians which can only be eliminated by using third-order moments. The steering of the minor semiaxis is given by $\mathbf{v}_2$ which is always orthogonal to $\mathbf{v}_1$.

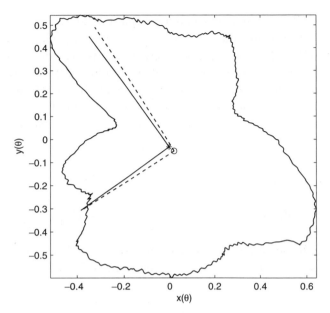

Fig. 8.　Center and semiaxes for the contour in Fig. 5(a) by means of the perimeter method (continuous line) and the area method (dashed line).

The corresponding angle given by that eigenvector suffers from the same ambiguity problem.

Figure 8 shows the center and the semiaxes for the contour in Fig. 5(a) using the perimeter method (continuous line) and the area method (dashed line). The center and the inertia matrix using the perimeter method are much influenced by the local variation of the contour due to noise, so the area method usually has higher accuracy and less variability in estimating both the center and the orientation and length of the contour axes.

## 2.2.6. *Affine transformations*

We will describe how affine transformations can be performed for discrete contours in the complex domain. We can start defining the complex form of contour $\mathbf{r}(j)$ as

$$Z_{\mathbf{r}}(j) = x(j) + iy(j) = \rho(j)e^{i\theta_j}, \tag{35}$$

where $x(j)$ and $y(j)$ are the Cartesian coordinates, and $\rho(j)$ is the polar coordinate of the contour.

The translation of the origin to point $Z_0$ is given by

$$Z_{\mathbf{r}}^1(j) = Z_{\mathbf{r}}(j) - Z_0. \tag{36}$$

This translation will lead us to a contour that does not have uniform samples in the angular coordinate. This is due to the fact that $\psi(j) = \angle Z_{\mathbf{r}}^1(j) \neq \theta_j$, and thus the phase of contour $\psi(j)$ is not equal to $\theta_j$ as defined in Sec. 2.2.1. In this case, function $\rho^1(j) = |Z_r^1(j)|$ is not enough to represent the new contour, as it will also be needed to take into account the phase function $\psi(j)$. The polar representation has increased from 1D to 2D. If this phase function $\psi(j)$ is *monotonic* (see Footnote d) for $1 \leq j \leq J$, by means of the method explained in Sec. 2.2.2 a new function $\rho_2(j)$ can be obtained for the uniform angular sites $\theta_j$ given by Eq. (3) by using linear or cubic interpolation using the polar data $\rho^1(j)$ and $\psi(j)$ for $1 \leq j \leq J$.

A scaling by a factor $r_1$ with respect to the origin gives rise to

$$Z_r^1(j) = r_1 Z_r(j). \tag{37}$$

A rotation $\varphi_1$ with respect to the origin is given by[h,i]

$$Z_r^1(j) = Z_r\left[((j + j_1 - 2))_J + 1\right] \quad \text{with } j_1 = \mathcal{E}_s\left[\frac{(\varphi_1 + \pi)J}{2\pi}\right]. \tag{38}$$

We can handle scaling and rotation simultaneously. If we define $Z_1 = r_1 e^{j\varphi_1}$, where $r_1$ is the scaling factor and $\varphi_1$ is the rotation, both with respect to the origin, then

$$Z_r^1(j) = |Z_1| Z_r\left[((j + j_1 - 2))_J + 1\right] = r_1 Z_r\left[((j + j_1 - 2))_J + 1\right], \tag{39}$$

with

$$j_1 = \mathcal{E}_s\left[\frac{(\angle Z_1 + \pi)J}{2\pi}\right] = \mathcal{E}_s\left[\frac{(\varphi_1 + \pi)J}{2\pi}\right]. \tag{40}$$

Finally, if the rotation and the scaling given by $Z_1$ are defined with respect to a point $Z_0$ different from the origin, we can write

$$Z_r^1(j) = |Z_1| Z_r\left[((j + j_1 - 2))_J + 1\right] + Z_0(1 - Z_1). \tag{41}$$

Hence, due to the translations, the contour has to be resampled to the uniform phases (whenever possible) as explained above. Figure 9 shows the result of the rotation and the scaling of the contour shown in Fig. 5(a) with respect to a point different from the origin.

We can also define the normalized form $(Z_c, Z_r^N(j))$ for the discrete contour, as defined in Sec. 2.1, to represent contour $Z_r(j)$, which yields

$$Z_r^N(j) = Z_r(j) - Z_c. \tag{42}$$

Here again resampling the contour will be needed using the uniform phases as stated above. In the discrete case, the center of that normalized and resampled contour $Z_r^N(j)$ in general will not be equal to $(0, 0)$ as it should. This is due to the fact that in the discrete case the determination of the center gives rise to an approximated result

---

[h] Operator $((\cdot))_J$ stands for an argument with modulus $J$. It wraps around $J$ to take into account the fact that the discrete contours are $J$-periodic.

[i] Operator $\mathcal{E}_s[\cdot]$ stands for the closest integer greater than or equal to the argument.

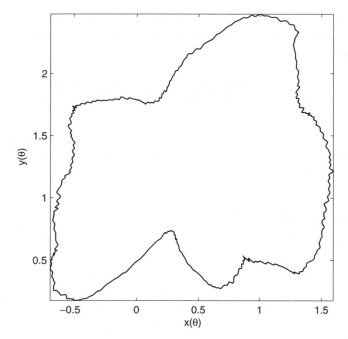

Fig. 9.   (a) Scaling by a factor of 2 and rotation of 90 degrees wrt point $(-0.4, 0.4)$ for the contour in Fig. 5(a).

and that the contour has been resampled (see Secs. 2.2.2 and 2.2.5). Nevertheless, the center of $Z_\mathbf{r}^N(j)$ will be closer to $(0,0)$ than center $Z_c$ will be for the original contour $Z_\mathbf{r}(j)$. If we *iteratively* repeat the normalization and resampling process, the final normalized contour $Z_\mathbf{r}^N(j)$ after a few iterations will be approximately $(0,0)$. The normalized representation will be given by that final normalized contour $Z_\mathbf{r}^N(j)$ with center $Z_c$ given by the accumulation of the resulting centers along the iterative process.

### 2.2.7. *Contour fitting*

The objective when matching contours is to find the *better fit* between two given closed contours by using the first- and second-order moments[j] defined in Sec. 2.2.5 and by using the complex affine transformations given in Sec. 2.2.6. We are interested in the better fit $(Z_{c3}, Z_3^N(j))$ for contour $(Z_{c1}, Z_1^N(j))$ onto contour $(Z_{c2}, Z_2^N(j))$. We can write

$$(Z_{c3}, Z_3^N(j)) = \left( Z_{c2}, \frac{a_2 Z_1^N \left[ ((j + j_2 - j_1 - 3))_J + 1 \right]}{a_1} \right), \tag{43}$$

---

[j]This will cause an ambiguity of $\pi$ radians in the fit, and third-order moments will be necessary to consider.

where $a_1$ and $a_2$ are the sizes of the major semiaxes of contours $Z_1^N(j)$ and $Z_2^N(j)$, respectively, determined by means of the inertia matrix method as explained in Sec. 2.2.5 and

$$j_1 = \mathcal{E}_s \left[ \frac{(\phi_1 + \pi)J}{2\pi} \right], \quad j_2 = \mathcal{E}_s \left[ \frac{(\phi_2 + \pi)J}{2\pi} \right], \tag{44}$$

where $\phi_1$ and $\phi_2$ are the steerings of the major semiaxes of contours $Z_1^N(j)$ and $Z_2^N(j)$ respectively, calculated by means of the same method.

## 2.3. *Contour homogenizations*

In many applications that use contours it is important for the discretization of the contour to be homogeneous in some sense. The segmentation methods that use contour regularization along the contour are based on the use of the first- and second-order derivatives which are sensitive to the contour discretization. An interesting approach following the AC ideas was first proposed by Friedland and Adam[19] — they proposed to use the polar coordinates under the monotonic phase constraint. In this case the optimization problem was posed as a stochastic approach using the simulated annealing algorithm.[21] These ideas have been further developed in Ref. 39 using a similar representation, which is based on the Bayesian theory and uses Markov Random Fields (MRFs) methods.[21] In this case, it is of paramount importance for the contour discretization to be homogeneous in the sense of constant arclength. Other statistical methods require to estimate the contour points from the content of an image.[40] In this case for the estimation to have similar properties, image data sizes must be homogeneous along the contour points. This means that the contribution to the total area of the contour by each point must be homogeneous. In the present section, we are going to introduce two iterative algorithms that resample the contour with uniform phase to obtain either constant-arclength or constant-area representations. As the phase will be distinct for each contour and for each method, the radial coordinate alone will no longer represent the contour. Both the radial and the angular coordinates will be needed in order to have the constant-arclength and the constant-area representations.

In a kidney contour defined by using uniform phases as given in Fig. 10(a), is the angular distance between adjacent points along the contour the magnitude that is uniform. However, that angle does not represent a metric property that leads one to properly define homogeneous smoothness constraints along the contour.[30] Fig. 10(a) shows that constraining the angular separation between adjacent points along the contour, the closer the points to the center, the more clustered and the farther the points, the more separated from each other. The contour representation by means of uniform phases is not adequate at all to represent a contour whenever a MRF in polar coordinates is involved, as proposed in Refs. 19 and 39.

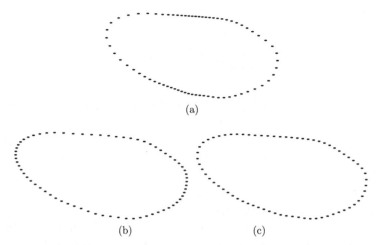

(a)

(b)                                    (c)

Fig. 10.    (a) Uniform phase representation for a kidney contour, (b) uniform area representation, and (c) constant arclength representation.

In Figs. 10(b) and 10(c) two different representations for a kidney contour are shown. In the former figure, the local contribution of each contour that points to the total area with respect to a given origin is uniform along the contour. In this case, the point distribution is more uniform, as it can be seen in the figure, though the points tend to cluster far from the center and to spread out close to the center. This effect is, in some sense, opposite to the one in Fig. 10(a) for uniform phases. This is due to the fact that the farther the points from the center, the more contribution to the area they have. This representation will be useful whenever for the determination of the contour points, the use of estimators that use data taken from the underlying image is required.[40] In this case, it is important to maintain the sample sizes for the estimators uniform along the contour, which means uniform area contributions. Finally, in Fig. 10(c), a third representation is shown. In this case, the arclength between any adjacent points is constrained to be uniform along the contour. Visually, the uniformity is better, as the human visual system employs the arclength as the metric, instead of angles or areas. That will be the optimum representation whenever a smoothing technique is applied by means of derivatives using polar coordinates as in the MRF approach presented in Ref. 39.

Equation (22) allows us to determine the perimeter (the total arclength) of the contour when the phases are uniform. If we modify the representation to be of constant arclength, the phases are no longer uniform, so we need to generalize the above-mentioned equation as

$$P_{\mathbf{r}} \approx \frac{1}{2} \sum_{j=1}^{J} \sqrt{\Big(\rho(j+1) - \rho(j-1)\Big)^2 + \Big[2\Big(\theta(j+1) - \theta(j)\Big)\rho(j)\Big]^2}, \qquad (45)$$

with $\rho(j)$ being the radial amplitudes, and $\theta(j)$ the contour phases for $j = 1, \ldots, J$. The same problem happens for the area that was given by Eq. (24) which can be rewritten as

$$A_{\mathbf{r}} \approx \frac{1}{2} \sum_{j=1}^{J} \rho^2(j) \Big[ \theta(j+1) - \theta(j) \Big].$$ (46)

In order to achieve the uniform area contributions given by each contour point, Algorithm 1 (see below) has been implemented. This algorithm usually converges in few iterations (less than 10). The goal here is to angularly reparameterize the contour by means of cubic interpolation in a way that the area contribution at each point is constant. The stopping criterion to finalize the algorithm is given by the variance calculated from the area contributions. Initially the variance decreases reaching a minimum and afterwards increases again. The algorithm detects this minimum in the variance to stop the iterations. If the contour in Fig. 10(a) is the input to Algorithm 1, the resulting output is the one given in Fig. 10(b). This contour can be converted back to uniform phases very easily using the uniform phases given by Eq. (3) by means of interpolation.

Algorithm 2 (see below) implements a method to obtain uniform arclengths along the contour. Remarks similar to those stated for the area method apply here too. If the contour in Fig. 10(a) is the input to Algorithm 2, then the resulting output is the one given in Fig. 10(c). This contour can be converted back to uniform phases using the uniform phases given by Eq. (3). The constant arclength representation can be converted to uniform area representation in two steps: first, the contour is converted to uniform phases using Eq. (3), and second, the contour is converted to uniform area representation using Algorithm 1. Similarly, a uniform area representation contour can be converted to a constant arclength representation contour using Eq. (3) followed by the application of Algorithm 2.

In order to avoid oscillations in the variances used as a termination criterion, it is sometimes required for the contour to be smooth and noise free. If that is not the case a periodic smoothing should be applied to $\boldsymbol{\rho} = (\rho_1, \rho_2, \ldots, \rho_J)$ prior to the execution of the proposed algorithms.

**Algorithm 1.** We begin with contour $\boldsymbol{\rho} = (\rho_1, \rho_2, \ldots, \rho_J)$ with uniform phases $\boldsymbol{\theta} = (\theta_1, \theta_2, \ldots, \theta_J)$. We proceed as follows:

(1)  Set the iteration counter to $n = 1$.
(2)  Set $\rho_j(1) = \rho_j$ and $\theta_j(1) = \theta_j$ for $1 \le j \le J$.
(3)  Build the augmented phase vector $\boldsymbol{\psi}(n) = \Big( \boldsymbol{\theta}(n), \theta_1(n) + 2\pi \Big)$, with $J + 1$ components.
(4)  Calculate the first difference vector $\boldsymbol{d\psi}(n) = \Big( d\psi_1(n), \ldots, d\psi_J(n) \Big)$ for the phase vector $\boldsymbol{\psi}(n)$ as

$$d\psi_j(n) = \psi_{j+1}(n) - \psi_j(n) \quad \text{for } 1 \le j \le J.$$

(5) Determine the area contributions $\mathbf{A}(n) = (A_1(n), A_2(n), \ldots, A_J(n))$ for the contour as

$$A_j(n) = \frac{1}{2}\rho_j^2(n)d\psi_j(n) \quad \text{for } 1 \leq j \leq J.$$

(6) Compute variance $\sigma_A^2(n)$ of the area contributions $\mathbf{A}(n)$ as

$$\sigma_A^2(n) = \frac{1}{J-1}\sum_{j=1}^{J}\left(A_j(n) - \frac{1}{J}\sum_{j=1}^{J}A_j(n)\right)^2.$$

(7) If $n$ is not equal to 1 and $\sigma_A^2(n) > \sigma_A^2(n-1)$, terminate the iterations.
(8) Determine the nonuniform cumulative area contributions $\mathbf{B}(n) = (B_1(n), B_2(n), \ldots, B_J(n))$ by means of

$$B_j(n) = \sum_{k=1}^{j}A_k(n) \quad \text{for } 1 \leq j \leq J.$$

(9) Determine the uniform cumulative area contributions $\mathbf{C}(n) = \left(C_1(n), C_2(n), \ldots, C_J(n)\right)$ by means of

$$C_j(n) = \frac{jB_J(n)}{J}$$

for $1 \leq j \leq J$, where $B_J(n)$ is the total area.
(10) Given the phase vector $\boldsymbol{\theta}(n)$ for the nonuniform cumulative area contributions $\mathbf{B}(n)$, compute the new phase vector $\boldsymbol{\theta}(n+1)$ for the uniform cumulative area contributions $\mathbf{C}(n)$ by means of cubic interpolation.
(11) Given the contour vector $\boldsymbol{\rho}(n)$ for the phase vector $\boldsymbol{\theta}(n)$, determine the new contour vector $\boldsymbol{\rho}(n+1)$ for the new phase vector $\boldsymbol{\theta}(n+1)$ by means of cubic interpolation.
(12) Set $n = n+1$ and go to step (3).

When the algorithm terminates, contour $\boldsymbol{\rho}(n-1)$ with phases $\boldsymbol{\theta}(n-1)$ has similar area contributions with minimum variance.

**Algorithm 2.** We begin with contour $\boldsymbol{\rho} = (\rho_1, \rho_2, \ldots, \rho_J)$ with uniform phases $\boldsymbol{\theta} = (\theta_1, \theta_2, \ldots, \theta_J)$. We proceed as follows:

(1) Set the iteration counter to $n = 1$.
(2) Set $\rho_j(1) = \rho_j$ and $\theta_j(1) = \theta_j$ for $1 \leq j \leq J$.
(3) Build the augmented phase vector $\psi(n) = \left(\boldsymbol{\theta}(n), \theta_1(n) + 2\pi\right)$, with $J+1$ components.

(4)  Calculate the first difference vector $d\boldsymbol{\psi}(n) = \Big(d\psi_1(n), \ldots, d\psi_J(n)\Big)$ for the phase vector $\boldsymbol{\psi}(n)$ as

$$d\psi_j(n) = \psi_{j+1}(n) - \psi_j(n) \quad \text{for } 1 \le j \le J.$$

(5)  Build the augmented radial vector $\boldsymbol{r}(n) = \Big(\rho_J(n), \boldsymbol{\rho}(n), \rho_1(n)\Big)$, with $J + 2$ components.

(6)  Calculate the first centered difference vector $d\boldsymbol{\rho}(n) = \Big(d\rho_1(n), \ldots, d\rho_J(n)\Big)$ for the radial vector $\boldsymbol{r}(n)$ as

$$d\rho_j(n) = r_{j+2}(n) - r_j(n) \quad \text{for } 1 \le j \le J.$$

(7)  Determine arclengths $\mathbf{A}(n) = \Big(A_1(n), A_2(n), \ldots, A_J(n)\Big)$ for the contour as

$$A_j(n) = \frac{1}{2}\sqrt{d\rho_j^2(n) + 4d\psi_j^2(n)\rho_j^2(n)} \quad \text{for } 1 \le j \le J$$

(8)  Compute variance $\sigma_A^2(n)$ for arclengths $\mathbf{A}(n)$ as

$$\sigma_A^2(n) = \frac{1}{J-1}\sum_{j=1}^{J}\left(A_j(n) - \frac{1}{J}\sum_{j=1}^{J}A_j(n)\right)^2.$$

(9)  If $n$ is not equal to 1 and $\sigma_A^2(n) > \sigma_A^2(n-1)$, terminate the iterations.

(10)  Determine the nonuniform cumulative arclengths $\mathbf{B}(n) = \Big(B_1(n), B_2(n), \ldots, B_J(n)\Big)$ by means of

$$B_j(n) = \sum_{k=1}^{j} A_k(n) \quad \text{for } 1 \le j \le J$$

(11)  Determine the uniform cumulative arclengths $\mathbf{C}(n) = \Big(C_1(n), C_2(n), \ldots, C_J(n)\Big)$ by means of

$$C_j(n) = \frac{jB_J(n)}{J}$$

for $1 \le j \le J$, where $B_J(n)$ is the total arclength.

(12)  Given the phase vector $\boldsymbol{\theta}(n)$ for the nonuniform cumulative arclengths $\mathbf{B}(n)$, compute the new phase vector $\boldsymbol{\theta}(n+1)$ for the uniform cumulative arclengths $\mathbf{C}(n)$ by means of cubic interpolation.

(13)  Given the contour vector $\boldsymbol{\rho}(n)$ for the phase vector $\boldsymbol{\theta}(n)$, determine the new contour vector $\boldsymbol{\rho}(n+1)$ for the new phase vector $\boldsymbol{\theta}(n+1)$ by means of cubic interpolation.

(14)  Set $n = n+1$ and go to step (3).

When the algorithm terminates, contour $\rho(n-1)$ with phases $\theta(n-1)$ has similar arclengths with minimum variance.

## 2.4. *Manual template adjustment*

### 2.4.1. *Procedure description*

In some applications a template needs to be manually adjusted to an object present in an underlying image. We will describe how to perform this task with the minimal user interaction and less complexity. Such a procedure will be needed to initialize methods to segment the kidney out of an US image sequence as described in Sec. 3 and 4. This adjustment can be performed with only two mouse clicks.

We will use the complex representation for the contour using the axial polar coordinate, assuming that the contour is closed and satisfies the monotonic phase property. We will use complex transformations to automatically scale and rotate the template using the two mouse inputs. This will be an illustrative and simple procedure which will show how to use some of the equations presented in the previous sections to help ease the affine transformations that otherwise will be rather involved. The template contour is first superimposed onto the image at a normalized size and position-centered with respect to the image boundaries. Then, the user must click both the left and right buttons at the estimated object axis ends, respectively, over the image. The contour template has two control points labeled as cross and circle that can be controlled, respectively, with the left and right mouse clicks as explained below. This procedure can be seen in Fig. 11 for a US kidney image.

We denote the normalized template with the radial vector $\rho^t = (\rho_1^t, \rho_2^t, \ldots, \rho_J^t)$, with $J$ components. This template is given for the uniform phase vector $\theta^t$ whose elements follow Eq. (3). The template is also normalized so as to have zero first-order moments using the area method as explained at the end of Sec. 2.2.6.

Figure 11(a) shows the contour template superimposed onto the image. The template is centered and located at a normalized position. The template has two control points — these control points correspond to the major axis ends of the template.

The cross control point can be controlled by the left button of the mouse and the circle by the right button. Thus, looking at the US image the user has to visually estimate the major axis of the kidney and put the mouse cursor over one of the axis ends and click with the corresponding mouse button. At this moment the template automatically scales and rotates so as to have the corresponding control point moved to the current cursor position, leaving the other control point unaltered. Proceeding similarly with the other control point, the final result is that the template has been adjusted to the kidney contour with only two mouse clicks. Figure 11(b) shows the result after clicking the left button of the mouse. The cross control point in the template has moved to that position, without affecting the position of the circle

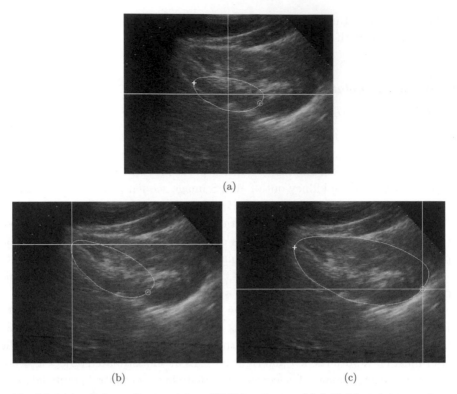

(a)

(b)                                      (c)

Fig. 11.   Manual template adjustment in a US kidney image. (a) Initial template superimposed
onto the US image. (b) Result after left-clicking the mouse. (c) Final result after right-clicking.

control point, forcing the template to scale and rotate correspondingly. Figure 11(c)
shows the result after clicking the right button of the mouse. In this case the
right button forces the circle control point to move to the mouse cursor position
without changing the position of the cross control point. The template automatically
scales and rotates. That completes the adjustment procedure achieving the fitting
in Fig. 11(c).

### 2.4.2. *Technical details about the rotations*

Given template $\rho^t$, in order to sketch the control points — the cross and the circle —
it will be necessary to determine the angular position for the major axis of the
template. In order to do that, the inertia matrix can be determined by means of the
centered second-order moments using the area method. As template $\rho^t$ has been
previously normalized (the template is centered), its first-order moments are zero; so
the inertia matrix can be directly computed by using the noncentered second-order
moments. We denote by $\lambda_1$ and $\lambda_2$ the eigenvalues of the inertia matrix. These
values can be easily computed as the roots of the characteristic function of the

matrix. The matrix is always positive definite,[k] so the eigenvalues are always real and positive. Let us assume that $\lambda_1 > \lambda_2$. Then, we can determine the eigenvectors. Let $\mathbf{v} = (v_1, v_2)$ be the eigenvector associated with the greater eigenvalue $\lambda_1$. If we call $\phi$ the major axis angle, it will be given by

$$\phi = \angle(v_1 + iv_2), \tag{47}$$

where $-\pi < \phi \le \pi$. As we have not used third- order moments, we have a $\pi$ radians uncertainty for the proper determination of $\phi$. In order to avoid that problem we can constrain the $\phi$ value to the $(-\pi/2, \pi/2)$ range: if $\phi \le -\pi/2$ we add $\pi$ to $\phi$, and if $\phi > \pi/2$ we subtract $\pi$ from $\phi$.

Once we know the angular position (in the right-sided semiplane) for the template major axis, we can determine index $j_o$ corresponding to the circle-shaped control point as (see Footnote i)

$$j_o = \mathcal{E}_s \left[ \frac{(\phi + \pi)J}{2\pi} \right]. \tag{48}$$

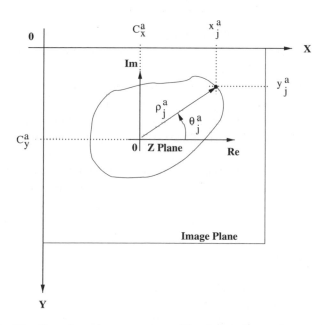

Fig. 12.   Complex reference system with origin in the contour center.

[k]Except in the degenerate case for which the contour becomes a line segment. In this case the inertia matrix is positive semidefinite.

If $j_o$ results to zero, we set $j_o = J$. For index $j_+$ corresponding to the cross-shaped control point we can write (see Footnote h)

$$j_+ = \left( \left( j_o + \mathcal{E}_s \left[ \frac{J}{2} \right] \right) \right)_J. \tag{49}$$

If $j_+$ results to zero, we set $j_+ = J$.

After the adjustment procedure the solution will be given by the new template center, denoted by $(C_x^a, C_y^a)$ (in the image coordinate system shown in Fig. 12) and by the adjusted (affinely transformed) template, denoted by the radial vector $\rho^a = (\rho_1^a, \ldots, \rho_J^a)$ (in the complex coordinate systems shown in Fig. 12 with origin in the contour center). As the operations that will be performed on the template vector $\rho^t$ to obtain $\rho^a$ are scalings and rotations (the translations will be done modifying the center $(C_x^a, C_y^a)$ value), the radial vector $\rho^a$ will remain normalized (its first-order moments by using the area method are zero) and will have uniform phases $\theta^a = (\theta_1^a, \ldots, \theta_J^a)$ given by Eq. (3). We have that $\theta^a = \theta^t$.

Initially, the template is placed at the US image center, i.e. we set $C_x^a = N/2$ and $C_y^a = M/2$, where $M \times N$ are the image dimensions in pixels. The initial value of the radial vector $\rho^a$ is set as

$$\rho^a = \frac{\min(M,N)\rho^t}{4\max(\rho_{j_o}, \rho_{j_+})}, \tag{50}$$

that is, we set the length of the major semiaxis to be equal to one fourth the minimum between image dimensions. An example for the initial adjustment $(C_x^a, C_y^a)$ and $\rho^a$ is shown in Fig. 11(a).

By clicking the mouse the initial template can be adjusted to the image contour. The left button controls the cross-shaped control point by means of Algorithm 3 (see below). The right button controls the circle-shaped control point by means of Algorithm 4 (see below). Figure 11 illustrates the whole procedure.

**Algorithm 3.** We begin with the current adjustment given by $(C_x^a, C_y^a)$, $\rho^a$, and $\theta^a$. $j_+$ and $j_o$ are the indices for the current control points. We assume that the user has clicked the left button on the cursor position $(P_x, P_y)$ (referred to the image coordinate system shown in Fig. 12). Figure 13 shows the complex coordinate system and the complex phasors used.

Do the following:

(1) Set $Z_1 = C_x^a + iC_y^a$ and $Z_2 = \rho_{j_o}^a \exp(-i\theta_{j_o}^a)$.
(2) Set $Z_3 = \rho_{j_+}^a \exp(-i\theta_{j_+}^a) - Z_2$ and $Z_4 = P_x + iP_y$.
(3) Set $\mathbf{Z}_5 = \rho^a \exp(-i\theta^a)$, $\mathbf{Z}_6 = \mathbf{Z}_5 - Z_2\mathbf{1}$, and $Z_7 = Z_4 - Z_2 - Z_1$.[1]
(4) The transformation (scaling and rotation) phasor is given by the expression $Z_8 = Z_7/Z_3$.

---

[1] $\mathbf{1} = (1, 1, \ldots, 1)$ with $J$ elements.

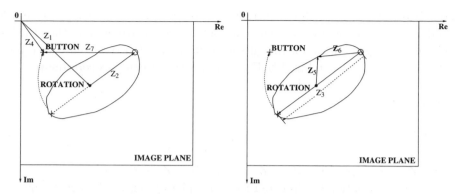

Fig. 13.   Coordinates system and phasors used in Algorithm 3.

(5)   The new center wrt the circle-shaped control point is given by $Z_C = -Z_2 Z_8$.
(6)   The new radial vector wrt the circle-shaped control point is given by $\mathbf{Z}_a = \mathbf{Z}_6 \mathbf{Z}_8$.
(7)   The new center wrt the image coordinate system shown in Fig. 12 is now $C_x^a = \mathsf{Re}\{Z_C + Z_1 + Z_2\}$ and $C_y^a = \mathsf{Im}\{Z_C + Z_1 + Z_2\}$.
(8)   The new radial vector wrt the complex coordinate systems with origin in the contour center shown in Fig. 12 is now $\rho^a = |\mathbf{Z}_a - Z_C \mathbf{1}|$.
(9)   In general $\angle\left[(\mathbf{Z}_a - Z_C \mathbf{1})^*\right] \neq \boldsymbol{\theta}^a$, and we need to shift $\rho^a$ in order to have the proper phase. We proceed as follows[m]:

(a)   Determine index $j_u$ for the new cross-shaped control point as[n]

$$j_u = \mathcal{E}_s \left[ \frac{\left\{ \angle\left[(Z_{j_+,a} - Z_C)^*\right] + \pi \right\} J}{2\pi} \right].$$

   If $j_u$ is zero, set $j_u = J$.
(b)   Determine the shifting index $j_d = ((j_u - j_+))_J$.
(c)   Set $j_+ = j_u$ and

$$j_o = \left( \left( j_+ + \mathcal{E}_s \left[ \frac{J}{2} \right] \right) \right)_J.$$

   If $j_o$ is zero, set $j_o = J$.
(d)   If $j_d$ is not zero, define the new radial vector $\rho^a$ as

$$\rho^a = (\rho_{J-j_d+1}^a, \ldots, \rho_J^a, \rho_1^a, \ldots, \rho_{J-j_d}^a).$$

---

[m]Operator $*$ stands for complex conjugation.
[n]$Z_{j,a}$ stands for the $j$-element of the complex vector $\mathbf{Z}_a$.

**Algorithm 4.** We begin with the current adjustment given by $(C_x^a, C_y^a)$, $\rho^a$ and $\boldsymbol{\theta}^a$. $j_+$, and $j_o$ are the indices for the current control points. We assume that the user has clicked the right button on the cursor position $(P_x, P_y)$ (referred to the image coordinate system shown in Fig. 12). Figure 14 shows the complex coordinate system and the complex phasors used.

Do the following:

(1)   Set $Z_1 = C_x^a + iC_y^a$ and $Z_2 = \rho_{j_+}^a \exp(-i\theta_{j_+}^a)$.

(2)   Set $Z_3 = \rho_{j_o}^a \exp(-i\theta_{j_o}^a) - Z_2$ and $Z_4 = P_x + iP_y$.

(3)   Set $\mathbf{Z}_5 = \rho^a \exp(-i\boldsymbol{\theta}^a)$, $\mathbf{Z}_6 = \mathbf{Z}_5 - Z_2\mathbf{1}$, $Z_7 = Z_4 - Z_2 - Z_1$.

(4)   The transformation (scaling and rotation) phasor is given by expression $Z_8 = Z_7/Z_3$.

(5)   The new center wrt the cross-shaped control point is given by $Z_C = -Z_2 Z_8$.

(6)   The new radial vector wrt the cross-shaped control point is given by $\mathbf{Z}_a = \mathbf{Z}_6 Z_8$.

(7)   The new center wrt the image coordinate system shown in Fig. 12 is now $C_x^a = \mathsf{Re}\{Z_C + Z_1 + Z_2\}$ and $C_y^a = \mathsf{Im}\{Z_C + Z_1 + Z_2\}$.

(8)   The new radial vector wrt the complex coordinate systems with origin in the contour center shown in Fig. 12 is now $\rho^a = |\mathbf{Z}_a - Z_C\mathbf{1}|$.

(9)   In general $\angle\left[(\mathbf{Z}_a - Z_C\mathbf{1})^*\right] \neq \boldsymbol{\theta}^a$, and we need to shift $\rho^a$ in order to have the proper phase. We proceed as follows:

    (a)   Determine index $j_u$ for the new circle-shaped control point as

$$j_u = \mathcal{E}_s\left[\frac{\left\{\angle\left[(Z_{j_o,a} - Z_C)^*\right] + \pi\right\}J}{2\pi}\right].$$

       If $j_u$ is zero, set $j_u = J$.

    (b)   Determine the shifting index $j_d = ((j_u - j_o))_J$.

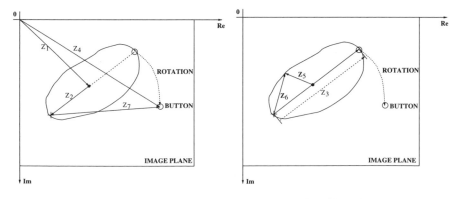

Fig. 14.   Coordinates system and phasors used in Algorithm 4.

(c)   Set $j_o = j_u$ and

$$j_+ = \left(\left(j_o + \mathcal{E}_s \left[\frac{J}{2}\right]\right)\right)_J.$$

If $j_+$ is zero, set $j_+ = J$.

(d)   If $j_d$ is not zero, define the new radial vector $\rho^a$ as

$$\rho^a = (\rho^a_{J-j_d+1}, \dots, \rho^a_J, \rho^a_1, \dots, \rho^a_{J-j_d}).$$

## 2.5. *Discussion*

We have extended the concept of polar representations for closed curves and discussed its implications for the estimation of metric attributes of the curve. We have focused on derivatives for contour regularization and attributes for shape analysis such as the perimeter and the area. Our results show that the area method outperforms the perimeter method in determining measurements such as the centroid and the orientation of the curve. In addition, a new complex representation for contours has been introduced and applied to affine transformations. This representation is very convenient to deal with transformations in the complex domain. Finally, a brief analysis of rigid contour fitting has been introduced. Our results on this issue have also disclosed that the area method is less sensitive to the noise present in the contour.

Discrete contours have been derived by means of the finite difference method for those contours for which the monotonic phase property holds. A brief introduction concerning contour interpolation and sampling has been presented for the sake of completeness. Contour wrapping and contour reparameterization have also been described. The former is necessary whenever rotation is involved, and the later is necessary whenever translation is involved. The scaling seemed to be the easiest affine transformation. The normalized representation served as a means of preserving, in most cases, the monotonic phase property by constraining to 1D any 2D shape analysis problem.

Contour homogenizations and manual template adjustment were presented in a detailed manner for US kidney images. For the former, three different contour representations have been compared: uniform phases, uniform area representation, and constant arclength. The constant arclength representation, although takes the problem back to a 2D domain due to the fact that the phases are not uniformly sampled, seemed to be the most homogeneous representation for 2D contours in the Euclidean sense and should be used whenever any metric is involved. This would be the case for contour regularization that has been considered in the literature during the last two decades. In this case the perimeter method is the one used, but having in mind the great sensitivity the perimeter has wrt noise, presmoothing is clearly encouraged.

Manual template adjustment deals with how to manually adjust a template to an underlying US kidney image with only two mouse clicks. The complex representation for the contour using the normalized representation is exploited throughout. All the details have been exhaustively presented disclosing the appropriateness of using both sorts of representations.

## 3. Solution Based on Shape Priors

An interesting methodology for kidney segmentation in US images has been recently proposed by Xie et al.[54] We will carry out a description of this procedure in order to highlight differences wrt ours (which will be described in the following section) as well as to let the reader know our perception of the pros and cons of this method.

This method is based on the following basic idea: for a correct segmentation, two pieces of information must be used, namely prior information about the shape of the object to be segmented and the image information surrounding the object sought. This, as it is well known, constitutes the base for the Bayesian processing philosophy as well. However, how this is exactly implemented in Ref. 54 departs from Bayesian ideas and goes through an entirely deterministic path.

We now explore the two modeling assumptions upon which the method is built.

### 3.1. *Shape modeling*

As for the first piece of information, the shape of the object, the authors propose a methodology that is closely related to the well-known Active Shape Model paradigm described in Ref. 13. The authors, completely aware of this work, indicate that they are following other more recent contributions.[35, 50] The method is basically as follows: the authors begin with a number of training images (say $B$ images, following their notation) known to contain similar shapes as the one of the object pursued. They perform some sort of segmentation of the object (either manual or automatic, which is irrelevant at this point) and they carry out a distance transform on the segmentation, i.e. a value 0 is given to the points on the contour and, for image points out of the contour, the (signed) distance of that point to the contour is given as the value function at this location. It is interesting to highlight that the objects in this set of $B$ training images are first registered so as to have a number of $B$ segmented objects that roughly overlap.

Once this is obtained, both the *mean shape*, say $\overline{\Phi}$, and the number (say $M$) of its associated eigenshapes $\Phi_m$ ($m = 1, \ldots, M$) are used to approximate the object to be segmented by means of

$$\Phi \approx \overline{\Phi} + \sum_{i=1}^{M} w_m \Phi_m. \tag{51}$$

It should be stressed that the approximated shape is, in the original reference, expressed in different coordinates — say $(x, y)$ — than both the mean shape and the eigenshapes (which are expressed in coordinates $(u, v)$). The function that converts one space into the other is a combination of rotation, scaling, and shift. Let this function be referred to as $T$. Therefore, the approximated shape should be actually written as $\Phi[W, T]$, where $W$ gathers the set of coefficients $w_m$ $(m = 1, \ldots, M)$ indicated in Eq. (51) and $T$ is the function just described. Notice that these two entities, $W$ and $T$, are the *free parameters* that the designer may tune in order to let the shape model in Eq. (51) match the object sought.°

## 3.2. *Image information*

The second piece of information consists of the model of the image pattern expected. The authors define a texture pattern that is sensitive to the contour position. To be specific, for each contour point the authors draw the tangent line to the contour at that point — this line divides the image plane into two halves, namely the *upper* half plane and the *lower* half plane. The information in these two planes will be dealt with independently of each other. The authors claim that this strategy (which is called a two-sided convolution for reasons that soon will be clear) circumvents some problems found elsewhere.[32]

Once these two planes are defined, two texture feature vectors are obtained for each contour point (one for each half plane). These feature vectors are the outputs of a number of Gabor filters, with some predefined orientations and spatial frequencies. The resulting number of components is 24, from eight orientations and three frequencies.[32]

The feature vectors are assumed to be a sample from a multivariate Gaussian mixture with a predefined number of distributions in the mixture (the authors claim that $K = 3$ Gaussians have drawn good results). The parameters of the mixture (i.e. the mixing weights as well as the mean vector and the covariance matrix of each of the K Gaussians) are obtained by well-known training procedures (the Expectation Maximization (EM) algorithm[15]) using a number of training images.

Once the model is trained, i.e. the mixture parameters are identified, the degree of membership of a certain feature vector to the population is determined by evaluating the probability density function at the position of this feature vector.

Finally, and in order to make things manageable, the number of orientations of the tangent lines to each image contour is discretized to six allowable values. Therefore, for each contour point, the orientation considered for its associated

---

°For brevity we are using letter $T$ both as a function and as the set of parameters that control the function. Needless to say, such a function is a matrix operation in homogeneous coordinates, and the parameters involved define the degree of scaling, rotation, and shift that the operation will carry out.

tangent line (as for finding the appropriate Gaussian mixture model to use) is the closest value, within the six values considered, to the real orientation.

### 3.3. *The algorithm*

The purpose is to tune the model indicated in Eq. (51), i.e. to find the optimum value of parameters $W$ and $T$ there defined, so as to make the perfect match between the feature vectors obtained for each tentative contour position and the mixture model described in Sec. 3.2. The term *perfect match* is quantified by the authors as an energy function which favors a *high average texture similarity* considering the feature vector calculated within the *inside* (wrt the contour) half plane, as well as high differences between texture variance similarities between regions inside and outside the contour.

To that end parameters $W$ and $T$ are iteratively adjusted by means of a gradient descent algorithm, and for the new tentative contour (say, contour at step $k$ in the optimization process) the feature vectors are recalculated and the process starts over until convergence (or some stopping criterion) is achieved.

The procedure described is applied to some real world images to illustrate performance as well as to two 2D US datasets. In the latter case, for the first US dataset, results are evaluated by visual inspection, while for the second dataset some numerical comparison between manually adjusted contours (performed by an expert) and the computer generated contours is carried out.

### 3.4. *Discussion*

The procedure just described is, by all means, a solid approach where the two main pieces of information that a designer may use to obtain a good segmentation are accounted for. Additionally, parameters in the model are identified by optimizing a well-defined mathematically consistent criterion. As for pros, it is clear that, provided that the training images and kidney models, respectively used for defining the Gaussian mixture and the shape model, are sufficiently relevant, the models will be able to find their way through a (probably large) number of test cases or even in clinical practice. Additionally, except for a number of predefined parameters (mainly, $K$ and $M$ described above), most of the modeling is fine-tuned on the run.

Having said this, we should also indicate some drawbacks inherent in the model. We understand that the model is not able to perform *local deformations* since parameters within function $T$ are global. The only way to proceed locally is by tuning the set of parameters $W$. But, once again, even though the locality here may arise due to some particular mode, the approach itself is global since raising the importance of some mode, generally speaking, will have a global effect. This is probably the main difference wrt the solution we describe in Sec. 4.

On the other hand the whole optimization process is grounded on image information — this may leave room for doubt about how the algorithm will behave when some sort of shading (due to, for instance, a rib that may be impossible to avoid) is observed in the data to process. We show in Sec. 4.7 how our algorithm deals with this situation, which may be encountered in practice with a non-negligible frequency.

Finally, given below are two additional comments that do not focus explicitly on the model, but on methodological aspects. First, the authors do not carry out an objective *validation* process; they do compare their segmentation with the one from an expert, but measuring variability within a set of experts and finding whether their algorithm is within the *interobserver range* (see Sec. 4.6 for an explanation of this concept) would have made their experiments more convincing. Second, the fact that their model is deeply based on training images and models makes the adaptation of their method to other organs a hard task. This is hard to avoid on methods so designed. The point is that the segmentation of kidneys, as well as other organs, is desirable to be executed directly in 3D. Adapting this method to an additional dimension is conceptually simple, but hard on practice.

## 4. Solution Based on Active Contours and Markov Random Fields

We now turn to describe the solution proposed by the authors of this chapter. The solution is grounded on the one originally from Ref. 39. However, additional material wrt this solution will also be provided, namely an extension to an entirely 3D model as well as a discussion about model parameter estimation. The method is grounded on the *star-like* object assumption (recall Sec. 2). The kidney interface detection problem is posed as an estimation problem by means of a Bayesian framework in which the prior distribution is built upon ACs (and surfaces, for the 3D case) and MRFs, and the likelihood model uses both the intensity image and the gradient image. Throughout the discussion we will bear in mind the 2D model; 3D ideas will be the topic of the section.

### 4.1. *Active contours*

ACs[7] and, particularly, *snakes*[30] are mechanisms that provide a way to obtain the contours of objects within an image by imposing some sort of prior knowledge. Specifically, they force continuity and smoothness in their solution as opposed to simply expecting that these properties may arise from the image data themselves. This idea was initially posed as *deformable templates*,[18] i.e. parametric models which could be deformed with relatively few degrees of freedom, and then snakes gained popularity after the seminal paper in Ref. 30. Snakes, however, are not designed to automatically extract the contours, but they refine solutions given by other segmentation methods. Therefore, by providing the snake with an initial contour estimate, the snake will evolve to the optimal contour solution, where optimality means minimizing an energy function that is a balance between internal forces (forces imposed by the model, such as smoothness in first- and second-order derivatives and the like) and external forces, i.e. forces toward salient features in the image.

Finding a local minimum in the energy function is not difficult, but this cannot be stated about finding the global minimum, since these functions are highly nonlinear, and therefore, they have many places in which the solution finding algorithm may get trapped. A possible turnaround to this pitfall is the possibility of discretizing the problem, and using a discrete spatial model together with a MRF and all the optimization theories developed hitherto.[21,53] This alternative approach is also based on energy functions, but the crucial difference is that the method falls within a probabilistic environment and makes use of a *Bayesian philosophy* in order to estimate the optimum contour, the existence of which is guaranteed, and a theoretical method of convergence to it has been reported.[21]

### 4.2. *Markov random fields*

A MRF is a probabilistic model of the elements of a multidimensional random variable in which the components have only local (as opposed to global) interactions.[53] It is defined on a finite grid, the sites of which correspond to each component of the random variable. Local interactions are defined in terms of neighboring variables, so a MRF is defined in terms of a neighborhood. Given a neighborhood, a *clique* is a subset of it in which all the components of the clique are neighbors.[21] From neighbors and cliques one can define potential functions to give rise to an energy function of the field. This function defines a Gibbs function — it turns out[26] that Gibbs random fields (GRFs) and MRFs are equivalent — so, both in theoretical and practical terms, a set of potential functions defined on the cliques of a neighborhood system induces a MRF.

About the use of MRFs in practical applications, it is interesting to highlight that even though MRFs suffer from a problem of dimensionality, the *Gibbs Sampler* (GS) algorithm proposed in Ref. 21 gives a constructive iterative procedure to get a realization of the field. In addition, in the case that the field defines a posterior probability function, one might be interested in finding the configuration that maximizes this field, i.e. in finding the *maximum a posteriori* (MAP) estimation. Once again, Geman and Geman[21] proposed the *Simulated Annealing* (SA) algorithm which, using ideas similar to that of the GS algorithm, converges to one of the maximizers of the field, provided a logarithmic *cooling schedule* is used.[25]

### 4.3. *State of the art*

In what follows, we will summarize published proposals that make use of both ACs and MRFs for segmentation purposes, and that are somehow related to our problem.

We have mainly focused on the medical imaging field, but some references will also be described from outside this field.

Friedland and Adam[19] developed a fully automated algorithm for the fast detection of the boundaries of the cavity of the left ventricle (LV) from a series of 2D echocardiograms. This is, to our knowledge, a pioneer work in defining a Markovian AC model in polar coordinates (the authors use as origin the center of mass of the contour). The procedure first adjusts an ellipse to the cavity by means of the generalized Hough transform — a region of interest is defined by means of two ellipses (inner and outer wrt the one just drawn). From the center of the ellipse a number of spokes are drawn. Hereafter the spokes will be called *rays*. The allowed contour positions within every ray are discretized, and a 1D (in the angular coordinates) MRF is defined so as to impose smoothness in the solution contour. The energy function of the field considers the image edges, the smoothness of the cavity, the maximum allowable volume enclosed within the ventricle, and the temporal continuity of the ventricle boundary. Notice that no Bayesian philosophy is used, but the MRF is just a means for optimization (using the SA algorithm). Model parameters are experimentally adjusted.

Friedland and Rosenfeld[20] proposed a model similar to the one just described, but, in this case, applied to infrared images. Specifically, the authors describe a procedure to recognize a rigid object as one of the objects within a predefined library. Their method has two stages: the first one is a contour detection stage which uses ideas similar to those of Friedland and Adam.[19] The second stage is a recognition phase in which a new energy term accounts for the differences between the segmented contour and the contour of every object in the library. The relative weight of the two energy terms is controlled by means of a parameter which changes dynamically as the algorithm evolves.

Figueiredo and Leitao[17] proposed a contour model similar to that proposed in Ref. 19 but, in this case, using the Bayesian philosophy. The method is fine-tuned to the segmentation of angiographies of the LV cavity. The authors, due to their imaging modality, propose an image model in which the intensity outside the LV is expected to be very different from the intensity in its interior. Independent Gaussian random variables are used, the mean values of which are conditioned to the contour position. About the prior model, they force smoothness by means of a multivariate Gaussian distribution defined in terms of the square of the finite differences of consecutive contour points. The joint optimization of both the contour and the parameters of the model is solved by means of an adaptive version of the *Iterated Conditional Modes* (ICM) algorithm.[6]

In 1994, Storvik[48] proposed a Markovian AC model in Cartesian coordinates, where the number of points along the contour is allowed to change. A contour is defined as a variable series of nodes, with the only restriction that the resulting contour is closed with simple connectivity. Nodes are allowed only on image pixels. In this case the potential that induces the field is not known. The prior is based on a fractal measure. The likelihood function consists of two terms: the first one assumes independent Gaussian data with different parameters inside and outside the current contour. The second term makes use of the image edges. Only data close to the current contour are used. Results are shown for an echocardiogram of the LV, and an MRI of the brain. Computational complexity is extremely high.

Dias and Leitao[16] resorted to the works of Figueiredo and Leitao[17] and Friedland and Adam[19] in their design of an estimation method of both the inner (endocardium) and outer (epicardium) contours of the LV cavity in a series of echocardiograms. The same polar representation as in Ref. 19 is used. However, this is the first approach in which some information about the US statistics is used, since the image model is Rayleigh, the reflectance of which depends on the current contour position. Contour sequences are modeled as a first-order MRF in 2D. Each variable has a temporal and a spatial index. The optimum (contour and model parameters) is obtained using dynamic programming ideas.[5] More recently, Haas et al.[24] have used these ideas to segment intravascular US images in 3D. In this case, the depth coordinate replaces the temporal coordinate used in Ref. 16.

An alternative approach to the traditional snakes modeling in which the image energy is defined in terms of image edges, i.e. image gradient, is the approach proposed in Ref. 11. In this work, the AC is defined out of region statistics. The problem faced is a detection problem, i.e. to detect the presence of a target on some background, the statistics of which are known to differ. The method is valid as long as both regions are homogeneous, and the hypothesis of approximate uncorrelation between pixels is used. The prior favors contour regularization. The transition model is built upon sufficient statistics, and parameters of the distributions are iteratively calculated with a *Maximum Likelihood* (ML) approach (closed-form expressions are found for several distributions). The MAP solution is obtained by an *ad hoc* multiresolution method with local contour site movements.

It is interesting to mention the effort of combining MRFs with deformable templates under a Bayesian approach made in Refs. 42 and 43. The methods described there are also region based. In Ref. 42, the authors aim at detecting cast shadows from sonar images of objects lying on the sea bed, while in Ref. 43, a similar procedure is employed to estimate the heart boundaries in echocardiographic images. In the former, the objects under analysis have a clear geometric shape, so the template is deformed globally and affinely. In the latter, on the other hand and due to the smooth properties of the heart, the template has to be deformed nonrigidly (the deformable template used by the authors is the one proposed in Ref. 28). In particular, the authors propose a MRF based on three types of deformations for the prototype template: global affine transformations, global nonaffine transformations, and local deformations. For this MRF, the prior is defined to constrain the deformations to be smooth, and the transition function favors smooth probability maps obtained from a labeling process, using blood and muscle classes. The MRF defined in the space of deformations is optimized by means of a hybrid genetic algorithm, an alternative method to the SA algorithm.

The results are satisfactory for ecocardiographies due, in part, to the clear statistical difference between blood and muscle.

The problem posed in Sec. 1, i.e. the *in vivo* segmentation of kidney contours out of a series of 2D echographies, differs from the segmentation of other organs, and so impedes direct application of the solutions described so far in this section. Specifically,

- the kidney is an elastic organ. Therefore its shape can be affected by the patient's posture during the scanning, as well as by other physiological conditions (state of stomach, bladder, intestine, and so forth).
- the kidney interior is not homogeneous due to the presence of numerous structures inside.
- a clear difference between the tissue of the kidney and other nearby tissues does not exist. As a matter of fact, in many situations it is not obvious even for specialist to tell where the contours are.
- as a consequence of the previous point, there will be areas with no gradients at all.
- some slices may show occlusions due to other organs. Such occlusions may be extremely severe in some cases.

We can therefore conclude that data to be analyzed will be incomplete, nonhomogeneous, and will show dependence wrt the contour only within a small neighborhood around the contour point. Solutions proposed so far in the literature are very application driven, so they do not constitute a complete and valid method when applied to scenarios other than those in the mind of the designers. However, these other proposals are a valuable starting point from which very useful ideas can be selected, developed, and fine-tuned.

### 4.4. *The model*

Before describing the details of the probabilistic model that will be used to carry out the segmentation process, we will give a high-level description of the procedure. This will also allow us to naturally introduce the basic terminology that will be used in the rest of this section (for an exhaustive repository of the terminology and notation see Ref. 39). In addition, we will include here some well-known expressions about MRFs for further reference.

As a general comment, contours will be defined within a discrete space and will be expressed as a series of points in polar coordinates.[19] Specifically, $J$ rays will be drawn from the contour center point $(C_x(p), C_y(p))$, and each ray will be discretized into $K$ points ($K$, an odd positive integer). A contour centered at that point will consist of as many points as rays, and for each ray, the particular point will be one out of the $K$ points indicated above. A contour is therefore uniquely defined by means of vectors $\rho(p)$ and $\theta(p)$ which denote the moduli and phases, respectively, of the set of contour points. Notice that these vectors have $J$ components. Index $p$ stands for the slice index within an US volume. Hereafter we will assume that the volume consists of $P$ slices, i.e. $1 \leq p \leq P$.

The basic segmentation procedure is as follows (see the diagram in Fig. 15 for reference throughout this section):

- The procedure assumes that a representative template of a kidney contour is available. This can be either hardwired in the computer application or user input at will. A brief description on how to create such a template is given in Sec. 4.5.
- For the US volume data under test (in which the kidney is known to be), the physician will select a slice, say, slice $p$, and will manually deform the template with the mouse — as physicians do in their clinical practice — so as to match the kidney contour within that slice. A brief reference on this is given in Sec. 4.5 (see also Sec. 2.4 for further details). The result of this action will be called *adjusted template*. In this case, the adjustment is performed manually. Consequently, the adjusted contour[P] will have center $(C_x^a(p), C_y^a(p))$ and contour vectors $\boldsymbol{\rho}^a(p)$ and $\boldsymbol{\theta}^a(p)$.

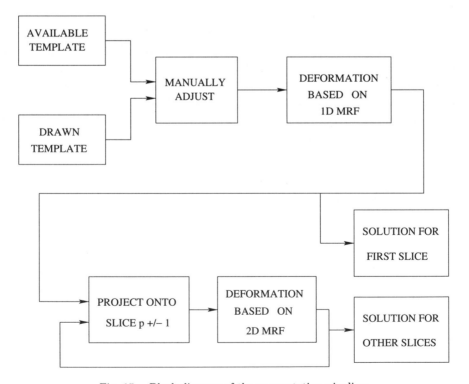

Fig. 15.    Block diagram of the segmentation pipeline.

[P]Superscript $a$ will stand for *adjusted*.

- The model will refine the adjusted template in the current slice. This procedure is unsupervised. To that end, the model will find the appropriate deformation vector, say $d\rho(p)$, to end up with a vector of moduli $\rho(p) = \rho^a(p) + d\rho(p)$. The contour phases do not undergo any deformation, hence $\theta(p) = \theta^a(p)$. These vectors have coordinates still referred to point $(C_x^a(p), C_y^a(p))$. Nevertheless, after the deformation the actual contour center will probably have moved (the center is the point which guarantees that the first-order moments — wrt the area — are zero as described in Sec. 2); we will denote the new center by $(C_x(p), C_y(p))$, and both the vector of phases and the vector of moduli should be referred to this point. For expository simplicity we will assume that this conversion is automatically done, so we will use no new notation to reflect this issue.

- Then the model automatically detects the kidney contours for the rest of the slices within the volume data. This is done in two steps. First, the solution contour of the previous slice is projected onto the current slice. We will also refer to this projected contour as *adjusted template*. In this case, the adjustment is automatic. Contour center for the current slice, say, slice $p$, will be $(C_x^a(p), C_y^a(p)) = (C_x(p-1), C_y(p-1))$, and as for contour vectors we do $\rho^a(p) = \rho(p-1)$ and $\theta^a(p) = \theta(p-1)$. Second, the model refines the segmentation as indicated in the previous paragraph.

As stated before, the objective is to determine for every slice the deformation vector[q] $d\rho$ using as starting information both center $(C_x^a, C_y^a)$ and vectors $\rho^a$ and $\theta^a$. To that end, we will define a *region of deformation* (ROD) as shown in Fig. 16. It will be within the ROD that a homogeneous deformation MRF will be defined in the angular direction. The configurations of this MRF are the possible values of the deformation vector $d\rho$ sought.

Denote by $d\omega_s$ the random variable *deformation wrt the adjustment in ray s*, with $1 \leq s \leq J$. Each angular position — indexed by $s$ — will be called a *site* of the field. We will refer to the set of angular positions by $\mathbf{S} = \{1, 2, \ldots, J-1, J\}$. The random variable $d\omega_s$ is discrete and assumes values within the state space $d\Lambda$, the cardinality of which is $K$, and the values of which will be denoted by $d\Lambda = \{dr_k : 1 \leq k \leq K\}$. The product space[r] $d\Omega = d\Lambda^{|\mathbf{S}|}$ represents the space of configurations (deformations) of the random vector $d\omega = (d\omega_1, d\omega_2, \ldots, d\omega_J)$. Since $d\rho = (d\rho_1, d\rho_2, \ldots, d\rho_J)$ is a realization of the field $d\omega$, $d\rho \in d\Omega$.

The values in $d\Lambda$ are defined within the ROD[s] shown in Fig. 16 and according to the expression

$$dr_k = 2\frac{k-1}{K-1}dr_{\max} - dr_{\max} \text{ for } 1 \leq k \leq K, \tag{52}$$

---

[q]Unless necessary, pointer $p$ that indicates the slice under inspection will be dropped.
[r]If $\mathbf{A}$ is a set, then $|\mathbf{A}|$ denotes the cardinality of the set.
[s]The ROD will be hereafter referred to as $\mathbf{ROD}(s)$ since, as Fig. 16 points out, $\mathbf{ROD}(s)$ is defined out of the point of the adjusted template on ray $s$. A formal definition is given in Ref. 39.

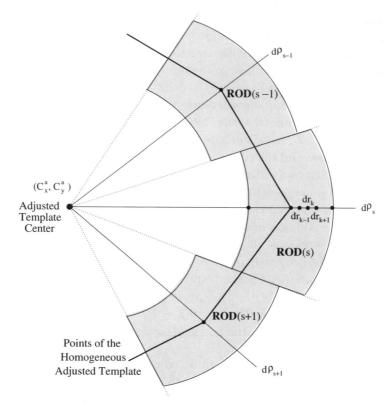

Fig. 16.   **ROD**($s$) and associated terminology. Quantity $\mu^{39}$ equals half the distance between $dr_k$ and $dr_{k+1}$ (see Eq. (52)) $dr_{\max}$ is the parameter to be set.

where $dr_{\max}$ is a parameter to be set.

For each site $s \in \mathbf{S}$ in Fig. 16 we have defined a cyclical and homogeneous neighborhood system $\boldsymbol{\partial}$ consisting of the four nearest neighbors. Specifically[t]

$$\boldsymbol{\partial}(s) = \{s - 2, s - 1, s + 1, s + 2\} \text{ for } s \in \mathbf{S}. \tag{53}$$

$\mathbf{C}$ denotes a clique induced by the neighborhood system $\boldsymbol{\partial}$. The relation $\mathbf{C} \subset \mathbf{S}$ is satisfied. $\boldsymbol{\mathcal{C}}$ denotes the set of all the cliques, i.e. $\boldsymbol{\mathcal{C}} = \{\mathbf{C}, \mathbf{C} \subset \mathbf{S}, \mathbf{C}$ clique induced by $\boldsymbol{\partial}\}$. The neighborhood system just defined induces four clique categories, which will be referred to as $\mathbf{C_I}$, $\mathbf{C_{II}}$, $\mathbf{C_{III}}$, and $\mathbf{C_{IV}}$. Figure 17 shows both the neighborhood system and the four clique classes.

A probability measure $\Pi$ in the product space $d\boldsymbol{\Omega}$ for the GRF $d\boldsymbol{\omega}$ with respect to the neighborhood system $\boldsymbol{\partial}$ is induced by clique potentials. The energy function of the field can be determined as the linear combination of such potential functions. Let $\mathbf{V}$ be the potential set. Then we will denote by $V_{\mathbf{C}}(\cdot) \in \mathbf{V}$ the potential function

[t]The operation must be applied cyclically. Therefore, the operation is $\mathrm{mod}(s + j - 1, J) + 1$.

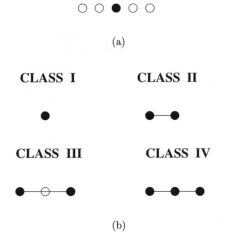

(a)

(b)

Fig. 17.   (a) Neighborhood system. (b) Cliques classes.

for clique $\mathbf{C}$, defined on space $d\Omega$. In order for the field to be a GRF we write

$$\Pi(d\omega = d\rho) = \frac{1}{Z} \exp\left\{ -\sum_{\mathbf{C} \in \mathcal{C}} V_{\mathbf{C}}(d\rho) \right\} \tag{54}$$

and the partition function

$$Z = \sum_{d\rho \in d\Omega} \exp\left\{ -\sum_{\mathbf{C} \in \mathcal{C}} V_{\mathbf{C}}(d\rho) \right\}. \tag{55}$$

Finally, the local characteristic of the field given by the Markov condition can be expressed as

$$\Pi(d\omega_s = d\rho_s \mid d\omega_t = d\rho_t, t \in \partial(s)) = \frac{1}{Z_s} \exp\left\{ -\sum_{\mathbf{C} \in \mathcal{C}/s \in \mathbf{C}} V_{\mathbf{C}}(d\rho) \right\}, \tag{56}$$

where $d\rho_s$ is an element of the vector $d\rho$ for all $s \in \mathbf{S}$. The summation in Eq. (56) is over all cliques $\mathbf{C} \in \mathcal{C}$ that contain site $s$. The local partition function $Z_s$ is defined[u]:

$$Z_s = \sum_{d\rho_s \in d\Lambda} \exp\left\{ -\sum_{\mathbf{C} \in \mathcal{C}/s \in \mathbf{C}} V_{\mathbf{C}}\left(d\rho_s d\rho_{\mathbf{S}\backslash\{s\}}\right) \right\}. \tag{57}$$

---

[u]If $\mathbf{A}$ and $\mathbf{B}$ are sets such that $\mathbf{B} \subset \mathbf{A}$, then $\mathbf{A} \setminus \mathbf{B}$ denotes the difference set, i.e. the set of all elements of $\mathbf{A}$ that are not in $\mathbf{B}$.

### 4.4.1. Prior model of the deformation field

The prior distribution in our scheme should model the *deformation smoothness*, i.e. it must *reward* with a higher probability those deformations that give the solution a shape of a membrane. To that end, potential functions will be defined in terms of first- and second-order derivatives. Derivatives will be carried out in polar coordinates, as opposed to Cartesian, in order to avoid the trend of ACs to vanish to a point if there is no image force[12] (see Sec. 2.2.3 for further details). Approximating derivatives by finite differences, we can write the first-order derivative at site $s$ as

$$d\rho_{s+1} - d\rho_{s-1} \tag{58}$$

and the second-order derivative at the same site as

$$d\rho_{s+1} - 2d\rho_s + d\rho_{s-1}. \tag{59}$$

A potential function will be defined for each derivative. Such potential functions correspond to the clique potentials $V_{\mathbf{C}}(\cdot)$. It is easy to see that the first-order derivative may define a class III clique potential function, and the second-order derivative a class IV potential (see Fig. 17(b)). Specifically, $V_{\mathbf{C}_I}(d\rho) = V_{\mathbf{C}_{II}}(d\rho) = 0$ and

$$V_{\mathbf{C}_{III}}(d\rho) = \vartheta_1 \Psi\left(\frac{d\rho_{s+1} - d\rho_{s-1}}{2dr_{\max}}\right), \tag{60}$$

$$V_{\mathbf{C}_{Iv}}(d\rho) = \vartheta_2 \Psi\left(\frac{d\rho_{s+1} - 2d\rho_s + d\rho_{s-1}}{2dr_{\max}}\right) \tag{61}$$

for $\mathbf{C}_I, \mathbf{C}_{II}, \mathbf{C}_{III}=\{s-1, s+1\}, \mathbf{C}_{IV}=\{s-1, s, s+1\} \in \mathcal{C}$ and for all $d\rho \in d\Omega$.

The probabilistic model so far described will be extended to incorporate an *in-depth* term to make it 2D. The key of the extension will be to favor solution contours in slice $p$ that are not too far apart from the solution contour in slice $p-1$. This can be easily done by adding an energy term that rewards small deformations in the current slice since, as previously stated, the solution on the previous slice is projected onto the current slice, so favoring small deformations leads to favor resemblance between consecutive solutions. This is equivalent to adding a class II clique potential between consecutive slices. However, since $\rho(p) - \rho(p-1) = d\rho(p)$, the net effect is the definition of a class I clique potential in the deformation field; the function we have used is

$$V_{\mathbf{C}_I}(d\rho(p)) = \vartheta_3 \Psi\left(\frac{d\rho_s(p)}{2dr_{\max}}\right) \tag{62}$$

for all cliques $\mathbf{C}_I \in \mathcal{C}$. Notice that this extended model will not be used in the slice on which the physician has manually adjusted the template. This first optimization uses a 1D MRF; subsequent slices do use a 2D MRF.

The prior distribution (but for the first slice) is characterized by the three-component parameter vector $\vartheta = (\vartheta_1, \vartheta_2, \vartheta_3)$, which allows the designer to weigh the influence of each term. Function $\Psi(\phi)$ does not need to fulfill any restriction. However, it is sensible that the function is even and monotonically growing on the $0 \leq \phi \leq 1$ interval, so that the restriction of low probability to sharp contours is maintained (or alternatively, when Eqs. (60)–(62) draw a low value, such configuration should have a large probability).

### 4.4.2. *Likelihood function*

In this section we will briefly describe the operative conclusions about the likelihood model that we propose and use here. The model is somewhat involved, so for technical details the reader is referred to Ref. 39.

The main modeling issue has to do with how a human observer recognizes the presence of a kidney within B-mode US scans. First, the kidney interior, even though it is not homogeneous, is frequently darker than its exterior. Second, the kidney contour, even though it might not be clearly visible along the whole organ, constitutes an important visual cue for determining its presence. Consequently, we have created a likelihood model that takes into account these two visual cues, namely an intensity model and a contour (gradient) model.

The likelihood function will be built upon a number of pixel sets that can be observed in Fig. 18. Even though precise definitions on these sets are given in Ref. 39, we will describe them here in natural language for easier reading:

(1) $\varepsilon(s)$ consists of the angular sector of pixels that are closer to the ray with phase $\theta_s$, taking point $(C_x^a, C_y^a)$ as the center. Figure 18 shows these sets for

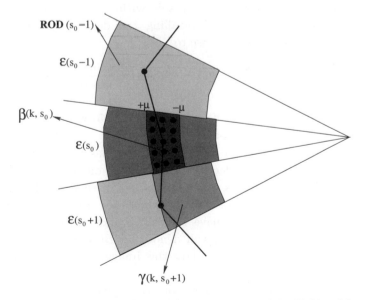

Fig. 18.    Regions involved in the modeling assumptions of the likelihood function.

rays $s_0 - 1$, $s_0$, and $s_0 + 1$. Notice that the set of all regions $\varepsilon(s)$ for $s \in \mathbf{S}$ constitutes a partition of the image pixels.

(2) $\boldsymbol{\beta}(k, s)$ is the subset of the pixels in $\varepsilon(s)$ that belong to an angular sector defined about the estimated contour point when this estimate is point $k$ on ray $s$. An example of this set is the darkest-dotted area in Fig. 18. The band width (the value of which is $2\mu$) is held constant for all $s \in \mathbf{S}$. Notice that sets $\boldsymbol{\beta}(k, s)$ turn out to be a partition of $\mathbf{ROD}(s)$, i.e. $\mathbf{ROD}(s) = \cup_{k=1}^{K}\boldsymbol{\beta}(k, s)$.

(3) $\boldsymbol{\gamma}(k, s)$ is the set of pixels belonging to $\mathbf{ROD}(s)$ in Fig. 18 and internal wrt the estimated point of the contour when this estimate is point $k$ on ray $s$. Clearly $\boldsymbol{\gamma}(k, s) \subset \varepsilon(s)$, and due to the fact that pixels within $\boldsymbol{\gamma}(k, s)$ are *internal* relation $\boldsymbol{\gamma}(k - 1, s) \subset \boldsymbol{\gamma}(k, s)$ also holds.

As for the intensity model, the probability density function of the intensity image $f(I(m, n) \mid d\omega_s = dr_k)$, with $(m, n) \in \boldsymbol{\gamma}(k, s)$, will be approximated by a *Beta distribution*.[34] Specifically, we will assume that the pixels within $\boldsymbol{\gamma}(k, s)$ are Beta-distributed with parameters $\alpha_1(s)$ and $\alpha_2(s)$. Formally, we can write[39]

$$f(I(m, n) \mid d\omega_s = dr_k) = f_B{}^{\alpha_1(s), \alpha_2(s)}(I(m, n)) \tag{63}$$

for all $(m, n) \in \boldsymbol{\gamma}(k, s)$, where $f_B{}^{\alpha_1, \alpha_2}(x)$ is the Beta probability density function with shape parameters $\alpha_1, \alpha_2$.[39]

Considering the probability density function $f(\mathbf{I}(k, s) \mid d\omega_s = dr_k)$ as a function of indices $k$ and $s$,[39] we can define the *log-likelihood* function $L_{\mathbf{I}}(k, s)$ as

$$L_{\mathbf{I}}(k, s) \propto -\ln f(\mathbf{I}(k, s) \mid d\omega_s = dr_k). \tag{64}$$

Assuming conditional independence of pixels within $\boldsymbol{\gamma}(k, s)$ (see Ref. 39 for a justification of this hypothesis) and recalling the density function of a Beta distribution, Eqs. (63) and (64) give rise to

$$L_{\mathbf{I}}(k, s) = \frac{1 - \alpha_2(s)}{|\boldsymbol{\gamma}(k, s)|} \sum_{(m, n) \in \boldsymbol{\gamma}(k, s)} \left[ \ln(1 - I(m, n)) + \frac{1 - \alpha_1(s)}{1 - \alpha_2(s)} \ln(I(m, n)) \right], \tag{65}$$

with $1 \leq k \leq K$ and $s \in \mathbf{S}$. We have normalized Eq. (65) with $|\boldsymbol{\gamma}(k, s)|$ in order to eliminate the influence of the size of set $\boldsymbol{\gamma}(k, s)$.

The second visual cue that we mentioned before has to do with the contours themselves which have a direct effect on the image gradient. However, US images are known to suffer from speckles which, regardless of their possible information content, show themselves as full of artifacts when they are converted to gradient images. To palliate this effect we have basically worked with a compressed and smoothed gradient image, which we will denote by $B(m, n)$ and will be referred to as *edge image* hereafter. Details on how this image is obtained can be seen in Ref. 39.

The probability density function of the pixels of the edge image $f(B(m, n) \mid d\omega_s = dr_k)$, for $(m, n) \in \boldsymbol{\beta}(k, s)$, is hard to determine. However, a turnaround, which turns out to be similar to Ref. 10, has been devised: the presence of a contour close to the pixels within $\beta(k, s)$ makes the values $B(m, n)$ in the set high. Thus, the higher the value, the higher the probability that an edge is at location $(m, n)$. We will employ an *exponential model*

$$f(B(m,n) \mid d\omega_s = dr_k) \propto \exp[B(m,n)] \tag{66}$$

for all $(m, n) \in \beta(k, s)$.[39]

Considering the probability density function $f(\mathbf{B}(k, s) \mid d\omega_s = dr_k)$ as a function of indices $k$ and $s$,[39] we can define the *log-likelihood* function $L_{\mathbf{B}}(k, s)$ by

$$L_{\mathbf{B}}(k, s) \propto -\ln f(\mathbf{B}(k, s) \mid d\omega_s = dr_k). \tag{67}$$

Assuming conditional independence of pixels within $\beta(k, s)$ (once again, see Ref. 39 for a justification of this hypothesis) and using Eq. (66) we obtain

$$L_{\mathbf{B}}(k, s) = -\frac{1}{|\beta(k, s)|} \sum_{(m,n)\in\beta(k,s)} B(m, n), \tag{68}$$

with $1 \le k \le K$ and $s \in \mathbf{S}$. To minimize $L_{\mathbf{B}}(k, s)$ wrt $k$ for each $s$ is equivalent to *maximize the sample mean* in subimage $\mathbf{B}(k, s)$. We have normalized Eq. (68) with $|\beta(k, s)|$ to get the same effect as in Eq. (65).

### 4.4.3. *Complete model*

The two pieces of probabilistic information described in Secs. 4.4.1. and 4.4.2. can be merged in the posterior function, the expression of which is

$$P(d\omega{=}d\rho \mid \mathbf{I}, \mathbf{B}) \propto \Pi(d\omega{=}d\rho) \prod_{s=1}^{J} f(\mathbf{I}(k_s, s) \mid d\omega_s{=}d_{k_s}) \prod_{s=1}^{J} f(\mathbf{B}(k_s, s) \mid d\omega_s{=}d_{k_s}), \tag{69}$$

with $k_s$ a generic index at site $s \in \mathbf{S}$ for which $d\rho_s = d_{k_s}$. Pixels within each angular sector $\varepsilon(s)$ have been assumed to be conditionally independent of those from the rest of the image (see Ref. 39 for a justification of this hypothesis). In order to get an equality sign (as opposed to the proportionality sign $\propto$) we define GRF $\Pi^\varrho$ — formally equal to that of Eq. (54) — as

$$\Pi^\varrho(d\omega = d\rho) = \frac{\Pi(d\omega = d\rho)}{Z^\varrho} \prod_{s=1}^{J} \exp(-\vartheta_4 L_{\mathbf{I}}(k_s, s)) \prod_{s=1}^{J} \exp(-\vartheta_5 L_{\mathbf{B}}(k_s, s)), \tag{70}$$

$Z^\varrho$ being a normalizing constant and $\vartheta_4$ and $\vartheta_5$ being two additional real parameters. Taking into consideration Eqs. (64) and (67) and the proportionality between $\Pi^\varrho(d\omega)$ and $P(d\omega = d\rho \mid \mathbf{I}, \mathbf{B})$, it is easy to see that configuration $d\rho$ that maximizes posterior $P(d\omega = d\rho \mid \mathbf{I}, \mathbf{B})$ also maximizes distribution $\Pi^\varrho(d\omega = d\rho)$

and vice versa. Hence, the objective is to determine configuration $d\rho$ for which $\Pi^\varrho$ is maximum.

Clearly, distribution $\Pi^\varrho$ is a MRF for the *a priori* neighborhood system $\partial$, and it is induced by a new potential set $\mathbf{V}^\varrho$. We can write

$$\Pi^\varrho(d\boldsymbol{\omega} = d\boldsymbol{\rho}) = \frac{1}{Z^\varrho} \exp\left\{-\sum_{\mathbf{C}\in\mathcal{C}} V_{\mathbf{C}}^\varrho(d\boldsymbol{\rho})\right\}, \tag{71}$$

$Z^\varrho$ being a posterior global partition function, and $V_{\mathbf{C}}^\varrho(\cdot) \in \mathbf{V}^\varrho$.

The local characteristic of field $\Pi^\varrho$ can be expressed by

$$\Pi^\varrho(d\omega_s = d\rho_s \mid d\omega_t = d\rho_t, t \in \partial(s)) = \frac{1}{Z_s^\varrho} \exp\left\{-\sum_{\mathbf{C}\in\mathcal{C}/s\in\mathbf{C}} V_{\mathbf{C}}^\varrho(d\boldsymbol{\rho})\right\}, \tag{72}$$

for all $s \in \mathbf{S}$, $Z_s^\varrho$ being the posterior local partition function.

As already stated, for the neighborhood system $\partial$, resulting cliques $\mathcal{C}$ could be classified into classes I, II, III, and IV (see Fig. 17(b)). Clique potentials $V_{\mathbf{C}}^\varrho(\cdot)$ are given by (recall Eqs. (60), (61)–(62)) $V_{\mathbf{C}_{\mathrm{II}}}^\varrho(d\boldsymbol{\rho}) = 0$, $V_{\mathbf{C}_{\mathrm{III}}}^\varrho(d\boldsymbol{\rho}) = V_{\mathbf{C}_{\mathrm{III}}}(d\boldsymbol{\rho})$, $V_{\mathbf{C}_{\mathrm{IV}}}^\varrho(d\boldsymbol{\rho}) = V_{\mathbf{C}_{\mathrm{IV}}}(d\boldsymbol{\rho})$, and

$$V_{\mathbf{C}_{\mathrm{I}}}^\varrho(d\boldsymbol{\rho}) = V_{\mathbf{C}_{\mathrm{I}}}(d\boldsymbol{\rho}) + \vartheta_4 L_{\mathbf{I}}(k_s, s) + \vartheta_5 L_{\mathbf{B}}(k_s, s), \tag{73}$$

with $\mathbf{C}_{\mathrm{I}}, \mathbf{C}_{\mathrm{II}}, \mathbf{C}_{\mathrm{III}}, \mathbf{C}_{\mathrm{IV}} \in \mathcal{C}$ and for all $d\boldsymbol{\rho} \in d\Omega$. The parameter vector $\boldsymbol{\vartheta}$ is enlarged by two components in the posterior, i.e. $\boldsymbol{\vartheta} = (\vartheta_1, \vartheta_2, \vartheta_3, \vartheta_4, \vartheta_5)$.

We can now face the optimization problem: in order to find out configuration $d\boldsymbol{\rho} \in d\Omega$ that maximizes field $\Pi^\varrho$ we can use the SA algorithm. In our case, we have resorted to a partially parallel visit schedule and a logarithmic cooling scheme.[25,53] The initial configuration $d\boldsymbol{\rho}_{(0)}$ can be arbitrary, but a faster convergence is achieved by starting from the ML contour,[16] i.e. the contour obtained by minimizing function $L_{\mathbf{B}}(k, s)$ in $k$ for each $s \in \mathbf{S}$.

Since the neighborhood system $\partial$ has five elements, it is necessary to define a five-element partition. The positions of each element of the partition are updated in parallel,[53] i.e. in each sweep five visits are carried out, one for each partition element.[v] The number of sweeps $N_s$ to achieve convergence is of order $10^2$. This gives very fast solutions in terms of computational time (see Sec. 4.7 for details) so we have not felt the need of analyzing other optimization procedures.[36]

### 4.5. Implementation details

We have created an environment that allows the user to create the template contour at will. The user clicks on several contour points on the real images, and the contour is drawn *on the fly*. Since it is expected that the expert outlined contour has just a

---

[v]This approach gives a natural way to an eventual high speed parallel implementation.

few points, we upsample the contour to have a modulus value for the set of *uniformly distributed* phases $\boldsymbol{\theta} = (\theta_1, \theta_2, \ldots, \theta_J)$, the components of which are calculated by

$$\theta_j = \frac{(2j - J)\,\pi}{J} \quad \text{with } 1 \leq j \leq J, \tag{74}$$

$J$ being typically much larger than the number of user-drawn points. Finally, the template is normalized so that its first-order moments (wrt the area) are zero (see Sec. 2), to obtain vector $\boldsymbol{\rho}^{nt}$ with $J$ components.[w] Two control points are added to the contour so that it can be manually adjusted as we now explain.

In order to mimic the clinical procedures we have created a second environment that allows a user to superimpose the template onto one slice of the real data, and by moving the two control points — as ultrasonographers are used to doing — the user can adjust the template to the kidney contour (see Sec. 2.4.2 for further details). An adjusted template defined by center $(C_x^a, C_y^a)$ and moduli $\rho^a$ for phases $\boldsymbol{\theta}^a = \boldsymbol{\theta}$ is thus obtained.

The result of the above procedure is an adjusted contour in which phases are uniformly distributed in the range of $2\pi$ radians. Figure 10(a) shows the spatial distribution of the contour points for a typical template when using uniform coordinates. It is clear that contour points closer to the center are closer to each other, while contour points farther from the center are more separated from each other. This is a side effect of the uniform phases, which should be avoided for a correct definition of the MRF, since, as we have described in Sec. 4.4, the field is homogeneous.

The solution adopted to solve this problem is to work in what we have called *homogeneous coordinates.* In this coordinate system — which is the one used throughout Sec. 4.4 — it is not the angle that is uniformly distributed in the range of $2\pi$ radians, but it is the area[x] enclosed within every angular sector. Therefore, points farther from the center of the contour should be closer to each other, while those points located closer to the center should be angularly more separated so that the areas of the two cases are equal. An example of this point distribution is shown in Fig. 10(b). Details of how to convert from one set of coordinates to the other are carefully described in Sec. 2.3.

## 4.6. *Validation*

In Ref. 9 the authors propose a methodology for evaluation of automatic boundary detection algorithms in medical images. One of their most interesting contributions is the proposition of two statistical tests that check whether a boundary detection

---

[w]The superscript $nt$ stands for *normalized template.*
[x]An alternative criterion would be to use a constant arclength. However, since our model is estimated from data within each angular sector, it is desirable to have the same data amount on each, which is approximately obtained by equalizing the sector areas. Other advantages have been reported for moments defined wrt the area for the case of spline curves.[7] See Sec. 2.3 for further details on contour reparameterizations.

algorithm can be validated. The authors pose the validation problem so as to check whether *the computer generated boundaries (CGBs) differ from the manually outlined boundaries as much as the manually outlined boundaries differ from one another.* This general idea is implemented by means of two different statistical tests, namely the William Index (WI) and the Percent Statistic (PS). The former is a ratio of agreements, with the numerator a mean agreement between the CGB and the expert outlined boundaries (EOBs), and the denominator a mean agreement between EOBs. The agreement is defined as the inverse of the distance between boundaries. If the CGB is identically distributed (ID) with respect to the EOBs, the expected value of this ratio is 1, so the test is passed if the upper value of the confidence interval (CI) of the statistic (calculated by means of a jackknife technique[2]) exceeds unity. About the latter, a statistic consisting of the fraction of times that the CGBs lie within what the authors call *interobserver range* is calculated, and a test is built to check whether this fraction is close enough to the expected value. For instance, with four experts, this expected value is $p = 0.6$, and the test is passed if the statistic exceeds $p - \epsilon$, where $\epsilon$ is a threshold that depends on both level $\alpha$ of the test (typically $\alpha = 0.05$) and the actual number of images to be tested.[y]

Finally, in both cases, a definition of the distance between the contours is required. The authors use two distances, namely the so-called *Haussdorf* and *average* distances. The former is a valid metric, while the latter is not. In our case, however, since corresponding points between contours are straightforward, we have created an alternative distance measure defined for contours $\rho_1$ and $\rho_2$, expressed in uniform phases, as

$$e(\rho_1, \rho_2) = \frac{1}{2J} \sum_{j=1}^{J} |\rho_{1j} - \rho_{2j}| \, (\rho_{1j} + \rho_{2j}). \tag{75}$$

Martin-Fernandez and Alberola-Lopez[39] show that this distance measure is indeed a metric.

### 4.7. *Experimental validation results*

All the kidney images shown in this section have been acquired by the authors with a piece of Hitachi EUB-515 US equipment (with a 2D US probe). In order to create volumes, the *freehand* modality was used, recording not only the video output but also the spatial location and orientation of the probe by means of a *miniBird* (Ascension Technologies, Burlington, VT) positioning system. Both the US slices and the probe position measures were matched using the Stradx freehand 3D US system (3D Ultrasound Research Group, Cambridge University, UK[46]). The

---

[y]Chalana and Kim[9] state that the expected value for four experts is $p = 0.8$, which has been shown to be incorrect.[1]

Table 1. Parameter setting for the experiments. In all the experiments $N_s = 250$, $J = 70$. SII stands for "slice index interval." The units of parameter $dr_{max}$ should be pixels; however, we give a normalized value with respect to the length of the adjusted template major semiaxis. The legend in the first column is Valid-1, first validation experiment; and Valid-2, second validation experiment.

| Exp. | | | Param. | | |
|---|---|---|---|---|---|
| | SII | MAT at slice # | $K$ | $dr_{max}$ | $\boldsymbol{\vartheta} = (\vartheta_1, \vartheta_2, \vartheta_3, \vartheta_4, \vartheta_5)$ |
| Valid-1 | [89, 122] | 106 | 15 | 0.05 | (35, 35, 10, 35, 35) |
| Valid-2 | [15, 30] | 30 | 15 | 0.05 | (35, 35, 30, 25, 35) |

calibration of the system was performed using a single-wall phantom as described in Ref. 47.

We will first present some results for a healthy adult kidney. In this experiment we use 34 slices. Table 1, second row (Valid-1), shows the parameters involved in this experiment. In particular, the second column indicates the indices of the slices and the third column indicates the slice number at which the operative to get a manually adjusted template (MAT) has been carried out (the MAT is shown in Fig. 19(a)). The algorithm has been run with the parameter setting indicated in the remaining three columns of this row. Four experts have manually segmented the dataset used. Figures 19(b)–19(d) show both the CGB (white) and the four EOBs (black) for slices 96, 100, and 116, respectively. The results for the two validation procedures (WI and CI) are indicated in Table 2, second row (Valid-1). Clearly, the algorithm performs for this example as the board of experts do.

A second experiment has been carried out on a normal kidney but with a severe occlusion caused by the presence of a rib.[z] Table 1, third row (Valid-2), indicates the parameters that define this new experiment. In this case the same four experts as before have manually segmented the 16 slices; in the occlusions the experts were kindly asked to delineate their expected boundary position. The MAT is shown in Fig. 20(a). Figures 20(b)–20(d) show both the CGB (white) and the four EOBs (black) for slices 21, 24, and 26, respectively. It is clear that the occlusion makes the EOBs as well as the CGB have more variability in that region. As for the validation procedures, results are shown in Table 2, third row (Valid-2). Once again, the algorithm performs as the experts do: CGB variability is similar to that among EOBs.

The solution proposed is feasible in a clinical setting. Results have been obtained, for all the experiments, in less than 1 s per slice with an average computer (specifically, with an 800 MHz Pentium III, with RAM 512 Mb running Matlab under Linux Red Hat 7.2) using, as reported, an SA algorithm. Other optimization methods (ICM, mean field annealing, and genetic algorithms) may give faster results, but this issue has not been dealt with due to the acceptable results obtained

---

[z]The echo from the rib does not appear in the image.

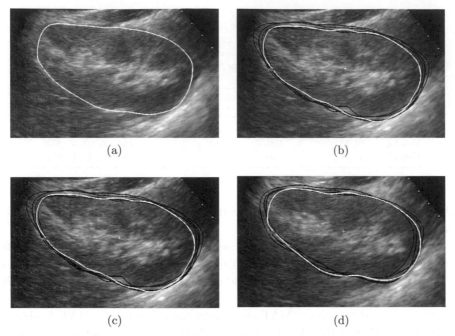

(a)            (b)

(c)            (d)

Fig. 19. Experiment Valid-1: (a) MAT on slice 106. (b) CGB on slice 96 (white) and EOBs (black) for four experts. (c) Same results for slice 100. (d) Same results for slice 116.

Table 2. Results of the validation experiments. The WI test is passed if the upper limit of the CI exceeds unity. The PS test is passed if $PS > p - \epsilon$, with $p = 0.6$ and $\epsilon$ is calculated to get a unilateral test at level $\alpha = 5\%$.

| Exp. | Param. | | |
|---|---|---|---|
| | WI-CI | $p - \epsilon$ | PS |
| Valid-1 | [1.0418, 1.0599] | 0.4618 | 0.6417 |
| Valid-2 | [1.0708, 1.1183] | 0.3985 | 0.75 |

with SA. It is clear that using such a simple (though robust) MRF model, i.e. a space with a small number of possible configurations, gives clear advantages as far as computational load is concerned.

### 4.8. *3D extension*

The presented model allows for a natural 3D extension. At the beginning of Sec. 4.4, where the main concepts of the model have been introduced, index $p$ denotes the slice under inspection. The key idea for the 3D extension of the model has to do with the introduction of this index in the *a priori* MRF model to favor the kidney

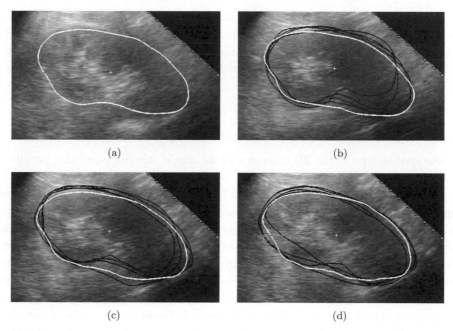

Fig. 20. Experiment Valid-2: (a) MAT on slice 30. (b) CGB on slice 21 (white) and EOBs (black) for four experts. (c) Same results for slice 24. (d) Same results for slice 26.

surface smoothness along the transverse direction. So in this case $dw_{\mathbf{s}}$, with $\mathbf{s} \in \mathbf{S} = \{1, \ldots, J\} \times \{1, \ldots, P\}$, denotes the random variable *deformation wrt the adjustment in ray $j$ and slice $p$*, with $1 \leq j \leq J$ and $1 \leq p \leq P$. Therefore $\mathbf{S}$ refers to the set of surface positions in which this variable is defined.

For each site $\mathbf{s} \in \mathbf{S}$ the neighborhood system $\delta$ consists of the neighbors

$$\delta(\mathbf{s}) = \{(j - 2, p), (j - 1, p), (j, p), (j + 1, p), (j + 2, p),$$
$$(j, p - 2), (j, p - 1), (j, p + 1), (j, p + 2)\}. \qquad (76)$$

This system induces two new classes of cliques, referred to as $\mathbf{C_V}$ and $\mathbf{C_{VI}}$, analogous to classes $\mathbf{C_{III}}$ and $\mathbf{C_{IV}}$, but now defined in the transverse direction.

So now, the finite differences of Sec. 4.4.1 are carried out by means of a discretization induced by the cylindrical coordinate system, in which differences are taken wrt the angular and transverse directions. These new spatial dependencies tend to favor those solutions with the form of a plate.[36] Additionally, it should be highlighted that we have not taken into consideration derivatives other than those contemplated in the cliques above (i.e. derivatives in the diagonal direction) as they add a high computational complexity and do not seem to improve the results.

Same considerations could be established wrt the potential functions of that section. In this approach, the potential that favors small deformations between consecutive solutions is no longer necessary.

Finally, we need to depart from an initial solution that adjusts the model as a whole. To that end, we have deviated from the procedure indicated above (the MAT used in the 2D model), and we approximate it out of several points introduced by the physician in a procedure with resemblances to customary clinical practice for the measurement of the renal volume.[4]

### 4.9. *Unsupervised parameter estimation*

For the specific case of the 3D extension of the model, the six weighting parameters of the Gibbs model, namely $\boldsymbol{\vartheta} = (\vartheta_1, \vartheta_2, \vartheta_3, \vartheta_4, \vartheta_5, \vartheta_6)$, which through this section refer to the weight of the first and second angular differences, the first and second transverse differences, and the intensity and edge log-likelihood factors, respectively, are difficult to determine manually. Moreover, the capability of the model to adapt to each particular case is highly dependent on the election of the parameter vector. Therefore, we need to devise a procedure for the estimation of these parameters, and it should be fully data driven and evolve as the segmentation result does so.

This topic is, by no means, new. One can find many results about parameter estimation in the literature.[36] The approach is different in the cases of causal and noncausal Markov models, as in the first case iterative procedures can be adopted naturally. Differences also arise for supervised and unsupervised scenarios. Clearly, the case of unsupervised noncausal parameter estimation is the most involved, and its complexity increases with the dimensionality of the field.

Generally speaking, the problem can be posed as jointly finding both the configuration and the combination of parameters

$$(d\boldsymbol{\rho}^*, \boldsymbol{\vartheta}^*) = \underset{d\boldsymbol{\rho}, \boldsymbol{\vartheta}}{\arg\max} \, \Pi^\rho(\mathbf{dw} = d\boldsymbol{\rho} \mid \boldsymbol{\vartheta}). \tag{77}$$

This maximization is intractable; therefore it is rewritten[33] as a procedure in which the two pieces of information are iteratively sought

$$\begin{aligned} d\boldsymbol{\rho}^* &= \underset{d\boldsymbol{\rho}}{\arg\max} \, \Pi^\rho(\mathbf{dw} = d\boldsymbol{\rho} \mid \boldsymbol{\vartheta}^*), \\ \boldsymbol{\vartheta}^* &= \underset{\boldsymbol{\vartheta}}{\arg\max} \, \Pi^\rho(\mathbf{dw} = d\boldsymbol{\rho}^* \mid \boldsymbol{\vartheta}). \end{aligned} \tag{78}$$

The method we propose here[aa] shares the weak convergence objective in Ref. 33, but with some differences:

- The *a posteriori* weighting factors are estimated too. In Ref. 33, the *a posteriori* factor is encoded by a Gaussian relation between the data and the model; so closed-form solutions for the weighting factor estimation exist.[36] This is no longer valid in our case, so we introduce the estimation of these factors in the overall procedure.

---

[aa]See Ref. 14, where the authors apply a similar approach in a different scenario.

- As the Gibbs model is a generalized linear model, it satisfies the property

$$\arg\max_{d\rho} \Pi^\rho(\mathbf{dw} = d\rho \mid \vartheta) = \arg\max_{d\rho} \Pi^\rho(\mathbf{dw} = d\rho \mid \beta\vartheta), \qquad (79)$$

with $\beta > 0$, so there is equivalence in the segmentation within a subset of parameter configurations; this is the reason why we impose the restriction

$$\|\vartheta\| = \sqrt{\sum_{l=1}^{6} \vartheta_l^2} = 1. \qquad (80)$$

Note that in the condition expressed in Eq. (79) the role of $\beta$ is the same as the one of the inverse temperature in the SA algorithm. So if we do not consider Eq. (80), the estimation procedure could alter the cooling scheme of the surface optimization. It is well known that the cooling schedule must be chosen carefully, so this restriction is necessary to decouple the segmentation optimization procedure from the parameter estimation task.[25,53] Note also that this restriction is a natural way to confine the parameter estimation to a bounded region. Moreover, it is also assumed that

$$\vartheta_l > 0, \quad l \in \{1, \dots, 6\}. \qquad (81)$$

This assumption tries to minimize the risk of detecting structures that we are not searching for. For instance, if we allow the inversion of the intensity log-likelihood, the restriction of a darker inner region is not longer fulfilled and the algorithm could detect another structure different from the kidney boundaries. One can argue that, once the correctness of the design is assumed, the result given by the true kidney boundaries should be the smallest energy configuration. This leads to the conclusion that the algorithm should evolve to this configuration. Nevertheless, in order to prevent practical troubles, we prefer to assume the positivity of the parameters given that the initial parameter selection could greatly influence the segmentation result.
- In practical terms it is interesting to interrupt the SA global optimization procedure more often in the first cooling steps than in the last ones. This is due to the fact that we need a fast estimation of the parameters to get away from its initial values, and once the model is well constructed, we only need to slightly refine it as the optimization progresses.

The method in Ref. 33 has many resemblances to the scheme we propose. As in our case, the optimization is driven by the cooling schedule provided for the SA algorithm, and the parameter estimation is inserted in this procedure by interrupting the SA algorithm at the end of some sweeps and to perform a Metropolis-Hastings based estimation of the parameters given the optimization result in that iteration. This allows for a direct insertion of the parameter estimation scheme in the segmentation procedure.

As we have pointed out, though the joint optimization process could provide a separate global optimum result for the configuration of the field given the parameter set and for the parameter set given the configuration of the field, this is hardly achieved in finite-time optimization procedures. It is well known that in EM-like procedures as the one presented so far there is a great dependence of the result on the starting optimization point. So there are two very important *a priori* choices to be made that have a great influence on the estimation and segmentation results, namely the initial configuration $d\rho^{(0)}$ and the initial parameter vector $\vartheta^{(0)}$. For the first choice, it is possible to take a configuration relatively close[bb] to the real result. Since this result is unknown we have resorted to the configuration that minimizes the edge image log-likelihood function in Eq. (68). For the second choice, the initial parameter vector proposed in Ref. 33, namely the $\mathbf{0}$[cc] one, is not valid in our case. We have observed that parameter vector components selected randomly within the $(0,1)$ interval — with joint dependence given by the restriction given by Eq. (80) — draws acceptable results.

### 4.10. *3D parameter estimation and validation*

The parameter estimation method presented in the previous section has been applied to the 3D direct extension of the method of Sec. 4.8, as in this case it is more difficult to perform a manual parameter setting due to the increase in the parameter space dimension. Moreover, the method has been implemented as a module in the 3D Slicer platform,[22] to take advantage of the facilities that this software provides for 3D data interaction. Finally, the freehand US data has been reconstructed in a way similar to that of Jose Estepar *et al.*[29] to give physical meaning to the transverse component.

The methodology of the experiments we have performed takes into account the random nature of the segmentation method we have proposed. For this reason, we have investigated the behavior of the algorithm for 30 realizations of the segmentation. The initial parameter vector is different for every iteration. There is a fast convergence of the parameters to consistent solutions. This is shown in Figs. 21 and 22 for 30 realizations of the first parameter adjustment. This is implemented as the initial step of the segmentation procedure and subsequently refined to provide the results in Table 3. It registers the mean relative difference in the parameter estimates. It can be seen that the edge log-likelihood term is the most unstable one. Some interpretations of this behavior could arise from the facts that it is the smaller parameter and that it is the one most closely related with the different segmentation evolution paths.

---

[bb]This closeness should be interpreted wrt a metric of the deformation space given by the transition probabilities between states.
[cc]$\mathbf{0} = (0, 0, \ldots, 0)$ with six elements.

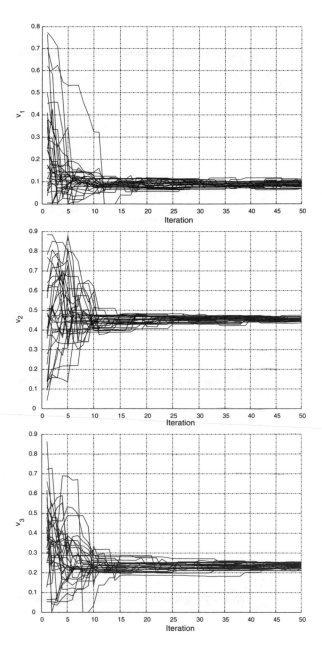

Fig. 21.  Convergence of the parameter components at the first step of the iterative procedure.

M. Martin-Fernandez et al.

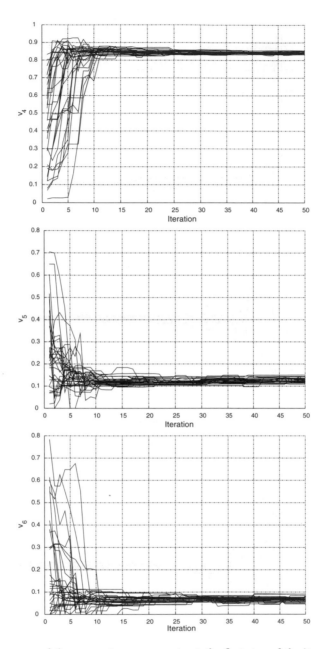

Fig. 22.   Convergence of the parameter components at the first step of the iterative procedure.

Table 3. Results of the parameter estimation. Relative differences were calculated as $\frac{|\vartheta_l^r - \hat{\vartheta}_l|}{\hat{\vartheta}_l}$, where index $r$ stands for a given realization and $\hat{\vartheta}_l$ is the mean value of the estimated parameters.

| Parameter | $\vartheta_1$ | $\vartheta_2$ | $\vartheta_3$ | $\vartheta_4$ | $\vartheta_5$ | $\vartheta_6$ |
|---|---|---|---|---|---|---|
| Mean relative difference | 0.0590 | 0.0275 | 0.0246 | 0.0160 | 0.0554 | 0.1675 |

The parameter estimation provides a more robust result than the one obtained by means of manual parameter selection. If the initial parameter vector is used to perform the segmentation, the WI validation test is satisfied only in 18 out of the 30 realizations (without parameter estimation and random choices of the parameters), whereas it is satisfied in 27 with the proposed parameter estimation method. We have found different results for the PS test. In this case, it is satisfied in 23 out of the 30 realizations without parameter estimation and in 30 with the proposed estimation method.

## 5. Conclusions

In this chapter we have dealt with an important and difficult problem, about which very few contributions have been reported in the literature. To the best of our knowledge, only two methods have focused on pursuing an automated procedure to detect kidney interfaces in US data. This necessarily means that there is much work to be done in this field. The validation techniques presented in Sec. 4.6 will hopefully serve as a framework under which algorithms to come could be evaluated and compared. Apart from the description and discussion of the two methods reported, we have also included a background section concerning discrete contour operations based on the monotonic phase property, which applies to the kidney problem. Several important issues as contour reparameterizations as well as complex and normalized representations were presented, and they may serve as useful tools for further developments.

## References

1. C. Alberola-Lopez and M. Martin-Fernandez, Comments on: A methodology for evaluation of boundary detection algorithms on medical images, *IEEE Trans. Med. Imaging* **23**(5) (2004) 658–660.
2. P. Armitage, G. Berry and J. N. S. Matthews, *Statistical Methods in Medical Research* (Blackwell Science, Oxford, UK, 2002).
3. J. Bakker, M. Olree, R. Kaatee, E. E. de Lange and R. J. A. Beek, *In vitro* measurement of kidney size: Comparison of ultrasonography and MRI, *Ultrasound Med. Biol.* **24** (1997) 683–688.
4. J. Bakker, M. Olree, R. Kaatee, E. E. de Lange, K. G. M. Moons, J. J. Beutler and R. J. A. Beek, Accuracy and repeatability of US compared with that of MR imaging, *Radiology* **211** (1999) 623–628.

5. R. Bellman, *Dynamic Programming* (Princeton University Press, Princeton, NJ, USA, 1957).

6. J. E. Besag, On the statistical analysis of dirty pictures (with discussion), *J. Royal Stat. Soc.* **48** (1986) 259–302.

7. A. Blake and M. Isard, *Active Contours* (Springer-Verlag, London, UK, 1998).

8. V. Caselles, R. Kimmel and G. Sapiro, Goedesic active contours, *Int. J. Comput. Vis.* **22** (1997) 61–79.

9. V. Chalana and Y. Kim, A methodology for evaluation of boundary detection algorithms on medical images, *IEEE Trans. Med. Imaging* **16** (1997) 642–652.

10. I. S. Chang and R. H. Park, Segmentation based on fusion of range and intensity images using robust trimmed methods, *Pattern Recog.* **34** (2001) 1951–1962.

11. C. Chesnaud, P. Refregier and V. Boulet, Statistical region snake-based segmentation adapted to different physical noise models, *IEEE Trans. Pattern Anal. Mach. Intell.* **21** (1999) 1145–1157.

12. L. D. Cohen, On active contour models and balloons, *Comput. Graph. Vis. Image Proc.: Image Unders.* **53** (1991) 211–218.

13. T. Cootes, C. Taylor, D. Cooper and J. Graham, Active shape models their training and application, *Comput. Vis. Image Unders.* **61** (1995) 38–59.

14. L. Cordero-Grande, P. C. de-la Higuera, M. Martin-Fernandez and C. Alberola-Lopez, Endocardium and epicardium contour modeling based on Markov random fields and active contours, in *28th Annual International Conference of IEEE Engineering in Medicine and Biology Society* (New York City, NY, USA, 2006), pp. 928–931.

15. A. P. Dempster, N. M. Laird and D. B. Rubin, Maximum likelihood from incomplete data via the EM algorithm, *J. Royal Stat. Soc.* **39** (1977) 1–22.

16. J. M. B. Dias and J. M. N. Leitao, Wall position and thickness estimation from sequences of echocardiographic images, *IEEE Trans. Med. Imaging* **15** (1996) 25–38.

17. M. A. T. Figueiredo and J. M. N. Leitao, Bayesian estimation of ventricular contours in angiographic images, *IEEE Trans. Med. Imaging* **11** (1992) 416–429.

18. M. A. Fischler and R. A. Elschlager, The representation and matching of pictorial structures, *IEEE Trans. Comput.* **22** (1973) 67–92.

19. N. S. Friedland and D. Adam, Ventricular cavity boundary detection from sequential ultrasound images using simulated annealing, *IEEE Trans. Med. Imaging* **8** (1989) 344–353.

20. N. S. Friedland and A. Rosenfeld, Compact object recognition using energy-function-based optimization, *IEEE Trans. Pattern Anal. Mach. Intell.* **14** (1992) 770–777.

21. S. Geman and D. Geman, Stochastic relaxation, Gibbs distributions, and the Bayesian restoration of images, *IEEE Trans. Pattern Anal. Mach. Intell.* **8** (1984) 721–741.

22. D. Gering, A. Nabavi, R. Kikinis, N. Hata, L. Odonnell, W. E. L. Grimson, F. Jolesz, P. Black and W. Wells, An integrated visualization system for surgical planning and guidance using image fusion and an open MR, *J. Mag. Res. Imaging* **13** (2001) 967–975.

23. O. H. Gilja, A. I. Smievoll, N. Thune, K. Matre, T. Hausken, S. Odegaard and A. Berstad, *In vivo* comparison of 3D ultrasonography and magnetic resonance imaging in volume estimation of human kidneys, *Ultrasound Med. Biol.* **21** (1995) 25–32.

24. C. Haas, H. Ermert, S. Holt, P. Grewe, A. Machraoui and J. Barmeyer, Segmentation of 3D intravascular ultrasonic images based on a random field model, *Ultrasound Med. Biol.* **26** (2000) 297–306.

25. B. Hajek, Cooling schedules for optimal annealing, *Mat. Op. Res.* **13** (1988) 311–329.

26. J. M. Hammersley and P. Clifford, Markov fields on finite graphs and lattices (Unpublished, 1971).

27. A. K. Jain, *Fundamentals of Digital Image Processing* (Prentice Hall, Englewood Cliffs, NJ, USA, 1989).
28. A. K. Jain, Y. Zhong and S. Lakshmanan, Object matching using deformable templates, *IEEE Trans. Pattern Anal. Mach. Intell.* **18** (1996) 267–278.
29. R. S. Jose-Estepar, M. Martin-Fernandez, P. P. Caballero-Martinez, C. Alberola-Lopez and J. R. Alzola, A theoretical framework to three-dimensional ultrasound reconstruction from irregularly sampled data, *Ultrasound Med. Biol.* **29** (2003) 255–269.
30. M. Kass, A. Witkin and D. Terzopoulos, Snakes: Active contour models, *Int. J. Comput. Vis.* **1** (1988) 321–331.
31. V. V. Kindratenko, On using functions to describe shape, *Int. J. Math. Imaging Vis.* **18** (2003) 225–245.
32. P. Kruizinga and N. Petkov, Nonlinear operator for oriented texture, *IEEE Trans. Image Proc.* **8** (1999) 1395–1407.
33. S. Lakshmanan and H. Derin, Simultaneous parameter estimation and segmentation of Gibbs random fields using simulated annealing, *IEEE Trans. Pattern Anal. Mach. Intell.* **11** (1989) 799–813.
34. A. M. Law and W. D. Kelton, *Simulation Modeling and Analysis* (McGraw Hill, New York, NY, USA, 1991).
35. M. Leventon, E. Grimson and O. Faugeras, Statistical shape influence in geodesic active contours, in *IEEE Computer Vision and Pattern Recognition* (Hilton Head Island, SC, USA, 2000), pp. 316–322.
36. S. Z. Li, *Markov Random Field Modeling in Image Analysis* (Springer-Verlag, Heidelberg, Germany, 2001).
37. S. Loncaric, A survey of shape analysis techniques, *Pattern Recog.* **31** (1998) 983–1001.
38. R. Malladi, J. Sethian and B. Vermuri, Shape modeling with front propagation: A level set approach, *IEEE Trans. Pattern Anal. Mach. Intell.* **17** (1995) 158–175.
39. M. Martin-Fernandez and C. Alberola-Lopez, An approach for contour detection of human kidneys from ultrasound images using Markov random fields and active contours, *Med. Image Anal.* **9** (2005) 1–23.
40. M. Martin-Fernandez, R. San-Jose and C. Alberola-Lopez, Maximum likelihood contour estimation using beta-statistics in ultrasound images, in *Proceedings of the IEEE-EURASIP Image and Signal Processing and Analysis* (Pula, Croatia, 2001), pp. 207–212.
41. K. Matre, E. M. Stokke, D. Martens and O. H. Gilja, *In vitro* volume estimation of kidneys using 3D ultrasonography and a position sensor, *Eur. J. Ultrasound* **10** (1999) 65–73.
42. M. Mignotte, C. Collet, P. Perez and P. Bouthemy, Hybrid genetic optimization and statistical model-based approach for the classification of shadow shapes in sonar imagery, *IEEE Trans. Pattern Anal. Mach. Intell.* **22** (2000) 129–141.
43. M. Mignotte, J. Meunier and J. C. Tardif, Endocardial boundary estimation and tracking in echocardiographic images using deformable templates and Markov random fields, *Pattern Anal. Appl.* **4** (2001) 256–271.
44. J. A. Noble and D. Boukerroui, Ultrasound image segmentation: A survey, *IEEE Trans. Med. Imaging* **25**(8) (2006) 987–1010.
45. N. R. Pal and S. K. Pal, A review on image segmentation techniques, *Pattern Recog.* **26** (1993) 1277–1294.
46. R. W. Prager, A. H. Gee and L. Berman, Stradx: Real-time acquisition and visualization of freehand 3D ultrasound, *Med. Image Anal.* **3** (1999) 129–140.

47. R. W. Prager, R. N. Rohling, A. H. Gee and L. Berman, Rapid calibration for 3D free-hand ultrasound, *Ultrasound Med. Biol.* **24** (1998) 855–869.
48. G. Storvik, A Bayesian approach to dynamic contours through stochastic sampling and simulated annealing, *IEEE Trans. Pattern Anal. Mach. Intell.* **16** (1994) 976–986.
49. G. Treece, R. W. Prager, A. Gee and L. Berman, 3D ultrasound measurement of large organ volume, *Med. Image Anal.* **5** (2001) 41–54.
50. A. Tsai, A. Yezzi, W. Wells and A. Willsky, Model-based curve evolution technique for image segmentation, in *IEEE Computer Vision and Pattern Recognition* (Kauai, HI, USA, 2001), pp. 463–468.
51. R. C. Veltkamp and M. Hagedoorn, State of the art in shape matching, in *Principles of Visual Information Retrieval*, 2001, pp. 87–119.
52. H. Wang, J. Kearney and K. Atkinson, Arc-length parameterized spline curves for real-time simulation, in, *Curve and Surface Design* (2002), pp. 387–396.
53. G. Winkler, *Image Analysis, Random Fields, and Dynamic Monte Carlo Methods: A Mathematical Introduction* (Springer-Verlag, Heidelberg, Germany, 1995).
54. J. Xie, Y. Jiang and H.-T. Tsui, Segmentation of kidney from ultrasound images based on texture and shape priors, *IEEE Trans. Med. Imaging* **24**(1) (2005) 45–57.
55. C. H. Yu, C. H. Chang, F. M. Chang, H. C. Ko and H. Y. Chen, Fetal renal volume in normal gestation: A 3D ultrasound study, *Ultrasound Med. Biol.* **26** (2000) 1253–1256.